Comments by Professionals

Smart, practical and effective! Parents and doctors will celebrate important insights the authors share from their experience ... helping thousands of children and families overcome one of the most challenging situations any child ever faces: Pain.

—Harvey Karp, MD, FAAP, creator DVD/book, *The Happiest Baby on the Block*

... impressed by comprehensiveness, accessibility and tone of this book. You treat readers with respect and give them a wealth of information, resources, strategies and coping techniques for themselves and their children.

—Leah Ellenberg PhD, Neuropsychologist, Beverly Hills, CA

... meets patients and families where they are at, hears their story, validates their pain ... while stressing normalcy as a fundamental context.

—Gary Walco PhD, Professor, U of Washington, Director,
Seattle Children's Hospital Pain Program

It shouldn't be a pain to take proper care of pain in children. This book steers the reader to proper multimodal treatment for painful conditions.

—Chris Giza MD PhD www.uclahealth.org/BrainSPORT/Pages/default.aspx

... an accessible, compassionate resource for young people coping with chronic pain and their families. Drawing on a wealth of knowledge from a broad range of experts in the study and treatment of pediatric pain ... presents up to date information to empower youth and families in making sound treatment decisions and developing the needed skills to manage chronic pain effectively.

—Deirdre Logan PhD; Director of Psychology Services, Division of Pain Medicine, Boston Children's Hospital, *Associate Professor, Psychiatry, Harvard Medical School*

... a landmark in elucidating current thinking about the nature of chronic pain in children ... perhaps more importantly provides a practical blueprint for making positive change to ... seemingly intractable problems.

—Michael Waterhouse, M.A., L.Ac., Acupuncturist, Beverly Hills, CA

... well-organized, easy to read ... many case studies bring clarity to the points that are being addressed. This should be a very useful and important guide for parents and practitioners.

—Margaret Bauman MD, Child Neurologist, Professor, Harvard Medical School

... invaluable in providing parents and children with the tools they need to better understand the causes and treatment of their chronic pain.

—David Ziring MD, Associate Professor Pediatrics, Director, Pediatric IBD Center, Mattel Children's Hospital, UCLA David Geffen School of Medicine

All too often experts write about people in pain, this book is for people in pain. ... a comprehensive, erudite ... highly accessible resource for parents and young people struggling to make sense of living with pain. One needs a guide book ... up-to-date, written in the right language, in tune with what people want. This is that guide book.

—Christopher Eccleston, PhD, Professor of Medical Psychology, University of Bath, UK. Director, Centre for Pain Research. 'Embodied: the Psychology of Physical Sensation' (Oxford University Press, 2016).

Without a doubt, an absolute "must-have" for every pediatrician's office!!

—Bruce Levine, Ph.D., ABPP, BCIA, Psychologist, Beverly Hills, CA

With clarity and insight ... unpacks complexities of chronic pain in young people ... vivid metaphors, clinical insight, up-to-date research, the go-to guide for parents and physicians.

—Subhadra Evans, PhD, Faculty of Health, Deakin University, Victoria Australia

Absolutely awesome! You two have nailed it! ... comprehensive, easy to follow, informative... great resource for families and health care providers.

—Diane Poladian D.P.T, physical therapist, biofeedback clinician, Granada Hills, CA

... beautiful and will be very helpful to patients' parents ... and might work well for ... mature patients themselves to read.

—Celia deMayo RPT, physical therapist, Santa Monica, CA

... clearly reflects ... extensive knowledge and detailed information on every aspect one confronts when experiencing chronic pain as the child or the parent ... reflects extensive experience of working with this population, who face so many unanswered questions and concerns.

—Kathryn dePlanque, PhD, Hypnotherapist, Santa Monica, CA

... a comprehensive look at the often-baffling circumstances related to chronic pain in children and teens ... Outlines traditional medical and alternative treatment options that are the key to unlocking chronic pain conditions. Parents and their children will finally find hope and solutions in the pages that follow.

—Karen Axelrod, MA, CST-D, CMT, craniosacral therapist, Redondo Beach, CA

... clear, up-to-date, research-based answers to just about any question one can think of. It even contains sample letters to send to teachers and friends explaining a child's pain. 'The Journey Back to Normal' will be an essential resource for parents and pediatric health care professionals. I used to keep a supply of the authors' 2005 book for ... parents in individual, family, and group treatment. This 2016 book is even more comprehensive ... in clinical use.

—Carl von Baeyer, PhD, Professor of Clinical Health Psychology and Professor of Pediatrics and Child Health, University of Manitoba, Canada.

Pain in Children & Young Adults is an indispensable tool for anyone wanting to understand pain and discover a path to a pain free life.

—Joe Garcia Program Director & Owner, Arena Fitness Training Centers, LA, CA

This is a book that speaks well to both patients and healthcare workers.

—Shahram Yazdani, MD Clinical Professor of Pediatrics, David Geffen School of Medicine, UCLA

... a truly wonderful resource for parents and families coping with chronic pain! It provides families with a detailed explanation of numerous chronic pain conditions (including rare conditions), and helps them to get organized, find help, and better use and implement effective treatment strategies. Parents will particularly appreciate the spectacular illustrations, the important comments included from leading experts in the field, and the voices of children and parents to tell their own stories.

—Tonya M. Palermo, Ph.D. Professor of Anesthesiology, Pediatrics and Psychiatry. University of Washington, Center for Child Health Behavior and Development, Seattle Children's Research Institute, Seattle, WA

Just the sort of book we all need on our desks-the only problem is to make sure it stays on my shelf - it's going to be very popular and I fear it will end up on someone else's shelf ...

—Tim Oberlander, MD, Pediatric Development Specialist, BC Children's Hospital, Professor, U of Vancouver, Canada

An outstanding, comprehensive guide for parents of children and teens suffering from chronic pain ... This unique book, based on current research and a wealth of highly successful clinical experience, is crucial for your child's road to wellness.

—Andrea Rapkin MD, Acting Chairman, Department of Obstetrics-Gynecology, Professor, David Geffen School of Medicine at UCLA

My only regret is that Pain in Children and Young Adults wasn't released when I was a young adolescent dealing with the trials and tribulations of IBS. Every parent of a young one dealing with chronic pain needs to read this book! The lessons are invaluable.

—Stacey Garcia, Nutrition Director, Arena Fitness Training Centers, Los Angeles, CA

Comments from Parents of our Patients

The path to recovery is filled with twists and turns ... Be honest and open toward identifying and resolving conflicts in the home that are contributing toward anxiety and pain in your child. Early-on in the road to recovery two very thoughtful physicians gave us some sage advice, "Watch her Feet, Not her Lips." We thank you LZ and PZ.

—Patty and Jan

This book is just as supportive as it is instructive, equipping parents with information from friendly, encouraging voices ...... insider knowledge and techniques to the confusing world of medicine ... stresses the importance of slowing down and taking a breath.

—Georgia Huston ga@teenpainhelp.org

I really like the way the book is laid out. Clear and easy to follow. The empathy and understanding that y'all offer felt really good to me as a parent with a kid who deals with pain. To know that someone else understands what I'm going through is extremely valuable.

—S.B., a parent

The CRPS section was so spot on and I love that it offered so much hope!!! Every single family who is going through this should read that chapter!! ... we appreciate you two. I really feel like you saved our family. The fact that you didn't rush into heavy meds was so key because I believe Duncan rewired those pathways.

—Chrissy, mom to Duncan

PAIN IN CHILDREN & YOUNG ADULTS:
THE JOURNEY BACK TO NORMAL

TWO PEDIATRICIANS' MIND-BODY
GUIDE FOR PARENTS

By

Lonnie K. Zeltzer, M.D.

Director, UCLA Pediatric Pain and Palliative Care Program,
Mattel Children's Hospital, Distinguished Professor of Pediatrics,
Anesthesiology, Psychiatry and Biobehavioral Sciences,
David Geffen School of Medicine at UCLA

Paul M. Zeltzer M.D.

Co-Director, WholeChild LA Inc.
Clinical Professor in Neurosurgery,
David Geffen School of Medicine at UCLA
Founder, *www.GoMedSolutions.com*
and *www.navigatingcancer.com*

Copyright © 2016 by Paul M. Zeltzer

Pain in Children and Young Adults: The Journey Back to Normal

All rights reserved. This book may not be reproduced in whole or part in any manner including Internet use, without express permission, except in case of brief quotation embodied in critical articles and reviews.

Illustrations and graphics: Paul M. Zeltzer
Book and cover design: wordzworth.com
Cover photography: Ishibashi by Greir

Printed in Canada on acid-free paper

Published by Shilysca Press (a Division of Shilysca, Inc.)
5041 Valjean Avenue, Encino, California 91436
Website: www.wholechildla.org
E-mail address: Drzeltzer@wholechildla.org

Shilysca Press
Encino, California

Questions about the book contents: Go to the Q and A section at www.wholechildla.org
Or UCLA Pain Program Site
https://www.uclahealth.org/Mattel/pediatric-comfort-care-program/Pages/default.aspx

ISBN 10: 0976017121
ISBN 13: 978-0-9760171-2-7

Library of Congress Control Number: 2015957045
Zeltzer, Paul M. 1942- Zeltzer, Lonnie K 1944-
Pain in Children and Young Adults: The Journey Back to Normal
1. Health 2. Illness 3. Pain 4. Child 5. Mind, body, holistic health

CONTENTS

A Message To Every Parent Of A Child In Pain   ix

SECTION A   BEGINNING THE PAIN(FUL) JOURNEY

Chapter 1	You Are Not Alone: What You Need To Know... First	3
Chapter 2	What Is Pain? Nine Lessons	9
Chapter 3	How Children Express Pain: What Do The Clues Mean? How Can A Parent Help?	29
Chapter 4	Chronic Pain Conditions (A): Sports Injuries, Pain In Extremities & Back	41
Chapter 5	Chronic Pain Conditions (B): Pain In The Head, Chest And Tummy; Menstrual Cramps, Fatigue And Sleep	59
Chapter 6	Diseases Associated With Chronic Pain: Arthritis, Crohn's/ Ulcerative Colitis, Sickle Cell And Cancer	87
Chapter 7	Diseases Associated With Chronic Pain: Autism, Communication Related Disorders, Cerebral Palsy & Rare Conditions	113

SECTION B   START TO TAKE ACTION

Chapter 8	How Do I Start The Pain Treatment Journey?	137
Chapter 9	The Web And Internet For Chronic Pain Information	147
Chapter 10	Getting Organized: The Key To Regaining Control	155

SECTION C   MY CHILD IS BEING TREATED... BUT NOT GETTING BETTER

Chapter 11	Emotions And Chronic Pain: Effects On Mood And Learning	167
Chapter 12	How Parents Can Help Their Child	187

SECTION D   TREATMENTS—WHAT ARE THEY? WHAT DO THEY DO?

Chapter 13	Physical Therapy, Massage, Cranio-Sacral Therapies, Personal Training: Healing The Body And Mind	207
Chapter 14	Psychological And Behavioral Therapies: Help For Parenting The Child With Pain	227
Chapter 15	Complementary Mind And Body Therapies	249
Chapter 16	Medicines For Treating Chronic Pain	283

SECTION E   GETTING BACK TO NORMAL...DAY-TO-DAY STUFF

Chapter 17	Getting Back And Staying In School	303
Chapter 18	HMO's, Benefits, Insurance & Family Medical Leave Act: Guidelines For Parents Of A Child With Chronic Pain	313
Chapter 19	The ABC's Of Receiving Good Care For Your Child	329
Appendix A	Pain Center Locator	331
Appendix B	Glossary-Useful Pain Terminology	345
Appendix C	Sample Letters & Tracking Forms	350
Appendix D	Selected Reading	356
Acknowledgments		361
Index		363
The Authors		379

A Message To Every Parent Of A Child In Pain

PAIN IN CHILDREN & YOUNG ADULTS: The Journey Back to Normal will guide you (and your child) in ways to take control of the pain—regardless of the cause(s)—and, ultimately, help your child to climb out of pain and get back to a normal life.

During our many years of treating children with chronic pain, we have learned much to share with you. One of the major things we learned is that, even for children with very different chronic pain conditions, **there are some common ways to reduce suffering**. It constantly amazes us that children who have chronic pain, often for such long periods of time, and who have gone through so many evaluations by different sub-specialists and diagnostic tests and treatments, have conditions that seem fairly easy to understand and treat…if the right framework is used and the right questions are asked. The **information in this book also includes sage advice from our colleagues who are some of the top pain professionals in the world.** This knowledge will help you become an effective advocate and obtain the best treatments for your child.

We have witnessed the frustration and helplessness of parents who are thwarted in their attempts to find effective treatment for their child's pain. Sadly, every year thousands of parents are told by their child's physician, ***"All the tests are normal…I can't find a cause for the pain."*** If the cause is not found, then parents worry how their child's physician is going to help get rid of the pain. Doctors may then refer the child to a psychologist. The mental health referral is interpreted by parents as, *"the doctor believes that the pain must be psychological"* (meaning *"not real"*). Children interpret the referral as ***"the doctor doesn't believe me and thinks I am faking it…that it's all in my head."*** Meanwhile, parents watch as their child endures debilitating chronic pain… day after day…. and becomes even more discouraged.

We see these children and their parents every day in our pain clinics. They come from many different cultures and socioeconomic groups and are racially, ethnically, and religiously diverse. Some are highly educated, others are not; they come from single and two-parent households. Some children have severe psychological problems, while others appear to have none. They are of all ages, shapes, and sizes. Their symptoms and the degree of pain they experience differ, but **what connects all these children is that the pain, regardless of its origin(s), is keeping them from living their lives.**

ix

Children with chronic pain don't have the luxury to be children—they spend a lot of time worrying, being afraid, and sitting in doctors' offices. None of us would want this for our child. But most parents simply don't know what else to do.

We also are struck by the degree to which **parental guilt is tied up in the pain**: *"I work too much." "My husband and I fight too much," "We shouldn't have moved out of our old neighborhood; she was so happy there."* These are sentiments heard again and again. Or parents blame themselves for how long the pain has affected their child. *"I didn't recognize the pain early enough." "I didn't believe her when she said she was in pain."*

Parental guilt may stem from a sense of helplessness —watching your child suffer. As parents, we blame ourselves when our child is in pain and we can't make it go away. These guilt feelings and distress at watching our child suffer is what pushes us as parents to want to do everything possible to take the pain away. However, while it is true that what we say and do—or don't do—can have an influence on our child's pain, it is not the "cause" of the pain.

Pain does not just affect the child. **Chronic pain moves into the home and invades the whole family—it exacerbates marital stresses and sibling rivalries.** The child with chronic or recurrent pain feels out of control, and parents feel helpless. While most parents learn how to parent by using their own life experience and common sense, **pain seems to defy both experience and common sense.**

Guilt spreads and infects many aspects of family life, especially when a child has been suffering over a prolonged period. For example, parents who feel guilty may become overprotective, inadvertently hindering their child's ability to feel competent and cope/overcome the pain. We say this not to give parents something else to feel guilty about but rather to point out how pervasive and destructive guilt can become. We will give you the tools to recognize and rid this unnecessary feeling and learn the best ways to help your child climb through and out of the limitations of pain.

Parents often fear that the doctors have "missed something serious." They worry that the pain is a signal of something terribly wrong with their child and that, if not properly diagnosed and treated, can cause irreparable harm, or even death. Thus, when doctors conduct tests and say that they can't find anything wrong, parents do not know what to do next. Should they take their child to more doctors… for more tests? Should they change doctors? Should they seek alternative therapies? If so, which ones? These are all important questions that we will address throughout this book.

We will explain how most common pain problems are rooted in the nervous system 'wiring' and 'signaling' and are thus 'electrical.' This is why checking out the 'plumbing' or 'carpentry' has not uncovered the problem. If your child's pain problem were evaluated by an electrical engineer, then the problem might have been identified. The problem for doctors is that we have many ways of evaluating the plumbing (e.g. gastrointestinal, gynecological, urological systems) and the carpentry (e.g. bones and muscles), but **we have fewer tools to examine the electrical system in our bodies.**

Most parents desperately want to know what is wrong with their child. In short, they want a diagnosis. Often a diagnosis is possible, such as complex regional pain syndrome (CRPS), or irritable bowel syndrome (IBS). **Most parents are frustrated by the lack of the concrete label to explain their child's pain.** This is understandable: if there is a diagnosis, then there might be a cure, a pill that will make it all go away. However, a diagnosis is only a part of the equation. **For most chronic pain conditions, there is no magic pill.** By the time it has become *chronic,* **pain has multiple factors that keep it going, add to its strength, and contribute to its impact on function.**

Pain takes on baggage as it gains strength with time. To stop it, the **baggage needs to be identified, disentangled, and dismantled.** This job is a joint effort on the part of clinicians, your child, and you. This task cannot be carried out by the doctor alone. However, it is natural that most parents want to be able to visit the doctor and have the doctor present them with a diagnosis and then simply give their child a medicine that will work immediately and completely, have no side effects, and require no effort on the part of the child or family. Why not? That is what we all would desire!

Living with a child in pain is difficult—but it need not be unbearable. We have seen amazing family triumphs in the face of severe chronic pain. Almost without exception, the families who flourish are those who find a way to take control of the pain instead of letting it control them. **We have learned a great deal from the families who have chosen to share their lives with us, as we worked together to help their child heal.** This book is the culmination of that partnership that allows us to share knowledge and experience with other parents and children.

PAIN IN CHILDREN AND YOUNG ADULTS offers you (and your child) specific strategies to take control of the pain—regardless of the cause(s.)

- We will guide you in understanding pain in general as well as specific types of pain conditions.

- We will explore how children express pain and how to interpret what they say.

- You will read in these pages the sage advice from some of the top pain professionals in the world.

- We will give you resources for finding the right doctor and other professionals, as well as tips for asking the right questions.

- We will teach you about breathing, muscle relaxation, and visualization exercises to help your child on a "bad pain day."

- We will describe ways to help your child sleep and how to get your child back to school.

- We will describe physical, psychological, complementary, and medical treatments for chronic pain.

- We will provide strategies for working with your insurance company to approve those therapies deemed helpful for your child.

- And in this process, lookout for bold phrases or sentences that we think are important.

Sections A-C will teach you about pain and why previous approaches have not worked. It will give you the information necessary to partner with your health team to find the pathway to pain relief.

Section A: Beginning The Pain(ful) Journey – Different Types Of Painful Conditions

Section B: How To Get Started: Getting Information And Getting Organized

Section C: My Child Is Being Treated…But Not Getting Better. Why?

Sections D and E will help you understand and learn the newer approaches to pain relief, why they work, and what questions to ask to make sure you are on the right track.

Section D: Beginning Treatment With Modern Approaches: What Are They?

Section E: Getting Back To Normal: The Future Starts With Day To Day Stuff

With information and guidance, you, the parents, can successfully take on these tasks above and also educate your child's doctors to help you achieve your goals. We can't stress enough how important it is to understand that in most cases **chronic pain responds best to some combination of medication, physical, psychological, and complementary therapies.** Patience and a positive outlook are your greatest allies.

Drs. Paul and Lonnie Zeltzer
Encino, CA
January 15, 2016

SECTION A

BEGINNING THE PAIN(FUL) JOURNEY

"Pain is inevitable… suffering is optional."

—UNKNOWN SOURCE

"Neither her pediatrician nor the other medical professionals we saw had the depth of understanding of what we were dealing with!"

—ALEX, MELODIE'S DAD

CHAPTER 1

YOU ARE NOT ALONE:
WHAT YOU NEED TO KNOW... FIRST

THE JOURNEY FORWARD

DIFFICULT DIAGNOSIS, UNPREDICTABILITY, COMPLEXITY: THAT'S CHRONIC PAIN

- Chronic pain can be difficult to diagnose correctly.
- Pain is not always predictable.
- Chronic pain treatment can be complex.

In this chapter we describe some lesser-known facts about pain.

PAIN IN CHILDREN AND YOUNG ADULTS

THE JOURNEY FORWARD

Here you are. Your child has a serious illness… maybe you have been given a diagnosis… maybe not. It could be a disease with a medical name that you may not recognize, something you thought only other people got: CRPS… Fibromyalgia… IBS… even 'chronic' headache: It's still P-A-I-N.

You feel frustrated, sometimes helpless and unsure of where or to whom to turn. Your family and friends don't quite understand. You hear, *"she needs to tough it out and not let it get her down."* Your primary care physician (PCP), on whom you trust and depend, is not satisfied with her response to the usual treatments in spite of his/her best efforts. So you could be sent to a specialist at a well-known medical center or institute, or maybe your PCP doesn't quite know what to do next. Now what?

To help you get started on the pathway to better understanding *Pain in Children & Young Adults* will help you—as a parent—accomplish the following five steps:

1 Feel more in control of the situation and less like a victim.

2 Organize your strategy for traveling the difficult road ahead.

3 Assess your child's current care… and identify if you need an "expert".

4 Understand your child's pain and its complexity so that the multifaceted treatment approach makes sense to you.

5 Be equipped to negotiate to get what your child needs: school, health insurance coverage, family support

You will need to develop a strategy and organize (more on that in Chapters 8, 9, and 10). But first let's use three illustrations to explain why you need to prepare and get organized.

DIFFICULT DIAGNOSIS, UNPREDICTABILITY, COMPLEXITY: THAT'S CHRONIC PAIN

Chronic pain can be difficult to diagnose correctly

Chronic pain affects over 100 million American adults—more than the total affected by heart disease, cancer, and diabetes combined. Pain also costs the nation up to $635 billion each year in medical treatment and lost productivity. And chronic pain in children and teenagers is a dramatically growing problem, with hospital admissions for youngsters with the condition rising nine-fold between 2004 and 2010[1]. Moderate

---

1   Inpatient Characteristics of the Child Admitted With Chronic Pain. Coffelt TA, Bauer BD, Carroll AE. Pediatrics, July, 2013. *http://pediatrics.aappublications.org/content/early/2013/06/26/peds.2012-1739*

YOU ARE NOT ALONE: WHAT YOU NEED TO KNOW... FIRST

to severe chronic pain is a problem for 1.7 million children, costing $19.5 billion annually in the United States alone[2].

The *average* number of doctors that patients in our outpatient practice have seen before us is 14… the record is 42. Other physicians or professionals had tried but healing did not take place in spite of expensive scans, Botox, nerve blocks, physical therapy, manipulations, a cabinet full of pills and often psychotherapy.

Why? **Pain in children is different than pain in adults.** Typically, the medications used for most types of adult chronic pain are either not approved for use in children, may not have been studied in children so side effects are unknown, or may not be effective for children. Also, rarely are invasive procedures such as nerve blocks/ epidural injections needed or effective for children, while they may be very effective for the types of pain adults most often get. There are increasing numbers of adult pain medicine clinics that function within the biopsychosocial model, but most still do not. Lonnie was a committee member of The Institute of Medicine (IOM) of the National Academies of Science that developed the IOM report on Pain in America[3] (2012). The IOM called **pain "a public health problem" and advocated for treating pain within a biopsychosocial model"**. As you read this book, you will have a clear understanding of what **"biopsychosocial model" means** and how it leads to more effective pediatric pain evaluation and treatment.

Pain is not always predictable

"How long 'til my child will be better?" We hear that question at every first clinic visit. We usually refrain from statistics because they apply to populations, not individuals. However, there is one fact that we want you to remember… no matter how smart any doctor or other clinician may be, **no one can predict how long any one person will take to recover!** We are capable of predicting what will happen to hundreds of people with chronic pain, but we cannot predict exactly how long it will take *your* child to recover. As a general rule, **it takes about as long to recover as it took to get to where you are today.**

Prognosis: What does that mean? It is what a doctor says *might* happen. It is the odds. This can be based on scientifically based statistics or on a physician's personal experience. However, when looking at one person, it's like flipping a coin. In 100 tries, the theoretical odds are 50-50 heads/tails each time. In actuality, we may get six straight heads.

---

2 Pediatric Pain Screening Tool (PPST): Rapid identification of risk in youth with pain complaints. Simons LE, Smith A, Ibagon C, et al *http://www.ncbi.nlm.nih.gov/pubmed/25906349.*

3 *www.iom.edu/Reports/2011/Relieving-Pain-in-America-A-Blueprint-for-Transforming-Prevention-Care-Education-Research/Report-Brief.aspx*

PAIN IN CHILDREN AND YOUNG ADULTS

Even with the same diagnosis, what evolves can be different between patients. An example:

> *Two of our 13 year-old patients, Evan and Jeanne, have irritable bowel syndrome (IBS). Evan was an elite level soccer player but, after he developed IBS and had diarrhea, he couldn't participate in soccer anymore because he was afraid he would need to 'poop' during a game. Jeanne was a skilled cello player who was chosen to travel with the USA Teen Symphony that was going on a three-week tour of Europe. She declined to go because of her intermittent belly pain, diarrhea and constipation. Both children had normal endoscopies, blood tests and time from when they first developed symptoms after the viral gastroenteritis that set it off for each. Jeanne also had a lot of general anxiety and some depression.*
>
> *After following our program, Evan got back into soccer in three months after responding to a medication he took at bedtime, called amitriptyline. It took Jeanne almost a year for her abdominal pain, diarrhea and constipation to resolve, and before she would even consider going on the next all-USA tour. She needed a selective serotonin re-uptake inhibitor (SSRI) called citalopram (Celexa™) and individual psychotherapy to help her anxiety and depression. This is one of many examples of how chronic pain can behave differently.*

Why is the course of the same type of chronic pain so variable? Until a few years ago, we did not understand how similar patients' courses differed so markedly. New research suggests that "messenger" molecules and cells called "microglia" in the brain and spinal cord are activated and they affect the strength of pain messages going up to the brain. And conversely these same messengers can affect how the brain sends "turn off" signals within the brain or back down to the affected arm, leg, or belly. **These negative "pain messengers" are activated by stress, anxiety or depression.** We also know more about activity that goes on within the brain itself, "neural connectivity," and how strength of connections between and among different parts of the brain can lead to increased or decreased pain. This information coming from modern brain imaging studies has informed us how emotions, thoughts, and stressors can impact brain interconnectivity to increase or decrease pain. This finding has opened the way to understanding the biological mechanisms of psychological interventions for pain. More about this in Chapter 2.

Chronic pain treatment can be confusing

> *"Nobody knows why...Their families can't help...Their doctors are baffled...They're alone, suffering... It just seems hopeless."*

—COURTESY GEORGIA HUSTON (*www.teenpainhelp.org*)

YOU ARE NOT ALONE: WHAT YOU NEED TO KNOW... FIRST

You may be thinking, "These guys are so calm, but we are the ones suffering with chronic pain… and I'm in panic mode!" Remember, this book did not spring from an ivory-tower view. It is **rooted in the real and successful experiences of many families.** We even include *nitty-gritty* examples of successful appeals to reverse health maintenance organizations (HMOs) or insurance claims and to other successes in coping from actual patients (See Chapter 18).

Don't just take our word for it. Go to the Internet, click on *www.wholechildla. org* or *www.wholechildcommunity.org* or our former patient, Georgia Huston's, book[4] (*www.teenpainhelp.org*) and read stories written by people who had chronic pain and traveled the path you are on right now.

In the chronic pain world, you may have exposure to a ton of professionals—not really… but it seems like a lot. You'll see radiologists, rheumatologists, orthopedic surgeons, sports medicine doctors, physical therapists, biofeedback specialists, neuropsychologists, rehabilitation doctors, nutritionists, psychotherapists and other healthcare providers. You will need excellent organization to ensure that correct, complete medical information is shared. This will establish you as the chief executive officer (CEO) of your child's treatment team (more on that in Chapters 9 and 10).

Okay, **you still may be feeling like this is some form of punishment and the whole experience has left you powerless and out of control.** Many of our patients have said their struggle felt like being in a torrent, tossed around, and hoping to find a place to get out from under the maelstrom. Akin to a cataclysmic flood, chronic pain changes our sense of stability and puts us in the middle of the torrent, out of reach from the shore. So, where is your Ark, a place of respite? How can you regain control? When we are ill, we want to find the key, unlock the Ark so we can climb to safety and wait out the storm. In the past, the medical system—the hospitals, doctors, nurses—could let us in. **Today's health care system has put us more on our own;** but we have ever increasing opportunities to help ourselves with knowledge. In this book, we will detail basic information about chronic pain—understanding what pain really is and how it gets expressed, common and uncommon pain problems, getting organized, beginning the treatment journey with understanding of its different parts. **Remember that your child was a person—not a patient—before pain symptoms alerted you to a problem**. Apart from doctors and the medical system, **he or she is still that before-pain person.** You and your family have choices. You can choose whether to get a second opinion, or travel to a major pediatric pain treatment center, for example. The power to make choices is yours.

Yes, chronic pain is serious, but take a deep breath and pause. You have time to learn and plan so that pain doesn't rule your family's life. You will learn to preserve

---

4   *http://www.blurb.com/b/6200329-pain-an-owner-s-manual*

wholeness and gain control over your situation through knowledge and awareness. Our hope is that this book, and the resources that can be accessed through it, will bring you to quieter, safer waters until the storm calms down.

It is time to begin and learn more about chronic pain in general and your child's pain specifically. Then you can ask the right questions and understand choices ahead.

Oh, and to help you on the way, as you may have noticed, **we'll highlight phrases that we think are important for you to pay attention to.** A Glossary of technical words and abbreviations can be found in Appendix B in the back of the book.

CHAPTER 2
WHAT IS PAIN? NINE LESSONS

"...we can absolutely relate to every word and concept you are imparting. When first confronted with Mel's pain syndrome (headache), our primary focus was alleviating her PAIN. The medical practitioners limited their efforts toward ruling out medical issues and prescribing traditional migraine medication."

—JAN: DAD TO MELANIE, AGE 11

LESSON 1   **PAIN IS NOT IMAGINED...IT IS REAL!**

LESSON 2   **PAIN IS BOTH PHYSICAL AND PSYCHOLOGICAL**

LESSON 3   **PAIN IS MODULATED BOTH UP AND DOWN BY THE BRAIN**

LESSON 4   **ACUTE AND CHRONIC PAIN: THE DIFFERENCE**

LESSON 5   **FEELINGS, THOUGHTS AND MEMORIES CAN INCREASE OR DECREASE PAIN**

LESSON 6   **PAIN CAN (AND WILL) BE CONTROLLED...BUT NOT BY MEDICATIONS ALONE**

LESSON 7   **TYPE OF PAIN DETERMINES TYPE OF SPECIFIC TREATMENT**

LESSON 8   **ALL TREATMENTS CAN FAIL**

LESSON 9   **YOU MUST BE PREPARED TO LEAD ON THE ROAD TO DIAGNOSIS AND RECOVERY**

PAIN IN CHILDREN AND YOUNG ADULTS

In this chapter you will learn:

• The most important features and types of pain
• The newest approaches and theories about how pain becomes chronic
• Myths and falsehoods about pain and its treatment
• To become an empowered parent to get the best care for your child

Pain can start quite suddenly.

> *It is September 2015, and your 7th grade daughter complains about a stomachache that you attribute to the fast food she gobbled down at a sleepover the night before. But you notice she has been complaining of similar aches in her belly every few days. A week or two later, she is limping and rubbing her leg. When you ask about it, she says her leg feels hot and prickly. The complaints seem unconnected, but you take her to the pediatrician for the stomach problems. The doctor attributes the stomach- aches to nerves. "After all," he says, "the new school year is here... and it is Middle School." The leg pain he attributes to normal "growing pains." "All children get them," he assures you.*
>
> *Flash forward: it is Fall, 2016 and ten doctors later. Your 8th grade daughter is still in pain. In fact, the pain is worse and has traveled to other areas of her body. She has missed half the school days this year and it is only October, and she shows little interest in the things she once loved—her friends and gymnastics. What's more, you are no closer to knowing the cause of the pain. Your nerves are frazzled; you are missing work, fighting with your husband, and you feel guilty. "How did this happen?" you ask yourself.*

LESSON 1: PAIN IS NOT IMAGINED, IT IS REAL

You may be just beginning the journey of understanding your child's pain, or you may have been struggling with it for years. Or maybe you're feeling the signs of what we call *Parent-Pain Burnout Syndrome ("P-PBS")*—fear, confusion, frustration, anger, and helplessness. You are not alone. **One in five children in this country is suffering from some form of chronic pain**[5]. And **5-10 percent of our youth have been significantly impacted or have disability related to the pain** in such areas as school attendance and academics, physical functioning, participation in social activities, sleep, emotional functioning and family functioning. And the same number of parents suffers right along with them.

One issue that complicates the diagnosis and treatment of chronic pain in children is **that nagging question: "Is the pain real or imagined?"** Though this question may arise in the treatment of adult pain, it is more frequently on the minds

---

5   *www.apadivisions.org/division-54/evidence-based/chronic-pain.aspx*

WHAT IS PAIN? NINE LESSONS

of physicians and parents when it comes to children's complaints. Why? Because children are considered to be less reliable than adults in reporting symptoms and degrees of pain they experience.

Pain, in one form or another, is a part of every child's life experience. Some children are fortunate to experience only common cuts and bruises while others experience more serious injury, illness, or disease. Some types of pain even can be useful, because they teach children what is dangerous (e.g. touching a hot stove) or alert parents to a condition that needs immediate attention (e.g. acute right lower belly pain associated with appendicitis). However, chronic pain *never* serves a useful purpose. **Pain is the most misunderstood of all childhood conditions for which parents seek help.**

Children who develop *chronic* pain are not pretending to have pain, even if it seems there is no reason for it. They are having real, honest-to-goodness pain and are suffering. Discovering the root of the problem and treating it sometimes means that doctors and parents must engage in challenging detective work; this will involve understanding the many factors that maintain and increase pain and suffering.

> *10-year-old Rita suffered with severe knee pain. Four doctors had been unsuccessful in treating her. The pain in her right knee had steadily progressed to the point where she was unable to straighten it. Rita said that the pain made her limp until she could no longer walk and it felt like "something was not right inside." After a 'misdiagnosis' by the pediatrician, she saw an orthopedist who said that an MRI showed torn cartilage (although Rita did not remember injuring herself). Rita had endoscopic arthroscopy to repair the cartilage. But the pain was worse after surgery. She described tearfully the "torture" that she experienced with physical therapy. Rita was referred to another orthopedist who gave her steroids and knee injections. Rita's mother said that, after no improvement and normal tests, the orthopedist told Rita, "Enough pillows, straighten your legs.... I have other patients with real pain... if you don't start moving your leg, I'll put it in a brace and crank it up at night!" She said that Rita cried throughout the visit and refused to return.*

We believe that if a child complains of pain, the pain is real and he or she is suffering. The job of parents and physicians is to figure out what might have started the pain and, more importantly, what is keeping the pain going. Typically, continuing pain is not due to one single thing like a torn cartilage, but more commonly from an array of factors. Rita's frustration and anxiety over not being believed only served to increase her pain. She was pushed to move her knee before she learned how to do that successfully and cope with the pain so that it wouldn't bother her so much.

PAIN IN CHILDREN AND YOUNG ADULTS

LESSON 2: PAIN IS BOTH PHYSICAL AND PSYCHOLOGICAL

In diagnosing the cause of pain, doctors typically first think about the common, disease-related possible causes. They will conduct tests or procedures to look for pathological evidence (e.g. inflammation, some bacteria, tissue injury, or mechanical obstruction). If their tests are negative for any identifiable disease, they may say that the cause of the belly pain is likely "functional." This means that the nerve signals between the brain and the intestines become functionally impaired. Your child's doctor may use the word "psychosomatic," meaning that the pain is "psychological" in origin. Many parents, children, and even some doctors think that this means that the pain is not "real" (that is, having no biological basis) and often the child is referred to a mental health professional. However, we now know that **there are biological and neurochemical processes that lead to the types of pain that are often called functional or psychosomatic**. In fact, in pediatrics we no longer even use the word "psychosomatic." When we use the word "functional," we are implying that the messaging or signaling mechanism between one part of the body and the brain is not working correctly. We use the term "dysregulated" to mean that the neural traffic between the brain and body part (e.g. intestines, leg) is not running smoothly and normally. Such abnormal nerve signal "traffic" causes increased sensitivity and pain in the body part affected, such as intestines or leg.

All pain is caused by a complex interaction between the brain and the rest of the body. **Just because doctors cannot find the "cause" of the pain does not mean it is "psychological."** Irritable bowel syndrome (IBS) has been called a "functional bowel disorder" by most gastroenterologists. We don't know exactly how or why IBS happens to some children. There may be genetic reasons (there is a higher incidence in twins than in non-twin siblings), familial reasons (there is an even higher likelihood of a twin having IBS, if a parent has IBS, rather than if the other twin has IBS), stress-related reasons, inflammation, and others. The bottom line is that **in functional pain, the pain signaling system is not working normally**. In most such cases, the current tests we have available to find a disease or illness will come back negative.

All pain has both physical (sensory) and psychological (emotional) components. In fact, pain is in the head... or really the brain—and not at the point of injury or where the pain is felt. We all have emotional reactions to pain. The brain registers both the *sensation* and emotional *suffering* of pain. **Emotions and beliefs directly affect (modulate) nerve signaling and neurotransmitters that underlie the physiology of pain and thus our perception of it and our behavior in response to it.** (Figure 2.1)

WHAT IS PAIN? NINE LESSONS

For example, your previously active and healthy young soccer player had a sports injury. Both the pain message *up* to the brain (from the local inflammation and torn ligament in the hand, "bottom up" pain) and its emotional reaction *down* ("top down" from the brain to the injured site) reaction to that injury join together to produce the effect of experienced pain and suffering.

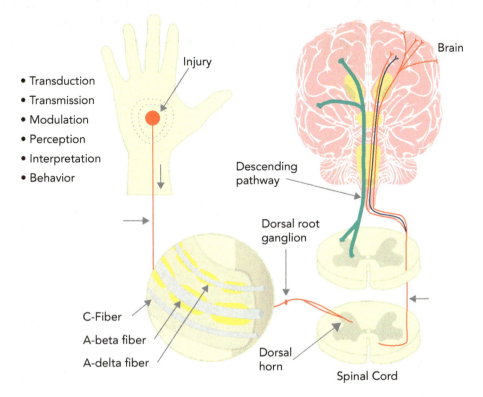

Figure 2.1. *The route of pain signals from periphery to the brain.*

A little history about pain: René Descartes (1596-1650), one of the most important Western philosophers of the past five centuries, believed that the mind and body were separate. This led him to argue that there was a 1:1 correlation between the pain stimulus and the amount of pain experienced[6] (see accompanying figures). That is, if you touched something hot (the stimulus), the pain would travel from your finger to your brain and register pain. He was only partially correct, but pretty good for 500 years ago!

---

6 "Descartes-reflex" by René Descartes - Copied from a 345 year old book, *Traite de l'homme*. Licensed under Public Domain via Wikimedia Commons –
http://commons.wikimedia.org/wiki/File:Descartes-reflex.JPG#/media/File:Descartes-reflex.JPG .
http://physiologyonline.physiology.org/content/nips/23/6/371/F1.medium.gif

13

The pain signal would indeed reach the brain. However, according to Descartes' theory, each person would experience the same amount of pain from the same amount of pain stimulus; and we know that isn't true. What Descartes didn't realize was that the mind and body are intimately connected neural networks (nerve signals and their connections) in many areas of the brain are active and communicate when we think and feel emotions (Figure 2.2 below) Through these *biological* processes of our thoughts and feelings, **we can *increase* pain by worrying about it and believing that it will get worse. Or… we can *decrease* pain by keeping our mind on other things and believing that it will get better.**

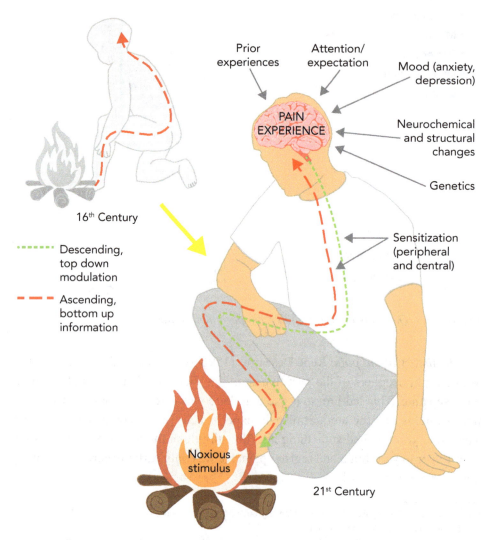

Figure 2.2. Changes in our understanding how the brain modulates pain perception.

WHAT IS PAIN? NINE LESSONS

What we think and feel changes our brain's neurotransmitters (chemicals). Depending upon what we are thinking or feeling, stress hormones, blood flow, and other physiological activities also change. For example, think of the last time you were frightened. Did you notice that your heart began to race, your hands became a little sweaty, and your breathing sped up? We now have brain imaging and other techniques to see which areas of the brain are active when we laugh, or are stressed, depressed, excited, scared, or in pain. These areas communicate and influence each other. This is why experienced pain is *both* biological and psychological.

So it is true when people say, "your pain is all in your head". Yes, it is also in your imagination. **And yes, biological, chemical processes are involved at all these levels.** That is far different from "faking it".

Dr. G. Allen Finley[7] offers this advice to children, whose family, friends, or doctors don't understand or believe they are in pain, "We tell patients, 'you know more about your pain than anyone else, you should think of these people as just needing to be educated… you are the expert.'"

LESSON 3: PAIN SIGNALS MOVE BOTH UP TO... AND DOWN FROM... THE BRAIN, AS WELL AS WITHIN THE BRAIN

There is a complex signal system of nerves and chemicals that come into play when your child feels pain. **This pain signal traffic is a "bottom up" and "top down" system between the site of the experienced pain, such as a bruised knee, and the brain.** Messages are carried between those two sites through the nerves in the spinal cord. While it seems obvious that you need a functioning brain to feel pain, if you are in a deep sleep or coma or under general anesthesia during surgery, you don't feel the pain. *But…* when you wake up, all of those pain signals reach your brain again and you feel the pain.

So how does this pain signal pathway get turned on and stay on? If there is ongoing tissue damage (e.g. as with inflammation in arthritis), there are signals going upward toward (Figures 2.1; and 2.3 below) the specific pain site area in the brain for that body part.

In fibromyalgia, however, and CRPS and IBS, the chronic pain develops as other pain centers in the brain becomes "activated" or turned on. **These activated pain perception areas continue on "automatic pilot."**[8] The damping, downward activity is reduced or inefficient. A familiar yet extreme example of this process is "phantom limb pain," or pain in an arm or leg that has been amputated… it's no longer there. When the painful leg or arm was there, pain signals were being sent to the parts of

---

7   Dr. G. Allen Finley , Professor of Anesthesia & Psychology, Dalhousie University, and the Dr. Stewart Wenning Chair in Pediatric Pain Management, IWK Health Centre, Halifax, Canada,

8   *http://quickhealthnotes.weebly.com/uploads/2/6/8/7/26878060/396395_orig.gif*

the brain receiving sensation/feeling data from that part of the body. After removal of that leg or arm that brain pain center is still "turned on", it has memory, and continues to register leg or arm pain. In this scenario, pain becomes a "top-down" process originating *from* the brain. The pain is real and originates as brain circuitry signals.

Almost all people who have a limb amputated "feel" phantom sensations such as touch, movement, and change in temperature for about a year or so. However, if these individuals had pain in the limb *before* the amputation, they are more likely to have phantom limb pain, since the primary signal in that area of the brain before the amputation was pain rather than normal sensations. It is similar with other types of pain, including IBS, chronic headaches, fibromyalgia and CRPS.

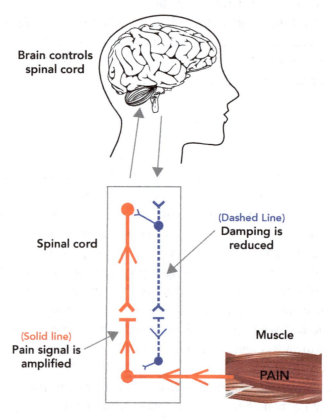

Figure 2.3. In chronic pain the pain's 'turn-off', top-down, system is inefficient.

LESSON 4: ACUTE VERSUS CHRONIC PAIN—WHAT IS THE DIFFERENCE?

Pain experiences can be roughly divided into two basic forms—acute and chronic. Approaching acute and chronic pain with the same mind-set has the result of

WHAT IS PAIN? NINE LESSONS

prolonging the pain experience for a child. Inadequate treatment of acute pain may actually worsen chronic pain or lead to its development.

Acute pain is the initial signal that there is tissue injury, inflammation, or infection that needs immediate attention. For example, your child burns his hand; he feels pain and withdraws it from the source of the burn. Thus, acute pain serves as a warning signal to "take action." This is what we often refer to as "pain that serves a purpose." Acute pain is brief and usually ends after the injury heals, the inflammation has subsided, or the stretch, contraction, or impingement on the body part has resolved.

Examples include a broken arm, post-surgery pain, most cases of gastroenteritis, a sore throat, pain from an ear infection, or muscle cramps from vigorous exercise. This type of pain can be mild to severe. Most acute pain conditions are readily diagnosable; the source is generally easily discoverable.

Chronic pain is **persistent and continuous for longer than expected periods of time.** It can also be recurrent, such as abdominal pain or backache. For other chronic pains, usually the first thought for parents is to find "the cause", so it can be treated and the pain stopped.

Recent research has also identified moderate to severe menstrual cramps in girls as a recurrent pain problem that needs to be addressed and mitigated. Typically period cramps are assumed to be "normal". Little attention is paid to it by parents or clinicians. However, menstrual cramps are significant sources of stress and school absences for some girls and may sensitize the nervous system to impact other brain areas of pain. See Chapter 5 for more on this.

Some types of chronic pain are related to an underlying disease, such as arthritis, cancer, sickle cell pain crises, nerve damage, or chronic infection, to name a few. But most chronic pains are *not* readily defined by a specific inflammatory, infectious or structural disease. Typically, the search for "the cause" brings the child to many doctors and tests, only to be told "the tests are all normal."

The problem is that the tests detect underlying *organ structure* in the diseases noted above. To identify the cause of chronic pain, you often need an "electrician," if the "plumber" or "carpenter" has not identified and fixed the problem. **If the organ-focused subspecialists have not readily identified and fixed the pain problem, then the cause of the pain may likely be within the *wiring* or *electrical connectivity* in the nervous system,** rather than in the specific organ being evaluated (e.g. intestinal tract or bones and ligaments). This type of "electrical signaling" pain persists long after the initial acute injury has healed or the infection has resolved (typically longer than three months, but may be shorter depending upon the situation) and clearly no longer serves a useful warning function. Examples of these pains include irritable bowel syndrome (IBS), fibromyalgia, complex regional pain syndrome (CRPS). In these situations, **the pain condition becomes the disease,** as is now recognized in the Institute of Medicine's report on "Pain in America," (2012. See bibliography in Appendix of book) [1]. Even when the cause is known, or associated with menstrual periods, for example, chronic pain hinders the body's ability to heal itself, and so the pain itself becomes a major problem.

With acute pain, physical movement, emotions, beliefs, and environmental factors (e.g. what doctors, nurses, and parents do and say) affect the child's experiences and even how long pain lasts. **With chronic pain, there is more opportunity for these factors to affect pain perception as well as the child's ability to function**—attend school, participate in athletics and engage in social interaction. (We discuss these factors in detail in Chapters 11 and 12.) For these reasons, even a pain initially related to known likely causes (e.g. arthritis or surgery) can become more severe or last longer than would otherwise be expected. This is when acute pain becomes the propagator of chronic pain.

LESSON 5: FEELINGS, THOUGHTS AND MEMORIES INCREASE OR DECREASE PAIN...AND A LITTLE NEUROANATOMY, PLEASE

We have three major subdivisions of our nervous system.

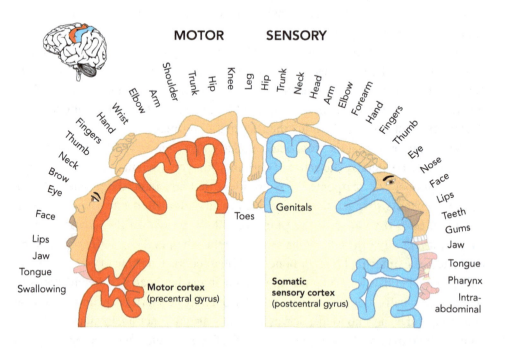

Figure 2.4. The body's Geo-location system in the brain's sensory & motor areas

1. Our **sensory nervous system** carries "feeling" information, such as temperature, touch, pain, sight and other sensations (e.g. itch). Each part of our body has a specific place in our brain that recognizes that part for sensation and makes it move with an action These locations are called motor and sensory cortex(es)... See Figure 2.4 above

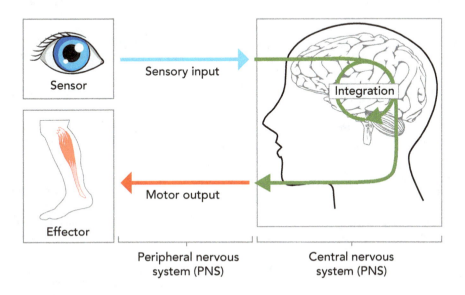

Figure 2.5.   Central nervous system: pathway from recognition (sight) to action (movement).

2. Our **motor nervous system** makes our muscles contract, allow us to move and do other things with muscles and bones. For example, motor signals to our legs influence our gastrocnemius muscles to contract and escape in response to something we see. Figure 2.3, 2.5 above

3. Our **autonomic (unconscious) nervous system** is made up of two sub-parts.
   - The **sympathetic nervous system (SNS)** is our "fight or flight" warning and protection system. When the SNS gets turned on, we are scared, angry, physically active, or excited; we feel our heart rate speed up; our breathing increases; we may become sweaty; and we are either "ready for action" or "frozen" like a deer in the headlights.
   - Our **parasympathetic nervous system (PNS)** balances the SNS and is our restorative system that helps us digest food, feel calm and positive, lower our heart rate, and feel peaceful. See Figure 2.6 below

PAIN IN CHILDREN AND YOUNG ADULTS

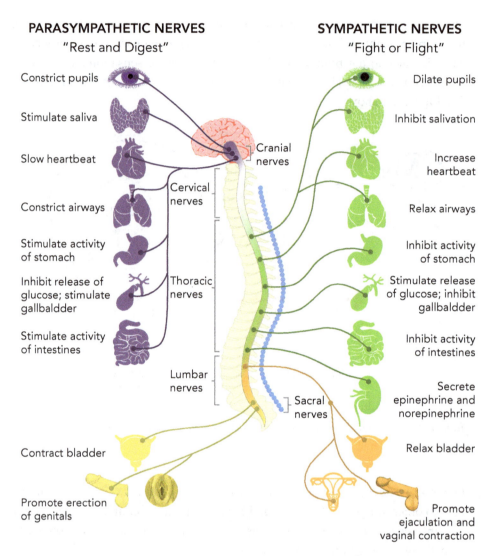

Figure 2.6   Actions of our two-part autonomic nervous system [9]

All parts of our nervous system can interact with each other. The brain is our central processing unit (CPU in computer terms) that integrates all the messages to and from connections that affect our experienced sensation, motor activity, and feelings of action and calmness. This brain connectivity includes our brain centers involved with thoughts, learning, emotions, and memory. This means that feelings and thoughts actually can increase or decrease the volume of pain signals, like turning up or down the volume control on the TV. When we feel anxious, our

---

9   Adapted from: *https://sites.google.com/site/anatomybody/calendar*

SNS becomes more active. This causes our heart to speed up and our hands to get clammy. Anxiety increases our pain experience by turning up the volume of pain signals and by increasing activity in the pain perception areas of that part of our brain that perceives the distress related to pain (cingulate gyrus).

Beliefs and thoughts also impact pain. Remember a time when you injured yourself, had a headache, or, for women, had menstrual cramps. When you focused your attention on the pain it got worse. This is because you cleared your brain of other things, leaving lots of room for pain signals. **If you then worried that the pain was a sign of something serious or that it was going to get worse, the pain probably did get worse.** This is because as you started to believe that the pain meant something serious or bad, these beliefs made you worry. **As you started to worry, the chemicals in your brain began to change, certain neural connections in your brain got stronger, and those changes increased the pain signals.**

Now remember a time when you were in pain, but **you were distracted by something else... you were on a date or at a concert/football game/child's recital. The pain moved from foreground into background** while you focused on where you were going and other things; the same pain *bothered* you less. If you are in pain and worried about it, just telling yourself that it will be fine and that you will get through it can lessen the pain by reducing the stress chemicals in the brain and you will change the brain connectivity pattern as you begin to relax.

Past memories of pain also play a role in the sensory feeling of the pain (how strong it is, for example) and how much it bothers you (the suffering component). **With each pain experience, memory circuits for that pain experience are created and can be recalled at a future time.** Which pain experiences get stored depends upon how your child is feeling at the time he experiences the pain.

If a child has a significant pain experience (an injury or surgery) and is also stressed, then their body will become more sensitive to pain. Anxiety increases the relationship between pain and memory of pain; that is, it helps lay down the memory pathway of pain so it can be recalled more easily later. This serves a protective function in the short-term but can be harmful if the stress continues.

LESSON 6: YOUR PAIN CAN BE CONTAINED... BUT NOT BY MEDICATIONS ALONE

We have a variety of mechanisms in our nervous system to control pain. We can reduce spinal cord sensory/pain traffic, and we can change connectivity between different parts of our brain, making them stronger or weaker. We have neurotransmitters that impact our emotions, thoughts, and physical feelings. For example, when we begin to worry that a pain will get worse and worse (this is called "catastrophizing"), we *decrease* the strength of the neural connectivity between the *prefrontal cortex* in the *frontal lobe* of our brain (our regulatory center) and our *amygdala* (fear center). **This allows the fear center to be turned on with less control or regulation by the prefrontal cortex, which in turn causes the sympathetic nervous system (SNS) to become activated; this increases the flow of adrenalin.** In turn the stimulated SNS increases the volume of pain signaling… and in fact the pain does get worse. This is the neurobiological mechanism underlying the self-fulfilling prophesy of "it will get worse… if you believe it will get worse."

Fortunately, **our "top down" pain control system can work just as effectively and efficiently as our neural systems that increase pain (Figure 2.3 above).** For example, your child has a stomachache in the morning before school. Maybe in the past, she would have catastrophized about being unable to go to school; she was convinced that the pain would become intolerable at school. However, **she learns how to use her "brain power" to reduce the tummy pain by a few strategies that can reduce or turn off pain.** Examples include breathing techniques, imagery, positive thinking, and others. (See Chapters 15 and 16 for more detail.)

> *12 year old Maria had been missing a lot of school because her stomach always hurt worse in the mornings. She would feel nauseated and not want any breakfast. She would spend a long time on the toilet to see if having a bowel movement would help her stomach feel better. He mother would tell her to hurry up or she would be late to school, but the longer Maria sat on the toilet, the more she worried that her stomachache would get worse, and the more she worried and catastrophized about her stomach pain, the worse the pain became until it was too late to go to school. Maria would continue to worry about her stomach and tell her mother that the pain was unbearable.*
>
> *I (LZ) saw Maria in my UCLA pediatric pain clinic, after a referral from one of the UCLA pediatric gastroenterologists who thought Maria had IBS. He had started Maria on nighttime amitriptyline, a common medication used in IBS, but her pain had not improved, neither had her school attendance. Mom was worried because the school had sent a note home about truancy. I didn't detect any major anxiety or depression but rather detected a fear about inability to control the pain.*
>
> *I referred Maria to one of our pain team psychotherapists, Azita Sachmachian, MFT, who taught Maria some breathing techniques as well as how to think about pain differently than Maria previously had. She provided Maria with some positive self-statements, like, "I know that I can lower this pain with my breathing," or "I know that this pain will go away soon." Maria saw Azita weekly and, after the first month, her stomach pain and nausea were controlled enough for Maria to attend school. Once Maria got to school, she became distracted by the schoolwork and friends. Over the next 3 months, her symptoms resolved enough for her to not be worried about them. She said that she used the breathing and thinking that Azita had taught her… and they worked.*

WHAT IS PAIN? NINE LESSONS

We have two major areas in the brain related to pain perception for a) *bother/distress/suffering* and b) *sensation* (where pain is located and what it feels like in the *cingulate* lobe). In treatment, the most important area to target first is the brain area of *pain suffering*. This is because if your child feels the pain, but it no longer bothers her as much as before, she will begin to function and do more, like go to school or play with friends. **The more she can function, even with pain, the more quickly the pain will go away or be reduced.**

Imaging studies have confirmed where these "transactions" take place. The emotional pain of social rejection activates two brain regions that are also important in the response to physical pain[10]. **Pain activates the anterior cingulate cortex,** which signals higher brain regions that impel an individual to act to stop the pain; social rejection similarly triggers activity in this region. **Activation of the right ventral prefrontal cortex appears to help dampen the distress of both physical pain and social exclusion. (Figure 2.3)**

A word about medications, opioids like **OxyContin™ or Vicodin™.** These are often thought of as the *only* medications for pain (often called "pain killers"), if Tylenol™ or Advil™ (ibuprofen) does not work. Early on in the course of Maria's pain problem, her local pediatrician had given her some Vicodin to help with the pain. However, this medication not only did *not* reduce the pain, but her nausea and constipation increased. The most effective treatments are those that help the body's pain control system work efficiently. While **opioids reduce some types of pain, they can work *against* the body's own pain control system by blocking your own natural *endorphin* (natural opioid) production.** Stopping the opioids can actually result in more pain, and that makes children need more opioids, etc. This is **why opioids alone, without any other pain control strategies, are ineffective in the long-run for most types of chronic pain.** Also there is evidence that chronic use of opioids for non-cancer pain can actually increase pain. This is called opioid-induced "hyper-algesia". In this seemingly paradoxical example, the pain gets better when the person weans off the opioids.

Medications that focus on the central neurotransmitters controlling *central* pain are far more effective than just taking analgesics, "pain killers". Similarly, many non-drug therapies like acupuncture or massage can influence natural neurotransmitters. Other non-drug treatments (e.g. biofeedback, yoga, and hypnotherapy) directly alter the brain's pain perception areas and neural connectivity. (See Chapter 14 and 15)

---

10   Reprinted from *http://jama.jamanetwork.com/article.aspx?articleid=197621*

LESSON 7: PAIN MECHANISMS DETERMINE TYPE OF SPECIFIC TREATMENT

Some pain is *neuropathic*, while other pain is *nociceptive*. What is the difference?

Neuropathic pain is caused by injury or damage to nerve tissue or by disordered nerve signaling without structural (physical) nerve damage or inflammation. **This kind of pain is often felt as burning or stabbing and typically is located in one part of the body.** Examples of neuropathic pain include sciatica or pinched nerve and shingles, and Complex Regional Pain Syndrome-Type I (CRPS-1). With shingles and CRPS-I, the skin and underlying tissue in the affected body part often feel super-sensitive and hurt. The pain is often described as "burning" or "stabbing."

Nociceptive pain is caused by an injury, inflammation, disease, or muscle spasms (stress on tissues). **Such pain is experienced by a child as an ongoing dull ache or pressure,** if the source is a solid organ such as the liver, spleen, kidneys, muscle, bone covering, or other tissues. **If the child complains of cramping, the source of the pain may be a hollow organ such as intestine, bladder, ureters, uterus, or fallopian tubes.** Examples of nociceptive pain include arthritis, gastroenteritis, menstrual cramps, or tension headaches. Typically pain from muscles, ligaments, and bones may be called "somatic" while pain related to internal organs is often called "visceral."

Irritable Bowel Syndrome (IBS) is an example of both pain types. A child with chronic pain may have pain that starts as nociceptive pain (if the problem begins with infection, injury, or inflammation), and then, after the initial problem resolves, the nervous system keeps misfiring and the pain becomes neuropathic. For example, **IBS may start with an episode of acute gastroenteritis. Typically, a viral infection** in the intestinal tract causes inflammation, with intestinal cramping and often diarrhea, nausea, vomiting, and perhaps fever. The inflammation goes away, but the pain remains: inflammation sets off the pain signals but after the infection clears, the signals between the brain and the intestines go on "automatic pilot" and keep firing. Additionally, because of the pain inside the belly, the muscles *over* the belly contract in response to the pain, thus adding somatic pain to visceral pain.

Arthritis is another example of combined neuropathic and nociceptive pain. Here, the child has ongoing nociceptive pain. However, if the pain continues and isn't addressed, the central nervous system and areas of the brain become sensitized and "turned on." The pain then becomes "louder," more severe, and even longer lasting than it might have been with just the arthritis alone. This is why, in some cases, after good treatment aimed at reducing the inflammation—even with documented evidence of no inflammation—joint pain continues.

WHAT IS PAIN? NINE LESSONS

It is important to differentiate between the types of pain, because **specific treatments depend on the mechanisms of and reasons for the pain**. If inflammation is the cause—e.g. ulcerative colitis or Crohn's disease in the intestinal tract, called inflammatory bowel disease (IBD)—then we need to treat the inflammation. This treatment will be different from that used, for example, in irritable bowel syndrome (IBS), where inflammation is not the major cause of the pain (electrical signaling is), even if the pain started with inflammation during a viral gastroenteritis. See Chapter 6 for more detailed examples.

LESSON 8: KNOW THAT ALL TREATMENTS CAN FAIL... AND WHY

There are two key reasons for treatment failures: A) Under-treatment and/ or B) ineffective choices.

A. Under-treatment

Despite advances in pediatric pain medicine, **children are frequently under treated, especially for acute pain.** Examples include post-surgical pain, trauma, and medical procedure pain. There are a variety of reasons for this:

- Misunderstanding/ underestimating seriousness of pain and its consequences,
- Individual and cultural attitudes,
- Complexities and effort in assessing pain in children,
- Inadequate education, under treatment by well-meaning adult specialists
- Insufficient research.

Furthermore, **some physicians and parents are hesitant to use common pain medications to treat children with acute pain, fearing these medications are *too strong* and that the child might become *harmed or addicted.*** But we know that acute pain, if not well treated, leads to chronic pain.

For example, your child has surgery with significant post-operative pain. He is not sleeping because of the continuing pain that increases his anxiety. The surgeon wonders why your child continues to have pain when, for most of his patients by this time after surgery, there is complete resolution of the pain. Instead, it is a month or more after the surgery, the surgical incision is well healed and there is no evidence of infection. Yet your child is bedridden with ongoing severe pain. Does this story of our patient James sound familiar?

25

PAIN IN CHILDREN AND YOUNG ADULTS

James, a 14 year old boy, had abdominal pain, now going on for three months after an acute viral gastroenteritis. Everyone else in the family had recovered after getting the same infection. After basic evaluation by the pediatrician, James was referred to a pediatric gastroenterologist who evaluated James for the most common, easily treatable causes of ongoing abdominal pain. But based on the history, physical exam, and first line testing, she decided that James had IBS and did not require an endoscopy or colonoscopy. She started James on amitriptyline, but two months later, even with increasing doses of the medication, James was no better and still not going to school, because of pain. His mom was concerned and asked the gastroenterologist to do more invasive testing with endoscopy/ colonoscopy. The gastroenterologist told mom that she truly did not think these invasive studies were indicated since all the blood tests ruled out any inflammatory, genetic, or metabolic conditions that could cause the pain. So, mom decided to take James to a different gastroenterologist who was willing to do these tests. The tests were done and were negative (normal).

James was still not sleeping or going to school. James became fearful of eating because eating caused him more abdominal pain. James' pediatrician then referred him to a pediatric allergist in case he might be allergic to certain foods. There he got more blood tests as well as skin testing and some tests came out mildly positive. James was put on a strict elimination diet, avoiding gluten and other foods that came out positive on testing.

Two months later, James was still in pain, was not sleeping, and was losing a significant amount of weight. James was having increased pain with eating and had developed "food aversion," meaning he was refusing food because of fear that it would make his stomach hurt worse. He found his strict diet unpalatable and told his mom that there was nothing in the diet that he even wanted to eat, even if he could. He was still not attending school and had become irritable and sullen.

If you were James' parents, what specialist would you take James to next? How long can this go on before the "cause" is found and treated and James is "cured?" In the "belly pain scenario" directly above, the following were *not* addressed:

- James' lack of sleep
- James' feelings of powerlessness/ helplessness
- James' isolation and lack of functioning
- The association of food with pain and thus food aversion
- James' mood, anxiety, or other stressors that contributed to his pain
- The brain-gut neural signaling problem and pain memory

26

WHAT IS PAIN? NINE LESSONS

We see many children with chronic pain who have been under-treated, and more of our patients have undergone unnecessary surgical procedures or are prescribed potent drugs simply because their doctor has run out of ideas… and feels pressured to alleviate the child's suffering by "doing more tests". Colleagues tell us that pressure to "do something" often comes from well-meaning parents who cannot bear to see their child suffer anymore. One of three things happens: a) children are subjected to unnecessary invasive testing, surgical procedures, and drugs, b) they go without adequate treatment, or c) their complaints are discounted. Unfortunately, the additional testing doesn't reveal anything helpful, surgery does little to stem the pain and in many cases makes it worse. As you are learning, there is neither an "easy fix" with a single cause, nor a single medication, to treat chronic pain.

Conventional treatments usually work for *acute* pain. For example, ibuprofen can reduce pain and inflammation for muscle aches, while morphine can be very effective for post-surgical pain. However, if acute pain is not well treated, the body's pain systems can become sensitized ("turned on") and then acute pain leads to chronic pain.

B. Ineffective choices in procedures or medications

The traditional medical model, with its emphasis on the doctor being responsible for "curing" patients, as well as its reliance on procedures such as surgery or other invasive procedures, and on pain medications, are often ineffective for ameliorating chronic pain, especially in children.

In most cases, the procedure, even if it helps short-term, doesn't continue to help, so that more and more procedures are needed until the procedure area itself becomes a new site for pain. And as we said in Lesson 6 above, not only do opioids (such as hydrocodone or morphine) not help many types of pain (other than to reduce some anxiety or put the child to sleep), they actually prolong the pain by decreasing the production of one of the body's key pain-fighting chemicals (neurotransmitters called enkephalins and endorphins).

LESSON 9: YOU MUST BE PREPARED TO TAKE THE LEAD ON THE ROAD TO DIAGNOSIS AND RECOVERY

You as the parent must *help* lead the way to get the right treatment for your child's pain. You never thought in the beginning that this was an option. But by now, you've probably guessed it's turning out this way. **The fact is most physicians are not adequately trained in dealing with chronic pain in children,** as they are with treatment of acute pain. We hope that by the time you finish this book, you

PAIN IN CHILDREN AND YOUNG ADULTS

will be more informed to obtain the needed expertise for your child, work together with that expert, and help educate your child's pediatrician along the way. And you and **your family will grow through the process, feel empowered, and become closer to each other.**

We end this chapter by restating four important points.

1　**If your child says that she is in pain, she is.** In our opinion, expressing the attitude that "the pain is all in your head" (…though it is really there… in her/his brain) should be avoided at all costs. Such a limited way of thinking leads to unnecessary tests, procedures, and treatments or, conversely, to a lack of empathy that may lead to substandard care. Ultimately, and most importantly, it may undermine your child's confidence in his ability to get better.

2　Your job is to understand which factors are contributing to your child's experience of pain, together with your child's primary care physician (PCP) or nurse practitioner (PNP):

- What has caused the pain to become chronic?
- What is increasing his suffering?
- What is maintaining the pain?

3　**Learn how to seek answers to these multiple factors—not simply by using an analgesic medicine to reduce the pain** itself as you would for an acute pain problem, such as an injury or a sore throat. As with any disease, there are emotional, cognitive, and environmental contributors to the pain, adding to the overall problem; each of these needs to be addressed for your child to get better.

4　**Understanding the general principles of pain** (how it is created, continued, or turned off) allows you to help your child cope better. You will be more successful at finding a specialist physician or primary care practitioner who has an understanding of current pediatric pain treatment.

Now it's on to Chapters 3, 4 and 5 where we will show you how pain is expressed and treated in many common conditions. See if you can find your child's story in them.

CHAPTER 3

HOW CHILDREN EXPRESS PAIN:
WHAT DO THE CLUES MEAN?
HOW CAN A PARENT HELP?

Not wanting to go out with friends because of the pain
Leaves you the hard job of friends to maintain,
Not wanting to go to school with the pain
Leaves you with a less knowledgeable brain
Having trouble coping with it
Doesn't leave you with much wit.

—EXCERPT FROM *As Simple as an Apple Tree*, BY ELLIE ROSS

DECIPHER THE CLUES

WHAT SHE OR HE SAYS

HOW DOES HE ACT?

OBSERVING YOUR CHILD

**HOW YOU LEARN BY COMMUNICATING WITH YOUR CHILD...
LISTENING**

HOW HER BODY REACTS

PARENTAL EXPECTATIONS AND HELPING YOUR CHILD

TOOLS TO MEASURE PAIN

PAIN IN CHILDREN AND YOUNG ADULTS

We all experience and express pain in different ways. Most children with chronic pain have no trouble letting us know that they are in pain. Even very young children —infants—express themselves when they are in pain. They may cry or become irritable; the child is not unsure of his pain. Rather, we parents sometimes have difficulty trying to interpret our child's behavior or understand what he's trying to tell us.

> *Annie is 2 years old when she was diagnosed with a painful form of juvenile arthritis. While most children begin to walk around the age of one, Annie refused to walk. She became increasingly irritable and withdrawn. Doctors initially thought she was developmentally delayed with a difficult temperament. In reality, she was just too young to articulate the excruciating pain she felt when she did try to walk. Putting pressure on her hips and knees was painful.*

DECIPHER THE CLUES

In pediatric training, we learned to listen to moms and dads, since they know their child best. As parents, Paul and I learned to "read" subtle cues that our three daughters provided when they were in pain. **(In this book we often say "he" or "she" but, in fact, the observations or recommendations apply to either gender.)** Interestingly, they were quite different from each other. One daughter was very vocal and demonstrative. With her, it was difficult to know how much pain she was in, since even lesser pain was displayed with all the gusto of an academy award-winning performance (she became a comedy writer). The second daughter was a challenge too, but in a different way; we had to pay closer attention to her physical cues since she just became quiet, withdrawn, irritable, but rarely complained (she became an attorney). The third daughter's pain was expressed verbally and clearly (she became a lead elementary school teacher and vice principal). Over time we learn to "read" our children. However, there are times when we are uncertain. This chapter is intended to help you "read" your child.

Dr. Christopher Eccleston[11] comments:

> *"The teenager who is being constantly alarmed [by pain] is going to be jumpy, nervous, find it difficult to concentrate, remember and communicate. He will become sleep-deprived, take on a pain face (sunken and darkened eyes, distracted look), and generally will become what psychologists call overly vigilant."*

---

11 Dr. Christopher Eccleston, Director of the Centre for Pain Research, The University of Bath, Bath, United Kingdom.

HOW CHILDREN EXPRESS PAIN

As parents, we all want to "do something" if we see our child suffering; *not doing something* seems like bad parenting, not to mention being cruel. But what if we do something that we believe makes the pain better and there is still no change in our child's behavior?

- Suppose she is still crying or acting out?
- What if she just becomes quiet and withdrawn?
- What do these signs mean?
- Does it mean that "something" we did to reduce the pain worked or didn't work?
- What was that something?

As you will see throughout this book, chronic pain often responds better to less—or at least, subtler forms of intervention. Your understanding of your child's pain will also play a role in which type of medical treatment he gets and whether or not the treatment "works." Doctors will differ in how well they understand and respond to your child's symptoms. Unfortunately, there is no single "objective" test to determine pain. Pain is simply what the child feels. However, there are four general indicators of how much pain a child is in. You will learn how to recognize the signs of pain by paying attention to these four clues:

- What your child says,
- How your child behaves or acts,
- How your child's body reacts.
- What you learn as you communicate with your child

That being said, in chronic pain we look at *function* rather than just words about pain. So we would add a fifth sign that may be more important than all the rest, borrowed from a basketball "head fake" allusion: **"Follow the feet... not the lips (or face)."**

WHAT SHE OR HE SAYS

Children describe their pain in many ways. Depending on her age, they may use words such as "achy", "sharp", "dull", "electrical", "burning", "throbbing", "pressure", or "stabbing". Such words can help you and your child's doctor understand the source of the pain and find the right treatment.

For example, Jimmie, a teenage boy with Complex Regional Pain Syndrome (CRPS-1), struggles to describe his pain, and offers lots of clues for parent and doctor:

> *Basically, anything that your nerves sense... really hurt. When my foot goes hot/cold it stings and goes numb, a bit like when you have been out in the snow... you get hot*

aches when you go back in the warmth. It goes super sensitive... feels like my bones and muscles inside are pushing out and stretching the skin.

The pain makes you jump. It feels like someone is pushing so hard they're piercing the skin; but you know that they are hardly pushing enough to push the skin down and make the skin around it bulge up. ... You don't know whether to laugh or cry. Your foot tells you "ouch" this really hurts and your common sense is saying don't be stupid, you should be laughing ... socks and sheets can hurt: it feels like the soft fibers have been replaced with blades of glass, scratching and digging into the skin.

Devin, Age 14 with CRPS-1, reports:

One of the strangest symptoms is when it changes color. My foot has been almost every color I can imagine. When this is happening, the pain is stinging and burning a bit like when you have blood drawn, only much worse. Sometimes when this happens, the stinging and throbbing pain builds up, to the point that you feel that you will scream till it eventually goes totally numb. This is really scary, like my foot has died, been frozen. It won't move at all. Then suddenly it defrosts and the pain builds up again.

Of course, not all children, even older ones, can articulate their pain as well as Jimmie and Devin. Younger children, those with cognitive or learning disabilities, or frustrated or highly distressed children, may tell you that the pain "just hurts" or they may simply groan or cry. Some become withdrawn and quiet. In such cases, you and your child's doctor will have to learn about the pain by honing your observation and communication skills.

I (Lonnie) remember during my residency, very early in my pediatric training, a mother brought Bailey, her 8-year-old daughter to see me. The mom said that Bailey had awakened that morning holding her belly and crying. The child had no fever but the mom was worried that something was terribly wrong and that she was in great pain. When I saw Bailey, she was curled up on her mom's lap. When I asked her what was wrong, she just buried her head deeper. I tried to make contact by commenting that she looked pretty upset.

As a relatively new physician, I was anxious about my performance. What if the child's reticence prevented me from taking an oral history, performing a physical examination, and determining what was bothering her; where, and to what degree? It all added up to failure. Meanwhile, the girl continued to whimper until finally, out of frustration, she yelled at me, "it just hurts!" She must have thought I was really dumb. But her outburst registered with me. How could I not know that she was suffering? Bailey knew!

HOW CHILDREN EXPRESS PAIN

Most physicians will not have the time or intimate knowledge of your child's specific history to make the leap from *"this child is complaining about something"* to *"I know what is causing the pain."* This is where your role as an advocate for your child comes in. **You need to find ways to make your child's doctor understand her pain**. If you have a good doctor, he may call on you to help your child express her pain, interpret her pain-related behavior, and determine when pain needs medical attention, or if it can be taken care of at home. If you have a less patient doctor, you may want to find another one, or, at least be ready to offer this information without being asked and see if you caught the doctor on a stressful day.

HOW HE ACTS

Most parents know that their child often acts differently from his "normal self" when they are in pain. There are, of course, the obvious signs that your child is in pain: crying, grimacing, groaning, or holding or rubbing their leg or stomach. But there are more subtle signs. **Your child may become less active, agitated, or sleep or eat less than usual.** They may show less interest in play or other activities or may just be grumpy. Thus, what the infant or child is *not doing* can be as important as what they *are doing*. How well you understand your child's pain will play a critical role in what type of medical treatment they get and whether or not the treatment "works."

Some children may magnify their behavior because they are aware that it makes their pain and suffering more believable. Thirteen-year-old Doug told me,

> *"I avoided going to school because I was afraid someone would accidentally bump into my arm." Doug had chronic arm pain (CRPS-1) that was "totally unbearable" when touched. When not at school he avoided contact with people and cradled his arm. Since the arm was not in a cast, bandaged, or swollen, he feared no one would believe he was in terrible pain; he had no "proof."*

A child's response to pain may be influenced by its severity, type, location, and duration. For example, if the pain comes on quickly, is of short duration, and of high intensity, the child's reaction is likely to be more dramatic. In this case it may be easy to recognize that your child is in pain. This kind of pain is usually the result of acute injuries such as when a child breaks his arm falling off a swing at the playground. And the child's behavior may match the severity of the injury. However, with pain that is less intense but lasts longer, the child may be in pain for some time before you notice changes in behavior. In this category, common sources of pain include headaches, achy joints, and muscle pain.

PAIN IN CHILDREN AND YOUNG ADULTS

As pain becomes chronic, children adapt by learning how to cope or deal with it unless their coping abilities are hindered by stress, or the pain escalates beyond what they can tolerate. Remember, **just because a child with chronic pain is not acting the same as a child in acute pain does not mean that he is not in pain.**

We are often frustrated by nurses or doctors who discount a hospitalized child's reports of pain after they see him playing videogames or interacting with visitors, declaring *"he doesn't look like he is in pain."* **Children who have chronic pain do not typically act like children with acute pain.** This behavioral difference is because they may have adopted effective approaches to cope—under certain circumstances and for limited periods of time. The challenge for parents is to figure out what a certain behavior means, since a behavior, such as crying, can express a variety of states of mind—anger, sadness, fear, frustration—not just pain.

Table 3.1. Pain: Questions to Consider: Is Your Child...	
1	...limiting their physical activities?
2	...more tired than normal or having trouble sleeping?
3	...more argumentative or irritable than usual?
4	...quieter than usual?
5	...having trouble concentrating and with school work?
6	...eating differently?
7	...not wanting to go to school?
8	...having trouble with other children at school?
9	...showing a change in appearance?
10	...not complaining, but is he still in pain?

While any of the above behaviors in Table 3.1 may be a sign that your child is in pain, be careful not to over-attribute specific behavior changes to the pain itself—there may be other reasons why your child is acting differently. A child who is sad, angry, upset, bored, hungry, or anxious might become clingy and irritable or avoid school and other social interaction.

You know your child better than anyone else. It's unreasonable to expect anyone, even your child's doctor, to know more about the causes of your child's pain than you do. Sure, the doctor may know the medical terminology and be able to prescribe the drugs and other treatments to make your child better, but you are the one who sees how she acts on a daily basis.

YOU LEARN BY COMMUNICATING WITH YOUR CHILD: *LISTENING & OBSERVING*

If your child is suffering from chronic pain and **if you feel like you don't know what to do, it's time for the two of you to start talking.** How do you maintain that balance between asking questions, being intrusive, and really listening? As parents we often have difficulty just listening. We may observe our child looking forlorn and pensive. We want to ask, "What's wrong?" We want to "solve" the problem. (This is especially true of fathers: the "male" brain.) If we have a child with a history of headaches or stomachaches, we may want to ask, "Are you in pain? Does your head (or stomach) hurt?" While such questions are rooted in good intentions, this approach may not be in the best interest of your child.

The problem is that once you ask your child if she is in pain, you have caused her to stop whatever she was doing at that moment and to *scan* her body to determine if she is in fact hurting. **Once the brain puts full attention on the body and on pain specifically, the pain is immediately magnified**: all the brain's perception areas become focused on the pain and the pain is felt more intensely.

While it may be difficult, you must trust that your child will tell you if they are hurting and want help—unless, of course, there is some underlying reason that they cannot tell you. For headaches or belly pain, the best approach is to tell your child that you will not ask if she is in pain, but that **she is free to tell you she is hurting and whether she wants your help or not.** Let her know that, even if she doesn't tell you and you don't ask, you realize that there may be times when she is in fact suffering.

Distraction Ideas

This doesn't mean you have to let your child sit and suffer in silence when you have a good idea he is in pain. How do we tie understanding with therapeutic action? See Table 3.2 for some ideas for distraction, anything to distract him or her, even if just for a few minutes. The goal is to reroute the nerve impulses that are misfiring and causing the pain, and, the less we focus on the pain, the quicker these impulses will become weaker.

Table 3.2. Distraction Ideas
1 Try asking him about his day,
2 Tell him about something that happened to you that day,
3 Talk about current events,
4 Make a plan for the next day,
5 Come up with a fun game or even a chore for him to do

PAIN IN CHILDREN AND YOUNG ADULTS

Elinor's eight-year-old daughter Marney developed chronic pain in her back and shoulders as well as severe headaches after an operation to remove a brain tumor. Elinor learned the hard way that, for Marney, focusing on the pain was debilitating.

> *The best piece of advice I got that immediately showed results was not to talk to Marney about the pain. She could really function up to a certain point, but if you asked her how she was feeling, she focused on the pain and would suddenly be aware of it again. So, as a family, we stopped asking her about it and that immediately showed a better quality of life for her. She was still in pain, but there was an improvement right away. She was able to be more easily occupied by other things, like her computer, that were more fun than focusing on the pain. The more she was able to be distracted, the more she was able to have fun and enjoy her life.*

Elinor points out another important issue: your child may be in pain but can still become distracted or even laugh. In fact, **laughing is a great tension releaser.** Elinor came up with other ways to help Marney cope with pain and she shares them here:

1 *Give as much control as possible over her pain and her life;*

2 *Improve understanding and control by giving her information about what is wrong with her and the ways you intend to treat it in a way that she understands;*

3 *Teach that what she knows, does, and feels, can influence her experience of pain; and*

4 *Teach simple ways of coping with and reducing pain, such as distraction.*

We who work with children in pain often ask them during the first meeting, "What helps you cope with your pain?" Often the response is, "nothing works." Dr. Carl vonBaeyer[5,12] heard this a lot so he brainstormed with kids to come up with a list of things that could help (Table 3.3). These are just a few ways to soothe the pain. You and your child can make up your own, and post them on the refrigerator as a reminder.

5,12 Carl von Baeyer, Ph.D., Professor Emeritus of Psychology and Associate Member in Pediatrics, University of Saskatchewan, and Professor of Clinical Health Psychology, Pediatrics, and Child Health, Faculty of Medicine, University of Manitoba, Canada:

HOW CHILDREN EXPRESS PAIN

Table 3.3. Kids list 14 things to help alleviate their pain	
Changing activities	Taking a hot bath
Listening to music	Rubbing the place that hurts
Changing position	Relaxing: getting all floppy
Doing physical exercises that strengthen the part that hurts	Breathing better
Listening to your body to see if it's telling you to change something	Talking to yourself about staying in charge
Listening to your thoughts to see if you're stuck on a helpless, negative one	Thinking about a really nice place to be
Telling someone about something that is giving you stress	Paying attention to the parts of yourself that don't hurt.

HOW HER BODY REACTS: SYMPTOMS AND SIGNS

When we talk about how the body reacts to pain, we use the words "signs" and "symptoms." *Signs* of pain are things the doctor notices in a patient, such as a response to touch, reflexes, an enlarged liver, or a rash. These are distinct from *symptoms* which are what your child tells you he is *feeling*. So, reported feelings of pain, nausea, or "bloating" are symptoms. **Pain is a stressor and the body can react to stress through a number of "stress systems" that include the nervous system, the hormonal system, the immune system, and the cardiovascular system.** Each of these systems when disrupted can affect any organ in the body, causing multiple signs and producing associated self-reported symptoms.

Objective signs of pain and stress: When a child is experiencing pain, his body often will respond with biological signs of stress like an increase in heart rate, blood pressure, breathing rate, temperature changes, sweating, dizziness and immune system changes. The pain can also cause symptoms such as pins and needles, muscle aches, and nausea. As a parent, you are not going to take blood pressures or measure stress hormones or immune proteins.

You *can* take a pulse to see if it is rapid (likely more than 80-100 beats per minute). One pulse point is at the wrist just below the thumb. You can also take note of other observable signs of stress such as whether your child is sweating or vomiting. You need to take into consideration what you notice physically about your child, what he is telling you, and what behavior he is exhibiting. Together, these tell a story. It is our job, as parents, to learn the story and make sense of it. This is what we do in a medical evaluation... notice the child's behavior, sometimes even in the waiting room.

The nurse takes "vital signs" (heart rate, blood pressure, height, weight, and, if the child looks ill, temperature). We also take a detailed history from the parent and child before examining the child. The history includes development, medical, social, and family related information. Based on the entire picture, we come up with what is called the "working diagnosis" or understanding of the problem. From this we develop a treatment plan.

Unfortunately, many of the biological signs of acute pain or stress on the body *are not* present in children with chronic pain. For example, more often than not, a child in chronic pain will have normal pulse and blood pressure. He will not be sweating or have changes in skin color or breathing. He may report severe pain, but may not "look" like he is in pain; he may even be able to smile or laugh. Pain is a subjective experience. Each child must be evaluated individually with information gathered about her, as opposed to using a standard guide.

PARENTAL EXPECTATIONS

Parents' expectations, whether stated or not, have a huge impact on how a child expresses his pain and even on his perception of it. Other factors that affect a child's pain-related behavior include context and the environment i.e. where the child is when he has pain.

> *After Shane was hit in the knee with a soccer ball, he played the rest of the game without any apparent change in behavior—not even a grimace. But he began to cry after the game and complained of knee pain as soon as he got into the car.*

Children often are reticent about reacting to pain in front of peers; it is much easier to do so with parents. Thus they may hold it in until they are in a "safe" environment when they can "let it all out." It is the same with chronic pain. Many years ago, Lonnie was managing the post-operative pain for children who had surgery at UCLA.

> *Marshall, 13 years old, had just had major hip surgery and would have been expected to be pretty uncomfortable without a significant amount of pain medicine, like morphine. I had set him up with what is called a "PCA" or patient-controlled analgesia device in which he could press a button and get a pre-set amount of morphine delivered to him via his intravenous line, so that he could get what he needed to be comfortable. I noticed, however, that he was not pushing his button and thus not getting any morphine. His muscles were pretty tense and his blood pressure was high, typical signs of pain; but he was denying any pain or need for pain medicine.*

HOW CHILDREN EXPRESS PAIN

The intern who was working with me told me that this boy must be doing well since he did not need any morphine. I asked the intern to talk with the boy's mom outside the room, while I talked with him alone. I discovered that the boy's father was in jail for selling narcotics; his mom was worried that if her son used the morphine (an opioid) he would become "just like his dad." Although she never told him not to push his PCA button to get morphine, he "knew" that it would upset her if he did, and so he pretended that he was fine without pain medication.

However, he clearly wasn't doing "fine;" his body was becoming increasingly tense, he was afraid to move, and his blood pressure was dangerously high. He was suffering, but his concern for his mother overrode his own needs. Children are acutely aware of what their parents and other figures of authority want or expect (even if we as parents and doctors do not realize it).

TOOLS TO MEASURE PAIN

Doctors quantify pain in order to prescribe the right treatment and know that it's working. To help treat children with chronic pain, pain measurement tools have been developed and confirmed to estimate the level of experienced pain.

Children as young as three years of age can quantify their pain, if they are offered the right tools. For children under age six, visual tools help in the understanding and explaining to others the concept of *"less... or more hurt."* For example, we can use poker chips, pain thermometers, pain ladders, and pictures of children's faces with expressions ranging from neutral to very distressed. A child is asked to point to the number of poker chips, place on the ladder or thermometer, or face that best shows how much pain she feels. For a child who is in the hospital, frightened and upset, as well as in pain, asking him how he is *feeling* is not going to be a reliable indication of his pain. To get the best results, it is important that whoever is conducting the test makes sure the child understands that he is being asked about his hurt or "owie". You are not asking how he "feels" because his mommy is out of the room, or because he is scared or hungry.

Children of ages 3 to 5 years can do the Faces scale. Typically, older children and adolescents starting at 10 years or so can use the same number rating scale that adults use. In this method, the child is asked how much pain she is in on a scale of 0 to 10, with 0 = no pain and 10 = the most pain possible.

We asked Teddy, aged 12, how much his head hurt on the 0-10 scale. He promptly told us, "It was a "25 !"" The message he was giving us was that the pain was so bad it was off the scale. We got that message loud and clear!

39

The Bottom Line

Earlier in this chapter, we stated that the best way to approach a child's pain is by *not* asking her about it. Because focusing on pain at home reduces opportunities for distraction, **we do *not* ask parents to have their children keep "pain diaries" or to have their children rate their pain**. We leave the rating systems for when the child is seen in the office. Children understand the difference between being asked about their pain in a doctor's office or hospital and having a parent ask continuously throughout the day. Children easily distinguish between two types—one with the doctor and the other at home.

That being said, newer technologies such as Smartphones allow an array of children's self-reporting of pain and other feelings, especially if the apps are linked with intervention tools. In this way the older child or adolescent can work on coping tools by themselves for practice and to learn which strategies are most effective.

Now that you have the basics down, in the next few chapters we'll explore how and why pain is expressed in many common conditions.

CHAPTER 4

CHRONIC PAIN CONDITIONS (A):
SPORTS INJURIES,
PAIN IN EXTREMITIES & BACK

wrap! Bandage bruised rib
strap! Shoulder-support cross-bib
whew! Winded, bending over
knock! Unconscious, quarter over
snap! Quick! Save front tooth
expletive! Shouts painful truth
rip! Cartilage strips at knee
ouch!
ANOTHER SPORTS INJURY.

—LEE EMMETT, AUSTRALIA[13]

CHRONIC PAIN CONDITIONS

SPORTS INJURIES

COMPLEX REGIONAL PAIN SYNDROME (CRPS)

MYOFASCIAL PAIN

JUVENILE FIBROMYALGIA (JFM)

BACK PAIN

_____

13 *www.voicesnet.org/displayonepoem.aspx?poemid=132368*

PAIN IN CHILDREN AND YOUNG ADULTS

CHRONIC PAIN CONDITIONS

There is a subtle, but important, distinction between "diseases that are associated *with* pain" versus "chronic pain conditions." Diseases associated with pain are illnesses in which pain stems from a "known" cause such as infection, inflammation, injury, or obstruction associated with the "disease." **Chronic pain conditions are illnesses in which the "cause" of the pain (whether headaches or muscle pain) is related to *dysfunctional pain signaling* and/or *muscle contractions* rather than specific structural or inflammatory causes.** We discuss chronic pain conditions involving the extremities and back in this chapter and other common pain conditions in the following three chapters.

Patient Stories: How they find us

We often call our UCLA Pediatric Pain and Whole Child LA clinics the "bottom of the funnel clinic" or "clinic of last resort." The average number of doctors seen *before* us is 14; the most was 42! The majority of children coming to us have common pain problems such as headaches, stomachaches, leg/arm/back pain, or they come with diagnoses such as "migraines," "IBS", or "CRPS" (pronounced "C-R-I-P-S"). They come with distressing symptoms that have caused them to miss school, be unable to engage in sports, not sleep, feel isolated, and mostly feel misunderstood. Doctor after doctor has listened, examined, tested, and finally parents are told, *"Nothing could be found to explain the reason for the pain."* Yet parents see their child still suffering. What do they do? Do they find more specialists; have their child undergo more tests or even surgery?

What are the first steps parents commonly take before they bring their child to us? They have gone to metaphoric "carpenters" or "plumbers," depending upon the site of the pain or what they believe to be its cause. In our opinion, what they needed at that point were "electricians." We are not demeaning the group we are calling "carpenters" (e.g. sports medicine physicians, orthopedists, rheumatologists, podiatrists) or "plumbers" (e.g. gastroenterologists, urologists, gynecologists). Often based on the history, after the primary care clinician (PCC) evaluates the problem, and if no solution is found, the PCC may send your child to one of those specialists. To which specialist depends upon whether the pain appears to be in the muscles, bones, joints or internal hollow organs such as bladder or bowel. Most of the time, these specialists do identify and resolve the problem. However, **when the basic tests and common therapies do *not* explain and resolve the pain and other symptoms, the next common path often is to seek additional specialists... for more tests.** But unfortunately, the pain persists, and becomes chronic and disabling so that it interferes with your child's day to day life.

42

CHRONIC PAIN CONDITIONS (A)

Does the following example of a foot injury sound familiar?

Vivien is a 13-year-old girl who was active in gymnastics and volleyball until she sustained an injury to her foot about 1½ years earlier. She had gone to the emergency department (ED) of her local hospital after she noted two days later that her foot was beginning to hurt more. At the ED, she had X-rays of her foot and there was a concern about a "possible hairline fracture" or "growth plate injury." She was put in a 'boot' and told to see a pediatric orthopedist. This orthopedist took more X-rays since the prior radiologic studies were not available for review, and he saw nothing abnormal. Because of the pain, he casted the foot and gave Vivien crutches. The recommendation was to stay off the foot for a few days. However, pain was getting worse and hurting constantly inside the cast. Her mother brought her to a Sports Medicine physician who removed the cast, and obtained an MRI of the foot that was normal. He referred Vivien to physical therapy (PT). Vivien had so much pain she could not bear pressure on her foot, either standing or walking and wouldn't let the physical therapist go near her foot.

Her parents brought her to a third pediatric orthopedic surgeon for an opinion. She reviewed all the prior radiological studies and confirmed that she also could not see a bone or joint reason for the pain, fitted the foot with a walking boot, and referred the child to a different PT. By this time, Vivien had been in pain for 7 months, missed a full semester of school, was behind in her schoolwork although she had been put on "home hospital"; her grades began to suffer. Formerly a straight 'A' student, Vivien began to stress about missed school and "catching up." She felt hopeless, was still using crutches and having difficulty in PT, refusing to do home exercises, and was now having difficulty falling asleep and staying asleep. She felt tired during the day, became more irritable and increasingly isolated from her friends who were athletes, as she formerly had been.

Because of the painful-to-light-touch foot, Vivien altered the way she walked and stood, causing muscle pains to develop in her knees and hips. Her arms and shoulders began to ache because of her crutches. Despite months of PT, she did not see any improvement.

Her parents took Vivien back to the Sports Medicine physician whom she had seen previously, and he diagnosed "complex regional pain syndrome" (CRPS). At this point, he suggested that Vivien go to a pediatric pain clinic because what he originally thought to be a foot problem that needed a "carpenter" actually needed an "electrician." The primary problem was not in the muscles, bones or joints but rather in the electrical signaling between the foot and the brain.

PAIN IN CHILDREN AND YOUNG ADULTS

She needed at this point an "electrician" not a "carpenter".

At the first pain clinic Vivien attended, one recommended by a friend of the parents, the anesthesiologist was used to treating adults and wanted to insert a catheter in Vivien's back to place an anesthetic into the space where the nerves come out along the spinal cord (epidural anesthetic infusion) to get rid of the pain. Her parents thought this seemed a bit drastic and returned again to the Sports Medicine physician for guidance. He then referred her to our pediatric pain clinic.

Understandably, parents take their child with foot pain to metaphorical "carpenters," doctors who have expertise in bone or joint problems and evaluate with exams, X-rays, MRIs and blood tests for conditions that could be associated with foot pain. When nothing specific is found that seems to be the likely cause of the pain, physical therapy, casting, or a boot is prescribed. However, for the child with a super sensitive foot that hurts when standing on it, physical therapy (PT) may be experienced as "too painful" to undertake. Then parents look for other solutions but often don't know where to find help.

SPORTS INJURIES

Tracy Zaslow, MD[14] gives her perspective on these childhood injuries. We will discuss specific extremity pains later on in this chapter.

What Parents of Kids With Sports Injuries Need To Know? Playing sports is a great way for children to develop confidence, self-discipline, improve physical fitness and coordination, and learn teamwork. But sports participation has changed dramatically over the past decades; now young athletes participate in significantly more hours of intense training than was previously known. Our youth regularly participate on multiple teams at one time and train at levels that rival professional athletes.

Injury is a risk for anyone participating in sports, but children have certain qualities that make them more susceptible.

- *Children are still growing. Bones, muscles, tendons, and ligaments are growing; they are still developing strength, balance and coordination.*

- *Children vary in size. Young athletes should be matched for sports according to their skill level and size. When kids of varying sizes play sports together, there may be more frequent injuries.*

---

14 Tracy Zaslow, MD, Clinical Assistant Professor of Orthopaedic Surgery, University of Southern California. She is a Sports Medicine expert affiliated with Children's Hospital of Los Angeles. *www.sportsmedicinela.com*

CHRONIC PAIN CONDITIONS (A)

- *Children can injure growth plates. Growth plates are areas of new tissue formation, present only in children and adolescents that are particularly vulnerable to injuries. Injuries to these areas can disrupt normal growth and development of the bone.*

- *Young athletes often do not get all the rest they need. This factor increases the chance they will sustain acute and overuse injuries.*

Types of Sports Injuries In Children And Teens *The most common sports injuries are overuse injuries, affecting different parts of the body depending on the particular sport, even more than acute injuries (sprains, strains, broken bones and concussions). Overuse injuries occur in every sport! It's not so much the sport that causes the overuse injury, but the repetitive micro-trauma — chronic use of a specific part of the body and inadequate time for rest and recovery. In soccer, basketball, volleyball (running and jumping sports) the knee is one of the most common sites of injury. The growth plates are the weak link in young athletes and are vulnerable to repetitive stresses. For example, the elbow is so commonly injured in young baseball players that it is even called "little league elbow".*

Presenting Symptoms & Common Treatments of Sports Injuries *Sports injuries present with pain in a localized area, often worse with, or soon after, activity and sometimes associated with swelling or bruising. Initial treatments for most sports injuries are rest, ice, compression and elevation (also known as RICE). Rest is key to success but it should be relative rest: this refers to stopping activity when there is pain and refraining from aggravating activities. However, relative rest does not mean complete inactivity as complete inactivity (unless prescribed for a specific purpose like a broken bone) can lead to stiffness, pain hypersensitivity and a slower recovery. Relative rest allows the injured area to recover without further trauma, and it encourages early range of motion, and supports cross-training to maintain fitness.*

A home exercise program and, sometimes, physical therapy are essential to recovery from both acute and overuse injuries. For acute injuries, these modalities enable early range of motion and speedy return to sport. For overuse injuries, home exercise programs help to improve underlying biomechanics and sports activity technique to prevent injury recurrence.

Surgery for Children/Teens With Sports Injuries *Surgery is rarely indicated for young athletes. However, acute fractures that are crooked or too out of place to heal on their own, stress fractures that have failed to heal with conservative care, and ligament/ cartilage tears (i.e. ACL tears, meniscus tears in the knee) do require surgery. When surgery is needed, current techniques are much improved and employ minimally-invasive procedures specifically designed to help the young athlete achieve a speedy recovery and expedited safe return to sport.*

PAIN IN CHILDREN AND YOUNG ADULTS

Psychological/ Family Issues Inhibiting Expected Time For Recovery What to do then? While most sports injuries heal quickly, recovery from a sports-related injury can be complicated by many psychosocial issues. Key signs of slow recovery include: pain out of proportion to the injury, prolonged recovery course, and the athlete's disinterest in rehabilitation programs.

Athletes who display these factors will first undergo appropriate testing/imaging modalities to confirm the injury and ensure no other physical injury has gone unrecognized. Then psychological and social stressors should be explored with the patient and his/her family (and often include coaches and teachers too). A comprehensive team approach is then employed to treat the pain.

From the psychological side, individual and family therapy is explored with or without pain and/or psychiatric medications. To target physical components of pain, physical therapy, acupuncture, and therapeutic massage are employed. The key to success is building a team including Physical Therapy, Professional Trainers and the PCP to address the issue from all sides and promote long-term health and well-being.

COMPLEX REGIONAL PAIN SYNDROME (CRPS)

When the pain associated with common sports or other injuries does not resolve in the expected time period, there should be consideration of the pain being prolonged by a *neural signaling mechanism*. Again, this is the "electrician" approach to understanding the cause of the pain and thus treatment. Typical sports injuries begin as a "carpentry-fixable" problem with casting, splinting, and/or boot-walking, followed by physical therapy. Treatments such as icing and perhaps mild analgesics such as acetaminophen or non-steroidal anti-inflammatory drugs (NSAIDS) like ibuprofen, if needed, are used for a short time following the injury. Rarely are stronger analgesics such as opioids needed.

However, if the nature of the pain changes to sharp, stabbing, shooting, pins and needles, burning pain, then the maintenance of the pain should be considered *electrical*. Thus, the initial injury or aching ("nociceptive") inflammatory pain has switched to nerve-signaling mediated ("neuropathic") pain.

Symptoms and mechanisms

If the skin over the painful area begins to be sensitive and painful to even light touch, such as bed sheets at night, shoes, or light touch of contact with water, then the local nerves transmitting the feeling of different sensations such as pressure, heat, cold, have turned into nerves that all transmit the sensation of pain. This latter

CHRONIC PAIN CONDITIONS (A)

condition is called "allodynia" and is a hallmark of CRPS. This change in the nature of pain means that the ongoing cause of the pain has changed from injured arm or leg (peripheral) to brain signaling (meaning central).

Rather than the primary neural signal traveling "upward" (e.g. from foot to brain), it is now "downward" (from brain to foot). **Thus the ongoing cause of pain has become a central electrical signaling problem and no longer a bone, muscle, or joint problem.** This is why the *carpentry* approach to treatment that works so well following a typical acute injury no longer is effective for treating an *electrical* problem that continues the pain.

> *Jack was an enthusiastic 11-year-old soccer player who sustained an injury to his right foot when he fell after being knocked over by an enthusiastic teammate running after the ball. After X-rays and an MRI were deemed normal, the foot was casted since it hurt to walk on it. After a short while, the foot became painful in the cast that was then removed because it was thought that perhaps it was applied too tightly. However, replacement of the cast by a walking boot did not reduce the amount of his pain, and Jack regressed to a wheelchair since any pressure on his foot was exquisitely painful. Jack was unable to engage in PT because he could not tolerate any pressure, no matter how light, on his foot that became slightly swollen and mottled (bluish spots) and sometimes turned red or blue. He couldn't bear any contact with his foot and his toenails grew long and hair on the lower leg began to diminish. Because he was unable to use the muscles of that extremity, his right leg became much smaller/thinner than the left. Soon the pain spread up his entire leg and in time moved to include the other foot as well.*

Jack had developed CRPS with continuance and magnification (central mediation) of the pain. Because the neural pathway between the foot and the brain was "turned on" ("excited" from a nerve signaling perspective), the neural excitability spread over time to nearby nerves in the foot/brain pathway up the spinal cord, so that the pain "spread" to affect the entire leg and soon even the other foot. **Treatment needed to change from the *"master carpenter"* to the *"electrical engineer"* approach.**

> *Tony, age 16, doesn't remember injuring himself at a family weekend out of town. When he returned home he noticed that the inner part of his left ankle began to hurt. As the pain continued and progressed in severity, his mother took him to the pediatrician wondering if he somehow had twisted his ankle and possibly had torn a ligament. The pediatrician referred him to a pediatric orthopedist who did not believe that there was any significant injury based on his exam; he thought that all ankle limitation was related primarily to avoidance of ankle movement because*

of pain. However, because the pain was so severe to the point that Tony could not even walk on that leg, the orthopedist ordered an MRI of the ankle; the study was normal. He recommended PT and provided a splint for the ankle if it was too painful to flex. The pain over the medial part of the ankle became sharp, stabbing, and sensitive to light touch so that Tony could not even wear a sock on that foot. The orthopedist recognized this condition as CRPS and referred Tony to our pain clinic for treatment.

In this case, there was no specific sport or other-related injury that could be identified as the initiator. This example points to the fact that **CRPS can begin following insignificant or minor injuries or even after no identifiable injury**, seemingly out of nowhere.

Prior to this "neural signaling" condition being recognized among physicians and other practitioners, these children were thought to have significant psychological problems and often were referred to mental health professionals, therapists. As you will see in the section on treatment, in fact, various brain/mind treatments are effective but not because of treatment for "serious psychopathology." Rather, we now know that learning **mind-based techniques,** such as imagery, biofeedback, cognitive-behavioral therapy (CBT), mindfulness, and breathing techniques, among others, **actually work by reprogramming the neural circuits in the brain that maintain the foot pain or expand it to other area of CRPS pain.**

Dr. Elliot Krane[15] describes the typical diagnosis and approach to treatment of CRPS in children and adolescents below.

Complex Regional Pain Syndrome CRPS describes a cluster of painful symptoms, almost always involving one or more limbs of the body. It is characterized by severe, unrelenting spontaneous pain in the affected body part, painful sensitivity to normally non-painful stimulation such as light touch, and changes in the appearance of the affected body part including color changes, and in later stages changes in skin, muscle and hair growth. Often there are temperature and color changes that imply changes in blood flow to that part of the body, and there may be changes in how that part of the body sweats as well. In spite of treatment, the pain rapidly leads to disability and disuse of the limb.

CRPS is the most common example of neuropathic pain in children, i.e. it has its origins in the nervous system, rather than pain that originates in damaged tissue such as bone or organs or skin. The name says it all: The condition is

---

15 Dr. Elliot Krane, Pediatric Anesthesiologist, Professor, and Director of the Pediatric Pain Program at Packard Children's Hospital at Stanford University, Palo Alto, CA. https://med.stanford.edu/profiles/elliot-krane

CHRONIC PAIN CONDITIONS (A)

- *Complex, i.e. it involves several different parts of human anatomy: several types of nerves, the central nervous system (brain and spinal cord), blood vessels, and also the inflammatory system;*

- *Regional, i.e. it affects part of the body but not the entire body;*

- *Of course, there is Pain;*

- *Syndrome and not a disease itself; it is the manifestation of a process that we have not yet identified or defined.*

What's In a Name? "Complex Regional Pain Syndrome" has been around for a very long time, first described and characterized in soldiers returning home from the American Civil War.

The condition was first thought to involve primarily the sympathetic nervous system and was called "reflex sympathetic dystrophy" (RSD). In the 1990s some specialists in the field of pediatric rheumatology, renamed this condition "Reflex Neurovascular Dystrophy," (RND) that correctly de-emphasized the theoretical involvement of the sympathetic nervous system and correctly emphasized the involvement of both neurologic and vascular systems. This term is accepted outside the specialty of rheumatology. Also in the 1990's the International Association for the Study of Pain (IASP) renamed this condition Complex Regional Pain Syndrome, a more descriptive and accurate term and the one that is most commonly used internationally.

CRPS is sub-categorized into Type 1 and Type 2. CRPS-1 refers to the syndrome occurring after an otherwise trivial surgery or injury and persisting after healing has occurred. CRPS-2 refers to a syndrome with symptoms identical to CRPS-1, but it occurs after an obvious nerve injury. Almost all cases of CRPS in children are Type 1.

What is CRPS? But what starts out as a routine fall or sprain, and which causes manageable somatic pain, soon changes into terrible neuropathic pain of CRPS. Often this seems to be the consequence of immobilization of the limb by an orthopedist or podiatrist, even though a fracture is not present. Somatic pain is characterized by pain that is deep and achy, and is clearly related to use of the limb, such as walking on the sprained ankle, and which responds well to conventional pain killers such as ibuprofen or narcotic painkillers such as hydrocodone. But neuropathic pain of CRPS is very different: the pain is spontaneous; it is not triggered by limb use but is present all the time. Rather than being deep and achy, it is often described as sharp and burning.

There are often electrical sensations in the limb. The hallmark of CRPS is allodynia, the word used to describe non-painful stimulation of the body as causing severe pain. With CRPS, the light touch of clothing or bed linens on or touching the skin, or even blowing one's breath on the skin causes excruciating pain. It's almost possible to diagnose CRPS over the telephone by having mom blow on the affected area.

CRPS also causes change in the appearance of the limb, usually swelling, although it can be very subtle and usually is not as severe as the swelling associated with a sprain or fracture. There are usually color changes. Early on the limb may turn red and at times may be pale or purplish, but later it appears purplish or blue all the time. Coincident with these color changes, the limb will be cold to the touch in comparison with the opposite limb that remains warm to the touch. In the latter stages of CRPS, something we usually do not see in children, other changes occur: hair growth on the limb is increased, the skin becomes dry and thickened, and the finger or toe nails become brittle and coarse.

Movement impairment occurs commonly in CRPS: there is diminished ability to wiggle wrist, fingers or the ankle and toes. CRPS continues and the limb is disused, muscles waste away (atrophy). In the latest stages, joints become frozen from lack of use, but this is rarely seen in children.

What Causes CRPS? *Why do 9,999 children sprain their ankle and nothing else happens; but 1 in 10,000 develops CRPS? We do not know. The probability is that it is not just a matter of bad luck, but rather that some individuals are genetically programmed to be susceptible.*

Previous decades held to a very simplistic theory of the cause of CRPS, but today we realize that it is a post-traumatic neurological and inflammatory condition of the several elements of the nervous system, including the somatosensory nerves, the sympathetic nerves, and even the brain and spinal cord. It involves inflammatory pathways out of proportion to the magnitude of injury that started the whole process in the first place.

How do we diagnose CRPS? *The diagnosis is "clinical."* ***There are no laboratory tests or X-rays that establish the diagnosis.*** *Commonly used are the "Budapest Criteria," so-named after a group of experts convened by the IASP in Budapest, Hungary in 2007.*

1   Continuing pain disproportionate to any inciting event

2   At least one symptom in 3 of 4 following categories

- *Sensory: Reports of hyperalgesia and/or allodynia;*

- *Vasomotor: Reports of temperature asymmetry and/or skin color changes and/or skin color asymmetry;*

- *Sudomotor/Edema: Reports of edema and/or sweating changes and/or sweating asymmetry*

- *Motor/Trophic: Reports of decreased range of motion and/or motor dysfunction (weakness, tremor, dystonia) and/or trophic changes (hair, nail, skin)*

CHRONIC PAIN CONDITIONS (A)

Must display at least one sign at time of evaluation in two or more of the following categories and there is no other diagnosis that better explains the signs and symptoms.

1 Sensory: Hyperalgesia (to pinprick) and/or allodynia (to light touch and/or deep somatic pressure and/or joint movement)

2 Vasomotor: Temperature asymmetry and/or skin color changes and/or asymmetry

3 Sudomotor/Edema: Edema or sweating changes and/or sweating asymmetry

4 Motor/Trophic: decreased range of motion or motor dysfunction (weakness, tremor, dystonia) or trophic changes (hair, nail, skin)

The Budapest Criteria have proven validity in adults, but not in juvenile forms of CRPS. Ultimately the diagnosis of CRPS relies upon the judgment of the physician: CRPS can be said to be present when a child has neuropathic pain (burning, electrical sensations, allodynia) that persists after healing or is present in the absence of any underlying injury or abnormality of the affected body part and in the absence of any other explanation.

How Is CRPS Treated? *The most important treatment in CRPS is frequent and high quality physical therapy (PT) and occupational therapy (OT). In spite of the pain signals going to the brain and telling the brain "don't use me," it is of utmost importance to begin to use the painful limb more and more. Because there is no underlying sprain or fracture, there is no danger of exacerbating an injury. Frequent means at least twice per week, augmented by a home exercise program (HEP), essentially "homework").*

Aggressive PT to remobilize a painful limb is frequently too painful for a child to endure. Furthermore, chronic pain is virtually always associated with sleep disturbance and exhaustion, mood depression, and excessive anxiety. Initiating weekly individual psychotherapy is of great value to help the child develop coping skills that will allow PT to progress, address depressed mood, low self-esteem, school absenteeism, and sleep disturbances. We always initiate our treatment protocol with twice or thrice weekly physical and occupational therapy and weekly psychotherapy. Most cases of CRPS in younger children respond to these measures alone.

Medications are useful in CRPS but it is important for the child and parents to acknowledge that no medication now available will take away all the pain. Opioid medications (that is, narcotic analgesics) are rarely useful. This is because neuropathic pain is almost always resistant to pain relief by opioids. The dose to obtain relief is so high the side effects and adverse events are practically universal. If opioids are to be used, they should be prescribed ideally by a pain specialist, and there should be close monitoring of effect, side effects and adverse events, usage, and the rationale for ongoing

PAIN IN CHILDREN AND YOUNG ADULTS

use: the determination that function has improved on opioids. If opioids do not result in functional improvement they should not be used.

Many drugs not designed as pain relievers have analgesic properties, including anti-depressants and some anti-epileptic drugs, that are very useful in CRPS. None will eliminate all pain. But many will reduce pain to some degree, improve the quality of sleep, and improve function. These include tricyclic antidepressants amitriptyline and nortriptyline and anti-epileptic drugs gabapentin, pregabalin, oxcarbazepine, and sodium valproate.

***Nerve blocks** In cases in which PT is too painful for a child to endure and medications do not adequately treat this pain, then nerve blocks are a rationale choice. The most effective and safest blocks are "peripheral nerve blocks." This is the injection of local anesthetics around nerves in the neck, trunk or limbs. Large studies of tens of thousands of patients in France, Great Britain, and the U.S. show that **the safety record of peripheral nerve blocks is much better than central blocks**. These techniques are amenable to continuous nerve blockade by leaving a small catheter near the nerve and pumping local anesthetics continuously for days or weeks.*

Blocks of the central nervous system, such as epidural blocks, may be effective but are less useful for several reasons: they require inpatient hospital admission for the duration, whereas peripheral nerve blocks can be maintained at home with a catheter in place near the nerve. Central blocks are associated with more severe side effects, including nausea and vomiting, sleepiness, weakness, and the risk of serious infections.

***Surgery** In cases in which CRPS becomes chronic and resists pain management by the techniques above, surgery may be warranted. The implantation of electrical stimulators to provide small electrical "shocks" to the spinal cord is sometimes performed (but rarely in children) and provides short-term pain relief for weeks to months. Seldom, however, are spinal cord stimulators effective for CRPS after one year, at which time most patients return to their baseline. Surgical disruption of the sympathetic nerves has been performed in past decades, but we have learned that the sympathetic nervous system is not the cause of CRPS, but rather it is the victim of CPRS as much as are the nerves and tissues out in the limb. Similarly, the evidence that spinal cord stimulation works is anecdotal and is not yet supported by good scientific proof.*

***What are the Short and Long Term Outcomes of CRPS in Children?** The short term outlook varies with the age and gender and the presence or absence of emotional and family problems. The younger the child, the faster and easier it is to stop CRPS symptoms.*

CHRONIC PAIN CONDITIONS (A)

- *Children younger than 10 are easiest to treat; those approaching their adult years the most challenging.*

- *Males with CRPS have better recovery rates and fewer recurrences than females.*

- *Bipolar disease, schizophrenia, personality disorders, etc. make treatment far more difficult and can lead to resistant CRPS.*

Success in reversing CRPS exceeds 80% in children, with perhaps 10-15% of children improving significantly but continuing to report some ongoing pain. In most children once the condition is successfully treated recurrences are infrequent.

We do not yet know what happens to children treated for CRPS once they reach adulthood, but we are studying this question now to determine how many become normal healthy adults, how many have had persistent or recurrent pain from the CRPS, recurrent CRPS, or other pain disorders.

*Our informal observations are that the prognosis is very good, with the majority of children returning to a pain-free, fully functional state. In this way, **childhood or juvenile CRPS differs significantly from "adult" CRPS.** We discourage our patients and their parents from reading and absorbing the disturbing data and anecdotal stories of CRPS that proliferate on the Internet. Instead, we ask parents to focus on this example on the web, a short video made by one of our young patients who responded completely to therapy and has been free of recurrences for a many years: http://tinyurl.com/ksl4w4p*

MYOFASCIAL PAIN

Not all extremity pain is CRPS. Sometimes pain persists because a group of muscles become stretched and go into spasm, whether in the jaw, shoulder, hips or back. Sustained contraction of these muscles can be very painful. Typically, they will feel tense, tight and are described as feeling like "ropes." They are tender to direct pressure and the muscles can have specific areas that are exquisitely painful with deep focused pressure. These areas are called "tender points" or "trigger points." The latter were named because these were the areas that many physicians used to believe that injections with anesthetic or even salt water or steroids would help to relieve the pain.

We now know that **repeated trigger point injections have no lasting positive effects,** but they can cause fibrous scarring in the areas of the injections and they then become a source of ongoing pain. Thus, at least in children and adolescents, pediatric pain specialists no longer carry out trigger point injections to treat muscle spasm pain (myofascial pain). See also Chapter 13.

PAIN IN CHILDREN AND YOUNG ADULTS

JUVENILE FIBROMYALGIA (JFM)

Chronic widespread pain—that is, pain in multiple muscles and joints in the body that lasts many months—affects 5% of school-age children. JFM is sometimes referred to by other names such as Juvenile Primary Fibromyalgia Syndrome (JPFS), Juvenile Fibromyalgia Syndrome (JFS), or simply Chronic Widespread Pain (CWP). Sometimes the pain is widespread, impacting much or all of the body. In particular, there are *tender points* noted at the neck, shoulders, arms and legs, even the chest, often at ligament insertion areas where the muscle connects to the bone.

This type of centrally brain-mediated, widespread musculoskeletal pain is called juvenile-type "fibromyalgia." It is worth noting that readers of the internet can find numerous stories about people with fibromyalgia and how it is a "lifelong" condition. However, this pronouncement is *not* true for children, adolescents, or young adults who have markedly greater neural plasticity/ flexibility compared with older adults.

The **origin of fibromyalgia is an electrical brain-signaling of central neural circuits that are "turned on"** causing the widespread pain. That is, various areas of the brain develop strong connections with each other, with fewer connections with specific brain pain and stress control areas, like the area near the front of the brain ("prefrontal cortex"). For this reason, mind-based treatments work to relieve pain by altering the inefficient pain-associated pattern of connectivity of neural circuits and by strengthening the connection with the prefrontal cortex. This type of **"brain-rewiring" through mind-based therapies reduces and can even eliminate the cause and experience of widespread pain.** The "brain-down" treatment works best with a "body-up" approach that includes an active program of physical therapy. **The goal is to "rebalance" the up and down normal sensory neural signaling process,** strengthen muscles, and change brain signal patterns.

Dr. Susmita Kashikar-Zuck[16] has carried out extensive research on treatment for fibromyalgia in adolescents and she describes her treatment approach below.[2]

Juvenile Fibromyalgia (JFM) in children and teenagers is a form of chronic widespread pain that is long-lasting and can become debilitating. JFM is typically diagnosed in the early teenage years and affects mainly adolescent girls who have pain lasting more than 3 months, is accompanied by sleep difficulties, fatigue, and multiple "tender" points across the body, and is not due to arthritis or other inflammations. The diagnosis of JFM is determined by the patient's description and a physical exam that includes a "tender point examination." Blood tests, X-rays, scans

---

16 Dr. Susmita Kashikar-Zuck, Pediatric Pain Psychologist and Professor, University of Cincinnati School of Medicine, *www.cincinnatichildrens.org/bio/k/susmita-kashikar-zuck*

CHRONIC PAIN CONDITIONS (A)

or other tests typically do not show abnormalities but they are performed to rule out other medical conditions. A pediatric doctor, usually a specialist in rheumatology or pain medicine, can assess for JFM.

The common presenting symptom of JFM is muscle or joint pain in at least three body areas. Teens with JFM can also experience headaches, abdominal pain, painful menstrual periods; sleep difficulty and fatigue are common. Some JFM patients experience problems with concentration. As a result, many have difficulty keeping up with their schoolwork. JFM is also associated with mood changes, like feeling sad or anxious. These mood issues arise from living with chronic pain and withdrawal from peers and social activities.

Common Treatments *Medications are often used to manage symptoms of fibromyalgia. While certain medications help reduce pain, others may have sleep benefits or help with mood regulation. Sometimes a combination of medicines is prescribed. Three major classes of medications are used for JFM:*

- *tricyclic antidepressants (e.g. amitriptyline)*
- *selective serotonin reuptake inhibitors (SSRI's) (e.g. citalopram) or selective serotonin and norepinephrine reuptake inhibitors SNRI's)(e.g. duloxetine), Cymbalta*
- *anti-convulsants (e.g. gabapentin, pregabalin)*

Most of these medications have been FDA- approved for fibromyalgia in adults but have not yet been specifically approved for JFM. Future pediatric studies will test whether these medications are safe and effective for children. Even if medicines are helpful, these alone are not a long-term solution, so often doctors recommend behavioral and lifestyle changes to help treat JFM in children and adolescents.

Non-pharmacologic treatments *Two types have been shown to be safe and effective for managing JFM: Cognitive-Behavioral Therapy (CBT) and physical exercise.*

CBT has been shown to be effective in improving daily function and mood in adolescents with JFM. CBT programs teach behavioral /cognitive strategies to cope with pain using: a) muscle relaxation, b) pleasant imagery, c) distraction and d) calming statements. CBT also teaches children how to make changes in their daily lives, such as scheduling activities to minimize pain and maximize productivity and fun. Teaching parents how to be good "coaches" for their child can also be very useful in helping children learn to cope well and not let pain interfere with their daily lives. See Chapter 14.

Moderate exercise helps maintain muscle strength (preventing injury) and may also reduce pain intensity. Recent studies have shown that adolescents with JFM may become sedentary and fearful of movement, resulting in deconditioning.

PAIN IN CHILDREN AND YOUNG ADULTS

Unfortunately, this means that when they do try to exercise, they are more prone to injury or pain due to poor body mechanics. Therefore, **carefully designed exercise programs are needed that improve body awareness and core strength while teaching safe movement skills** *that should be part of any vigorous form of exercise. One study of teenagers with fibromyalgia also found that* **graded aerobic exercise was helpful***. Maintaining a regular exercise program is necessary to reap the full benefits; many patients find this quite challenging.*

Why Is There Pain In JFM? *Patients and families are always concerned about the underlying cause of JFM and whether a cure can be found. Research has made it clear that patients with JFM have a higher sensitivity to pain - some of this may be due to genetic causes, but it may also be due to other reasons such as disturbances in the immune system. Some adults with fibromyalgia have a small-fiber polyneuropathy of sensory nerve fibers that carry pain signals from the body to the brain. There is the possibility that if the cause of this neuropathy is found, it may point to a treatable cause for pain. This research is not definitive in children or youth with JFM; more research is needed. With regards to therapies, there is good evidence that behavioral and lifestyle-based treatments including CBT and aerobic exercise can be very useful to manage JFM.*

New Research in JFM *Until recently, it was not known if children and teens with JFM simply "outgrow" their symptoms or whether they will have fibromyalgia for the rest of their lives. A recent study reported that 50% of youth treated for JFM will not have fibromyalgia when they reach young adulthood (i.e., their early 20s). This means that symptoms should be treated early so they do not result in negative physical, emotional and social consequences over time. The other half reported that their pain improved, but other symptoms like fatigue and sleep difficulties continued into adulthood. Many young adults manage and cope with their symptoms so they go on to college, get married, have children and lead a normal life. The good news is that JFM can get better or remain stable over time; the physical symptoms are unlikely to have a worsening or deteriorating course. Preventing JFM patients from becoming discouraged and inactive is important, as this can cause worsening disability.*

Neuromuscular Training *This novel exercise approach derived from Sports Medicine and injury prevention is a promising technique for helping JFM patients gain confidence in movement and core movement skills when they need to participate in moderate-vigorous activity. Neuromuscular training has been combined with well-tested CBT in a new program called FIT Teens (or Fibromyalgia Integrative Training for Teens) and is now being studied through a project funded by the National Institutes of Health. Many of these specialized programs are only available in a few Children's Hospitals across the country. However, as more studies are done to find the most effective approaches, it is hoped that the best treatments will become more widely available.*

CHRONIC PAIN CONDITIONS (A)

BACK PAIN

Common causes of back pain relate to contracted muscles (see also myofascial pain). Most of the time, the diagnosis can be made with history and a good physical examination, evaluating status of muscles, ligaments, bones, and joints. **Rarely in children and adolescents is there a spinal problem with bones of the spine (vertebrae), discs between them, or the nerves coming out from between the vertebrae.** However, **if 100 normal adolescents with no back pain all had spinal X-rays and magnetic resonance imaging (MRI)'s, there would be some abnormal discs noted in about 33% as 'incidental findings'3.** This is to say that finding an abnormality in the spine MRI, depending upon the finding, *does not necessarily mean* that "the cause" of the back pain has been found. **Most back pain problems in children and teens are related to poor posture, weak core strength of back and abdominal muscles, and often, carrying heavy (book) backpacks.**

Children are not getting the amount of physical exercise that they need to maintain good posture and core strength with reduction of physical education requirement in many schools. Often more focus is on sedentary activities (videogames and texting). Observe your child/teen standing in front of you.

- Are his shoulders at the same height?
- Does he slouch forward with his shoulders or does he stand with his pelvis back, chest forward, and shoulders back, a correct standing position?

Body posture in standing is often a good indicator of likely reasons for both headaches and back pain. Poor posture with weak core strength puts strain on other muscles such as neck and shoulders, and then neck and shoulder muscles try to compensate and become contracted; this causes head, neck, and upper back pain.

Slouching of the lower back with weak abdominal muscles allows the abdomen to pouch out forward. This posture leads to more strain on lower back muscles and low back pain. Physical therapy, increased exercise, working with a knowledgeable personal trainer, yoga, and mindfulness about bodily posture and physical movement will reduce back pain.

There are other, rarer causes of back pain. Some relate to rheumatological (joint) disease and are discussed in Chapter 6. Also discussed in that chapter are diseases such as sickle cell disease that cause thinning of the vertebrae and sometimes fracture. These bony changes in turn cause squeezing of the nerves coming out between the vertebrae. Children on oral or injected, intravenous (IV) steroids for other diseases, such as asthma, may have spinal fractures, causing back pain too.

PAIN IN CHILDREN AND YOUNG ADULTS

Children with abnormal pouching of the lining into the spinal cord can have abnormal cerebral spinal fluid (CSF) flow which puts pressure on the nerve outlets themselves causing pain in the back or extremities, a condition called "syringomyelia." This condition, also discussed in Chapter 7, is often accompanied by a defect at the top of the spinal canal that connects to the brain through the opening at the base of the skull. This condition is called a "Chiari malformation" and may be another cause of headaches and may indicate other such cord covering abnormalities as in syringomyelia. Scoliosis or curvature of the spine can lead to misalignment of back muscles creating abnormal torque, pull, and strain on different muscles and thus back pain.

This chapter has discussed features of pain in extremities. In the next chapter we will discuss pain and its mechanisms from head to tummy and important points about fatigue and sleep.

CHAPTER 5

CHRONIC PAIN CONDITIONS (B):
PAIN IN THE HEAD, CHEST AND TUMMY; MENSTRUAL CRAMPS, FATIGUE AND SLEEP

Today I have a headache - Is it because I ate that extra piece of cake?
Maybe it was the jumping up and down, or the night I had on the town?

Today I have a headache - It is pounding its way in like a stake.
It feels like a drill is in my head.
I need to rest; I will go to my bed.

Today is a new day and the sun is aglow,
The headache is gone, no more lying low.
I can do what I want; I know it's a sign.[17]

Oh What a Day

—BY SHEILA VANDENBERG, ARIZONA. HEADACHES

HEADACHES

ABDOMINAL PAIN AND IBS

CHEST PAIN

MENSTRUAL PAINS (DYSMENORRHEA)

FATIGUE—AND MITOCHONDRIAL DYSFUNCTION

SLEEP PROBLEMS

---

17   *http://www.headaches.org/2007/11/05/submitted-poetry-oh-what-a-day/ National Headache Foundation website*

PAIN IN CHILDREN AND YOUNG ADULTS

In this chapter we continue our discussion of chronic pain, but how it gets *expressed* depends on the organ and locations that are affected. The mechanisms in the brain are similar for severe menstrual cramps or chest pain; but obviously, their expression changes. Children still miss school, are unable to engage in sports, have insomnia and feel misunderstood. And if organ/ site-focused evaluations come up empty and the usual treatments are not working, we need to consider the *electrical wiring* as the problem.

HEADACHES

While many parents worry that something dangerous like a brain tumor is causing their child's headache, in fact the three most common types of headaches in childhood are those associated with a) head trauma (e.g. post-concussion headache), b) chronic daily headaches, often associated with myofascial (muscle tension) contributors, and c) migraines. **Headaches are the most common chronic pain problem of childhood.**

When children have headaches, **parents are often worried that their child has something serious that needs to be taken care of immediately or something drastic will happen.** For example, **they may worry that their child has a brain tumor**, especially if they knew someone who died from a brain tumor or other cancer. Brain tumors in children are rare, occurring in fewer than 1 out of 10,000 children. The symptoms of a brain tumor are those of increased pressure in the head causing headaches associated with morning vomiting with or without nausea. Brain tumors often have other neurologic findings but **headaches associated with morning vomiting should definitely be evaluated by the primary physician**, typically with a brain MRI or referral to a child neurologist who likely will get this study.

One common cause of increased intracranial pressure (ICP) is called "*pseudotumor cerebri*" in which there is evidence of increased cerebral spinal fluid pressure in the ventricles (canals within the brain and connecting to the spinal cord). Typically, the finding in the child with headache related to *pseudotumor* is evidence of increased ICP on fundoscopic exam in which the doctor looks into the pupils of the eyes with an ophthalmoscope to visualize the margins of the optic nerve and the pulsations of the veins in the background of the eyes (venous pulsations). If pulsations are absent or the margins of the optic disc are blurred, there is concern for increased ICP. A brain MRI or computed tomographic (CT) scan is obtained to make sure that there is not a brain tumor causing the increased ICP.

There are other causes of increased intracranial pressure (ICP), such as hemorrhages or strokes, (cerebral bleeds) in the brain. However, these are typically acute and cause rapid onset of a severe headache and should be evaluated immediately via an ER visit. They often are associated with mental confusion.

CHRONIC PAIN CONDITIONS (B)

In the old days, physicians would perform a lumbar puncture (LP) or spinal tap to measure the pressure, although now that is rarely done to diagnose *pseudotumor cerebri,* if the brain imaging studies are negative and there is no mental confusion. If there is significant increased ICP, an LP could remove too much fluid from below, causing part of the brain to dip below the base of the skull (herniation) with disastrous consequences. There may be times when there is a need to measure cerebrospinal fluid (CSF) pressure, such as in a child who has hydrocephalus, a condition associated with increased CSF pressure that is often the result of birth-related conditions or illnesses during early childhood, like meningitis.

When the hydrocephalus is first diagnosed, these children typically have a ventriculo-peritoneal (VP) shunt placement by a pediatric neurosurgeon. The shunt acts as a release valve or drainage system so pressure does not remain elevated. When these children with functioning VP shunts develop headaches, the neurosurgeon may have to measure the pressure but does so in the hospital with a special valve placed in the head into one of the ventricles to determine if the shunt needs revision.

Pseudotumor cerebri can be caused by medications. Tetracycline-derivative antibiotics (e.g. minocycline) used by dermatologists to help treat acne are a common cause.

The different types of headaches can actually morph into one or the other. For example, a child playing soccer has multiple mild "head vs soccer ball" connections during games, but one slightly more intense bump on the head might mark the time for beginning a chronic daily headache. This may be initiated as a head trauma headache, but over time, as the headache continues, it becomes a chronic daily headache. **With ongoing head pain, shoulders and neck muscles develop spasms and pull on the muscles of the scalp adding more pain to the already existing headache**. The headache then develops *muscle tension* contributors to the pain. As the headache continues, life becomes disrupted with reduced sleep, concentration, missed school, decreased or avoidance of physical activity… and athletics. Increased isolation occurs, since the former athlete typically had athlete friends who are busy doing athletics, and mood changes occur. Then stress, worry, depressive symptoms all may contribute further to the chronic headache. These didn't cause the headache but over time the headache picks up "baggage" that contributes to the pain's chronicity.

Migraine Headache

Migraines tend to have a stronger genetic contributor and often there is a history of migraines in other family members. These headaches occur intermittently and are intense. Unlike in adults, migraines may not be located on just one side of the head (unilateral) but can be on both sides (bilateral). They are usually associated with phono- and photo-phobia (sound and light sensitivity, respectively) that worsen the

PAIN IN CHILDREN AND YOUNG ADULTS

headache. Typically, the child wants to sleep in a quiet, dark room until the headache goes away. In some children there are "auras" or visual cues such as flashing lights or other feelings associated with the upcoming onset of a migraine. These cues can be useful in the timing to take "abortive" medication such as the category known as "triptans." However, some migraines continue in a prolonged state and are layered intermittently on top of chronic daily headaches. For these latter daily headaches, the typical migraine medications are often ineffective.

Not uncommonly, headaches of any of three above can be associated with nausea and vomiting. Treatment of these side effects can be carried out with the category of medication called "anti-emetics" (Phenergan™, Zofran™, Compazine™). However, if sleep improves and activity increases, and headaches begin to become less disabling, the nausea and vomiting typically disappear.

Common headaches, including migraines and chronic daily headaches, are described by Dr. Jason Lerner[18], a Pediatric Neurology specialist in headaches.

Headaches in children are more common than most people realize. Studies have shown **almost half of children report having had a headache and by the age of 18 over 90% report having had at least one headache.** *Frequent and severe headaches have the greatest impact on overall quality of life, causing missed school days and enjoyed activities. In the United States, 20% of children report frequent and severe headaches within the last year.* **Before the age of 12 the frequency of headaches is similar in boys and girls; however, the prevalence increases in girls with age.**

Types *Migraine and tension type headaches are the most common types described in children. Migraines tend to be more severe, unilateral (although often bilateral in children), throbbing, worsened by physical activity and accompanied by nausea, vomiting, and light or sound sensitivity. Migraines can also be preceded by a change in vision or sensation called an aura. In comparison, tension type headaches tend to be mild to moderate in intensity, bilateral, described as a tightening or squeezing, not aggravated by physical activity and not associated with nausea, vomiting, light or sound sensitivity or an aura.*

There are other less common headache disorders seen in children. Chronic migraine or chronic tension type headache fulfill the criteria for either a migraine or tension type headache and occurs 15 or more days per month for more than 3 months. New daily persistent headache is a persistent headache that occurs every day from a very specific onset. This headache may have characteristics of either migraine or tension-type headaches.

---

18   Dr. Jason Lerner, UCLA Associate Professor in Pediatrics and Neurology, UCLA, Child Neurologist
www.uclahealth.org/provider/jason-todd-lerner-md

CHRONIC PAIN CONDITIONS (B)

Diagnosis and treatment *The diagnosis of headaches in children is primarily clinical. Imaging studies such as MRI and CT scans, blood tests and spinal taps are typically not required unless there is a concern for infection, increased pressure or focal findings on a neurological exam. Headaches have a variety of causes and triggers and there is frequently a strong family history.*

There are 4 primary ways of treating headaches in children:

- *Lifestyle changes*
- *Abortive medications*
- *Prophylactic medications or therapies*
- *Bio-behavioral modalities.*

Lifestyle changes *Various triggers when avoided prevent most and in some cases all headaches. Regular exercise does help reduce the frequency of headaches and 60 minutes of physical activity per day as recommended by the Physical Activity Guidelines for Americans is suggested for best effect. Stress should be avoided or controlled when possible. Children report common stressors as: sports performance, acceptance to college, homework, bullying, and excessive after school activities.*

*Skipping meals is a common cause of headaches that occur in the afternoon. When interviewed, many children admit to skipping breakfast and/or lunch. Eating 3 healthy meals a day plus snacks can make a huge difference in reducing headache frequency in some children. There are often certain foods that may trigger headaches. These include: chocolate, citrus fruits, aged cheese, processed meats and monosodium glutamate (MSG) to name a few. However, everyone is different and a headache diary is required to find individual food triggers. Dehydration is another typical trigger. Children should be drinking water throughout the day and intake should be increased when participating in sports and during hot months over the summer. While caffeine use at the time of a headache may assist in aborting a headache, chronic use may be linked to sleep and mood disturbances and rebound headaches. Finally, sleep hygiene is very important. Many children get erratic sleep and too few hours. 8-10 hours are recommended with a regularly scheduled bedtime and wake-up time. **A 3-month rigorous headache diary documenting all of these triggers is essential to the comprehensive treatment of headaches.***

Medications *When lifestyle changes alone do not prevent headaches, a number of medications are used to abort a headache or can be taken on a daily basis to prevent them. Abortive medications include non-steroidal anti-inflammatory medications, acetaminophen, and triptans. The key to taking abortive medications is to use the appropriate dose based on age and weight and to take the medication within 20 minutes of the onset of the headache. Currently, **excessive use of abortive medications***

PAIN IN CHILDREN AND YOUNG ADULTS

is a hotly debated topic. Reports indicate that use of abortive therapies more than 4 times per week may or may not lead to rebound headaches.

Headache Prevention Three main classes of medications have been used: antihypertensive, antiepileptic and antidepressant medications. Research has shown that nutritional supplements may be as successful as medications to prevent headaches. These include: magnesium, riboflavin (Vitamin B2), CoenzymeQ10, and butterbur. Finally, useful bio-behavioral therapies include counseling, relaxation techniques, biofeedback and cognitive behavioral therapy.

Head Trauma and Concussions

Headaches associated with head trauma and concussions are described below by UCLA pediatric head trauma specialist and Child Neurologist, Dr. Chris Giza[19]. Dr. Giza's Takeaway 'Pearls of Wisdom' for Post-traumatic headaches in children are the following:

- *Headaches are common early symptoms of traumatic brain injury and concussion*
- *"When in Doubt, Sit it Out"*
- ***There is no single test or checklist to diagnose concussion; see someone knowledgeable!***
- *Most post-concussive headaches are self-limited*
- *Management of chronic post-concussion headaches or other symptoms should be individualized – "It's Not One Size Fits All"*
- ***Not every headache that occurs while playing sports is a concussion***

Traumatic Brain Injury (TBI) is any biomechanical force applied to the brain that results in brain dysfunction. Common mechanisms of TBI include motor vehicle accidents, falls, sports and recreation, being struck by an object or assault. TBI can range from mild (concussion) to moderate to severe (coma). It is important to distinguish between mild TBI/concussion and moderate-severe TBI.

Mild TBI or Concussion is a brain movement injury that occurs without there being a 'hole in the brain'. It is an injury of brain dysfunction rather than destruction. This means it is largely a recoverable injury. Headache is the most common symptom of concussion, occurring more than 90% of the time. Other common early signs of concussion include confusion, disorientation, dizziness, nausea, memory disturbance, incoordination, light and noise sensitivity, sleep disturbance and fatigue. Most (90%)

---

19 Christopher C. Giza, MD, Professor of Pediatric Neurology and Neurosurgery, UCLA Brain Injury Research Center. Director, UCLA Steve Tisch BrainSPORT: Sports Concussion - Mild TBI Program. Interdepartmental Programs for Neuroscience and Biomedical Engineering. David Geffen School of Medicine at UCLA. Mattel Children's Hospital – UCLA. *www.uclahealth.org/provider/christopher-giza-md*

CHRONIC PAIN CONDITIONS (B)

*of concussions occur without loss of consciousness. For student-athletes, it is not necessary to formally diagnose a concussion at a sporting event – **if there is suspicion for a concussion the athlete should be removed from contact risk** – "When in doubt, sit them out!" There is no single test to diagnose concussion, so concussion is a clinical diagnosis and should be made by an experienced medical professional.*

In the vast majority of concussions, symptoms are maximal at or within hours of the injury, but occasionally the symptoms may begin later. Post-concussive headaches may also be associated with nausea, vomiting, light sensitivity and noise sensitivity which are also common symptoms of migraine. "Red flag" symptoms that warrant immediate evaluation include unresponsiveness, persistent confusion, seizure, paralysis and progressive or worsening severe headache, vomiting, lethargy or incoordination.

*After a concussion, a child is 3-6x more likely to get another concussion, due to incoordination, slowed reflexes, poor judgment and a brain energy crisis. Therefore, **the most important initial care for a concussion is to remove the child from activities that have a risk for concussion,** particularly contact or collision sports. Because anxiety and stress prolong symptoms, it is important for the injured individual to be evaluated by a clinical care provider with experience in concussions, and for that provider to educate and reassure the patient and family so they know what to expect. These relatively simple interventions have been shown to shorten recovery times.*

*While some rest may be necessary during the first days after a concussion, studies have shown that strict **rest longer than a few days results in greater symptom reporting and can prolong symptom recovery.** With bad symptoms, missing a day or two of school, but after that an individualized return to learn plan should be implemented with the student's instructors, parents and medical team. Over-the- counter pain relievers can be used, but care should be taken to avoid repeated daily use of pain medication.*

***Most concussion symptoms that persist longer than a few weeks are attributable to other diagnoses or risk factors,** such as migraines, chronic daily headache, anxiety, depression, medication overuse, pre-existing learning disability or ADHD and/or a prior history of concussions. Neck strain, eye movement impairments and problems with the inner ear balance organ (vestibular) may also be associated with longer symptoms. Those with prolonged headaches or other symptoms after a concussion should seek medical attention and initiate the appropriate individualized treatment for their particular condition.*

***A small percentage (10%) of individuals with a concussion may develop chronic headaches or symptoms.** For them, treatment includes anti-migraine medications, headache prevention medications, a headache diary, reducing overused medications, neck stretching/strengthening, physical therapy, gradual aerobic conditioning and exercise, psychological intervention, cognitive behavioral therapy, anti-anxiety medication, anti-depressant medication, better sleep hygiene, avoiding dehydration and/*

or low blood sugar and even exercise. Multidisciplinary evaluation and treatment may be particularly beneficial for those with chronic symptoms.

*Moderate-Severe TBI is also a biomechanical brain injury but with more overt neurological symptoms. This will usually manifest as **persistent confusion, memory disturbance, seizure or even coma.** These patients will be brought directly to medical attention right away – usually to an emergency room or hospital. **Severe headaches with nausea, vomiting, memory loss and confusion are all "red flags" for possible moderate-severe TBI,** and will generally merit CT scanning to rule out a brain bleed as the cause. Some patients with moderate-severe TBI will require breathing support with a ventilator, EEG monitoring to look for seizure activity and a monitor implanted to measure brain pressure.*

*Headaches can also occur chronically after moderate-severe pediatric TBI; however, they may be harder to diagnose in individuals with persistent unresponsiveness, limited ability to communicate and/or significant cognitive-behavioral impairment. The causes of persistent or worsening headaches in patients recovering from moderate-severe TBI may warrant neurological consultation and additional diagnostic testing such as brain scans. Treatment for these headaches after moderate-severe TBI, like those after milder injury, will depend upon the underlying diagnosis. In general, those with moderate-severe TBI report headache as a major symptom less often than those with mild TBI/concussion. For more info about concussions see: **www.aan.com/concussion** www.cdc.gov/headsup www.neurosurgery.ucla.edu/concussion*

ABDOMINAL PAIN AND IBS

Abdominal pain is the second most common pain problem in children, with the most common being headaches. About 15-35% of children have episodic abdominal pain with about 10% of this group having stomachaches serious enough to miss school. Boys and girls are equally likely to have stomachaches up to adolescence when the prevalence shifts toward the females. Sally and Jordan present typical stories of children with problematic tummy pain.

Sally, 13 years old, was an active soccer player and straight-A student. She developed a viral gastroenteritis with abdominal pain and diarrhea, as did other members of her soccer team. However, after missing soccer and school for two weeks because of abdominal pain, even after the diarrhea resolved, Sally's mother took her to her pediatrician. He found that other than abdominal tenderness to palpation of the belly, Sally's exam was otherwise normal. Sally had reduced her food intake since eating made her belly hurt more, and her mom was still very concerned that "something must be wrong," so the pediatrician referred Sally to a pediatric gastroenterologist.

CHRONIC PAIN CONDITIONS (B)

The gastroenterologist examined Sally and found normal bowel sounds and some tenderness to palpation of the belly. She ordered some urine and blood tests that came back normal. She then provided reassurance that the pain would resolve and encouraged Sally to go back to school, indicating that she did not believe that further invasive testing was needed. Three days later when the belly pain seemed to be getting worse, mom re-contacted the gastroenterologist who recommended that Sally take peppermint gel-tabs before meals and prescribed amitriptyline, a tricyclic antidepressant, in a low dose to take at bedtime.

Sally's mom was worried that something "had been missed" and didn't want to "mask it" with medication. She took her daughter to another pediatric gastroenterologist and urged the gastroenterologist to do more tests. This gastroenterologist did further testing, including an endoscopy, but all was found to be normal. He suggested that Sally might be helped by a psychologist. By this time, yet another week had gone by, Sally was further behind in school, not doing any physical activity, was isolated from her friends, had difficulty sleeping, was tired all day, and her belly still hurt! She was becoming discouraged that the doctors did not believe that her pain was real and her mom was worried that the cause of the pain had not yet been discovered. Their pediatrician encouraged them to return to the first gastroenterologist and explain their frustrations.

The gastroenterologist diagnosed functional abdominal pain and referred Sally to our pain clinic, since she knew that we had a variety of treatment modalities to offer. Sally and her mother arrived to our clinic feeling despondent, with Sally not believing that we would have anything new or helpful to offer. In fact, she was sick of going to doctors and was resistant to the idea of coming to see us.

Jonathan had a different presentation.

Jonathan, 14 years of age, had a history of intermittent stomachaches when he was younger but nothing that kept him out of school. His father also had recurrent abdominal pain that none of his gastroenterologists were able to cure, although it hadn't stopped him from working. Jonathan's abdominal pain seemed to be getting worse since he started middle school and he developed intermittent diarrhea and constipation, as well as nausea. In fact, he was as upset by his nausea as he was by his belly pain.

His parents tried different remedies that had been used for his father: Lomotil™ for diarrhea, Miralax for constipation, and increased dietary fiber. They also eliminated dairy and gluten from Jonathan's diet, but he was becoming increasingly miserable, sullen, not attending school, and crying in the evening when his pain was at its worst. His parents brought him to his father's gastroenterologist who performed a number of tests, as well as an endoscopy and colonoscopy, with all tests and biopsies found to be normal. Jonathan's pediatrician suspected that Jonathan had irritable bowel syndrome (IBS) and referred Jonathan to our pain clinic.

PAIN IN CHILDREN AND YOUNG ADULTS

While acute belly pain can occur with viral gastroenteritis, a bacterial infection ("food poisoning"), consuming MSG, or acute appendicitis, among other less common conditions, **the most common causes of recurrent or persistent abdominal pain is functional abdominal pain (FAP) or irritable bowel syndrome (IBS).** Inflammatory bowel diseases, such as ulcerative colitis and Crohn's disease, and other conditions like gluten enteropathy (Celiac disease), and enzyme deficiencies, occur less commonly and are identified based on presenting characteristics noted in the history of the illness, physical findings, and specific tests. We discuss these in more detail in the following chapter on pain associated with different diseases. In this chapter, we focus on more common abdominal pain conditions known as FAP and IBS.

Abdominal pain in these conditions may be episodic and recurrent or there may be continuous background pain with intermittent "flares" of intense pain. If there is just isolated abdominal pain with no other GI symptoms, and no identifiable inflammation, food intolerance/ metabolic condition, or structural problem, then this condition is called **Functional Abdominal Pain (FAP), is an "electrical" not a "plumbing" problem.** And this is because there is a "functional" problem with the electrical wiring (neural system) between the intestinal tract and the brain. **Dysfunctional brain-gut neural signaling causes the intestinal tract to become sensory-sensitive** with a low threshold for sensory neurons to signal pain.

The condition is called irritable bowel syndrome **(IBS) when there are additional gastrointestinal symptoms such as nausea, vomiting, diarrhea, constipation, and feelings of being bloated,** among others. (Figure 5.1). The brain-gut wiring dysfunction can cause many muscular events in the intestinal tract, such as contraction of the stomach involved in digestion of food and bowel wall stretching associated with constipation or bowel gas, to be painful. *There may be alterations in the motor contractions of the intestinal tract, with slowed motility associated with nausea, delayed gastric emptying, and/or constipation, and increased contractions of the intestinal tract* to cause diarrhea. **Not uncommonly children with IBS have both diarrhea and constipation at different times.**

16-year-old Ellie reflects on her own experience with IBS starting at age 6:

I have had chronic pain (IBS) for a little over ten years. My pain had me missing a lot of activities, including school. In the middle of 4th grade my stomach pain became chronic and started truly affecting my life. I switched doctors at age 10 and doctors' appointments became a regular thing. Skipping ahead, for the first month of Middle School I was there every day even with the pain. But after I made that first call home to my mom to pick me up, I had chronic stomach pain and chronic absences from school. They put me on an

CHRONIC PAIN CONDITIONS (B)

IRRITABLE BOWEL SYNDROME
(Pathophysiology)

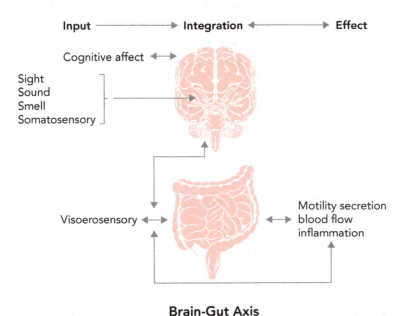

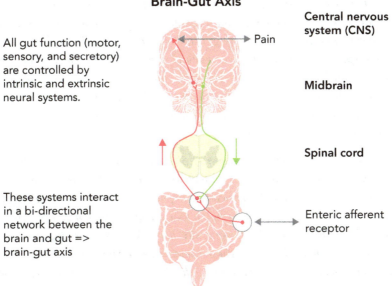

Figure 5.1. Why IBS is a neural and not primarily an intestinal disease

PAIN IN CHILDREN AND YOUNG ADULTS

independent study in all my classes, and accommodated me the best they could. Missing all that school made me scared to return to school because of all the work I had missed and all the social forming I had missed. That year I tried out a lot of the pain clinic programs: therapy, biofeedback, visual therapy, and acupuncture. Although I was adamant at the time of this working, the best thing for my chronic pain was distracting myself from it. The best way to do that was by going to school and making some friends.

Now, as I will be entering my sophomore year of high school in the Fall of 2015, I stand by that. Although I still get the pain, going to a busy school day everyday helps not think about it. Also being nervous or anxious makes your pain worse, so make sure you have someone to talk to, even if it's just a friend because it's the little things that can make a big difference!

Ellie's mom provides perspective on the parental experience:

My daughter has IBS. She is the youngest of three children and overall, she is characteristically bright, high achieving, happy-go-lucky, and fringed with a sense of humor. Before she was diagnosed, she had setbacks. Not major, but parentally worrisome nonetheless. She already had chronic ear infections.

Without lacking sympathy, she began showing signs of abdominal discomfort around five years old. She had constipation causing her unimaginable pain; she would use the bathroom crying and screaming. I took her to a specialist, as I was certain this was not typical, certainly not a five-year-old. I began feeling like the mom who ran to specialists and frankly, it did not feel right; not with my family; not with my friends, not intuitively, not in any way. It wasn't that our daughter's pain wasn't real, it really was. We had her tested for everything. There were some positive results, but nothing worth shouting at a mountaintop...

Ellie's pain waned in intensity and severity. She missed school- weeks at a time. Her social growth stymied- she was tired of explaining to friends why she wasn't in school, and that it was not contagious. It had a tremendous impact on the family, trusting whether it was "real" or "not real" and consequently it took an emotional toll on everyone, but most particularly on Ellie. To add to the intensity, her older sister was diagnosed with uveitis and juvenile rheumatoid arthritis. The medicinal stress on the household was extreme. The parental patience sometimes worn, her medical specialist referred us to a pain specialist.

Over time, Dr. Z led mostly our daughter, at times the two or three of us, her dad too, OR all of us, her siblings included, to different resources to learn and re-learn how to take control of the pain. Ellie tried and enjoyed biofeedback and psychotherapy. We were all vested, my husband and I, and most often just I went on my own as I learned to deal with the emotional pain. Hypnotherapy she tried for four or five weeks and

CHRONIC PAIN CONDITIONS (B)

said it wasn't working her; it wasn't worth the time or the money. She tried yoga. She went with an older friend who was also trying to find ways of becoming pain free. Her brother also thought joining her would benefit her. When the yoga teacher took a seasonal break, our daughter opted to wait; she hasn't re-started. Ellie found writing and photo-essays as a favored way to express her pain. She would meet with other students and share scripts. She definitely found her release through technology, shared ventures, and assisting the pain clinic team.

We have found that meeting with other families in similar situations doesn't make the stress go away, but it helps to know we're not alone. Some are starting out in this journey, some are in the middle, and some feel they have conquered it. Us? We're still learning, but every step forward we have become masters of controlling pain. It takes a long time to heal with your child, but it happens. Ultimately, you, your child, and your family have to find the right methodology that works for you and your child to own and control the pain, allowing the family to function normally and with control. The key is control: Learning and enjoying the method for you.

In summary, children with this abdominal pain condition may have just abdominal pain (FAP) or have other gastrointestinal symptoms (IBS), such as diarrhea and/or constipation, nausea, vomiting, bloating, pain after eating. They might develop decreased food intake and weight loss because of the fear of eating causing more pain. **In IBS, there are intestinal motor responses to this dysregulated brain-gut neural signaling; this problem can cause rapid intestinal muscle contractions and diarrhea, or slowed-down or non-functional contractions associated with constipation.** Sometimes there are both "speed up" and "slow down" motor events. **When pain is located in the upper abdomen and is worse after eating, the condition is called "functional dyspepsia"** (this resembles indigestion or gastro-esophageal reflux of acid but is related to abnormal electrical signaling), and when symptoms appear as acute and severe, they may be labeled "abdominal migraines."

We are learning more about these "functional" gastrointestinal conditions. Initially, IBS was thought to be a problem solely in the intestinal tract that was "causing pain through intestinal spasms." Then we learned that the problem does not lie directly within the intestinal tract, but in the brain/gut neural signaling. More recent research by Dr. Emeran Mayer at UCLA and Dr. Robert Shulman at Baylor Texas Children's Hospital implicates a critical role for intestinal bacteria (gut microbiome) in the brain/gut neural signaling relationship[4]. This research on childhood abdominal pain is further discussed below by Dr. Robert Shulman[20]:

---

20 Dr. Robert Shulman, Professor of Pediatrics, Director of the Center for Pediatric Abdominal Pain Research at Baylor College of Medicine, and Chief of the Division of Gastroenterology and Nutrition at Texas Children's Hospital in Houston. *http://texaschildrens.org/Locate/Doctors/Shulman,-Robert*

PAIN IN CHILDREN AND YOUNG ADULTS

Despite the fact that 10-15% of all school age children around the world suffer from recurring abdominal pain that is not easily explained by laboratory or other types of testing, there has been confusion around what causes the pain and how they should be described. Originally, the term 'functional' was meant to describe a condition where the 'function' of the gastrointestinal tract was not normal but the usual types of testing (for example, blood work, X-rays, biopsies, etc.) did not show any abnormalities.

Unfortunately, to many people, including some physicians, nurse practitioners, and physician assistants, the word 'functional' came to mean psychological – implying that the abdominal pain is at best, caused by psychological problems and at worst, made up to avoid school and/or other stressful situations. This could not be further from the truth in the vast majority of cases.

Current research has shown us that there are abnormalities of function that can be identified using specialized methods. As a result, we are beginning to understand how the gastrointestinal tract, the bacteria contained within, and the brain interact with each other on a daily basis – what has come to be called the "brain-gut axis." We are now starting to see how disturbances in one or more of the parts of this axis, or in how the parts talk with each other, can cause 'dysfunction' and manifest as a functional abdominal pain, FAP, disorder.

Previously, we could only group these children by their symptoms. For example, children with abdominal pain and changes in stooling pattern were classified as having irritable bowel syndrome (IBS); those with just pain as suffering from functional abdominal pain (FAP); those with upper belly pain often occurring after meals as having functional dyspepsia; and finally, those (rare children) with a pain onset and course like migraine headaches as having abdominal migraines. As we move away from symptom-based diagnoses to ones built on understanding the dysfunction(s) occurring in some or the entire brain-gut axis, I anticipate that over time, we will learn there are a number of different types of IBS, FAP, etc.

Most important and exciting are that better treatments will come with greater understanding of the causes of these disorders. These therapies are very likely to be more effective than what is currently available because they will target the specific dysfunction found causing and/or associated with the condition. For example, in one child, this might be a treatment that reduces the amount of low-grade irritation (inflammation) in the gastrointestinal tract. In another, it might be training the brain to be more effective in suppressing signals coming from the gut; in a third, it might be removing something in the diet upsetting the normal balance of bacteria in the gastrointestinal tract.

It is an exciting time in the care of children with functional abdominal pain disorders. If continued support is provided to researchers, both in the laboratory and at the bedside,

CHRONIC PAIN CONDITIONS (B)

and we keep an open mind to the scientific possibilities, the next decade could see a sea change in our understanding and ability to treat the multitude of children worldwide with these often debilitating disorders.

So what happened to Sally, the first case history in the section?

In our initial three-hour meeting first with mom, dad, and Sally, and then Sally alone, we found that both parents were very concerned that Sally would need to have her colon removed for ulcerative colitis, a condition that dad's stepmother had. They had been careful to not tell Sally this but Sally knew anyway. In our meeting with Sally alone, it was obvious that she was both depressed and anxious about ever catching up in school. In addition, Sally had been thinking about suicide a lot but did not have a plan and had not acted upon it; mom, but not dad, was aware of this.

The Diagnosis *On her exam she had a slightly elevated blood pressure, elevated heart rate and her pulse rate jumped from 78 to 120 when going to a standing from sitting position. So, we were learning that abdominal pain from what was thought to be a clearly uncomplicated case of IBS was getting really complicated. The pain was severe enough to affect her autonomic nervous system that was out of balance with pulse and blood pressure changes often diagnosed as paroxysmal orthostatic tachycardia, also called POTS. The pain was not going to clear up if the anxiety about school and feeling isolated continued. Also there was unrecognized depression.*

The Plan *In our plan, we worked with the pediatrician, parents and Sally. First, we needed to explain to Sally's parents that there was no way her diagnosis was ulcerative colitis and that worry needed to be 'off the table'. Sally was to start seeing a psychologist to deal with the peer issues, loneliness and isolation and develop some CBT-based strategies for lowering her anxiety about scary thoughts, studying, catching up, and concerns about needing to repeat her sophomore year.*

To address the depression and her depleted serotonin status contributing to clinical depression and its effect on upping the perception of pain, we started her on citalopram. This medication is in the category of anti-depressants called SSRI's and there has much experience with this medication in adolescents; citalopram also has a sleepiness side effect so it is often taken at bedtime and can help with sleep. We also suggested 5 mg of Melatonin to help Sally fall asleep more easily. We explained that the citalopram often takes 2-4 weeks to get an effect that Sally would notice. We cautioned mom and dad to not ask about pain, but listen if Sally wanted to offer an update on how she felt. We referred Sally to a psychologist on our team who was also going to help

Sally with a plan for a gradual return to school, starting with just a lunchtime appearance. Thirty minutes was spent explaining to the family why Sally had the pain she

PAIN IN CHILDREN AND YOUNG ADULTS

did, why it had not gotten better with the previous approaches, and the approximate timeline for feeling better (likely as long as it took for her to get to this point). We also told her we see 3-4 new patients a month with almost identical symptoms and concerns and that almost all get better and become stronger for the awareness they attain working through this problem.

***The Outcome** Four weeks later, at the follow-up clinic visit, the parents noted that Sally had called her friends on the previous weekend to come over and hang out, even though she still complained of pain every day. She was attending school for one hour a day. On our examination, Sally's heart rate changes from sitting to standing only increased by 20 beats/ minute rather than the 42 found at the initial appointment, an improvement; and now she did not feel dizzy on standing. Six months later she had caught up with her studies, occasionally had some belly pain, mostly before exams but used her breathing exercises and 'safe place' imagery to calm herself down. Sally was seeing the psychologist twice a month.*

CHEST PAIN

Whenever a child has chest pain, parents are naturally alarmed that something may be wrong with the child's heart, since in adults, sudden onset of crushing chest pain may signify a heart attack and this needs immediate attention. However, unless your child has a medical history of a congenital heart disease or has had cardiac surgery in the past, or there is a family history of heart rhythm problems, **a problem with the heart is unlikely to be the cause of chest pain in a child.**

The most common cause of chest pain relates to tenderness at the ligament insertions of the muscles along the rib cage where they attach to the breastbone (sternum) in the middle of the chest. The easiest way to find if the likely source of the chest pain is inside or outside of the chest wall is to press on the areas between each rib next to the sternum. If those areas are tender to pressure, then the most likely cause of the pain is muscle/ ligament tenderness (myofascial) and not a heart event. Usually massage, mentholated creams, and NSAIDs will relieve the pain.

If the pain persists and is associated with widespread pain, then consider central pain in the brain as the cause of the chest pain. In this case, both physical therapy (PT) and a brain top/down mind-based treatment approach will be needed.

Sometimes if the chest pain comes on suddenly and severely, it may be related to esophageal sensitivity and spasm. This can be identified as the cause by having your child take TUMS™ (advertised for "heartburn" relief) or other antacids and drink a lot of water. If the pain is related to a spasm of the esophagus, the acute pain should go away.

CHRONIC PAIN CONDITIONS (B)

Gastroesophageal reflux of acid from the stomach up into the esophagus can cause irritation and, if significant and long-lasting, can cause esophageal inflammation that can be the source of chest pain. In that case, the pediatrician will typically recommend a trial of a medication to reduce the stomach acid for a month or more to see if that relieves the pain. If not, then a referral to a pediatric gastroenterologist is warranted.

MENSTRUAL PAINS (DYSMENORRHEA)

"I mean if there was any justice in the world you wouldn't even have to go to school during your period. You'd just stay home for five days and eat chocolate and cry."

—ANDREA PORTES, ANATOMY OF A MISFIT[21]

Dysmenorrhea is one of the least acknowledged recurrent pains that many girls experience after their menarche (the first menstrual period). Rarely do doctors ask girls about menstrual cramps, and rarely do girls seek relief for menstrual pain. There is an assumption that menstrual pain is expected and must be borne and "toughed out" by all girls. Over-the- counter medications, such as "Midol" and ibuprofen, and heating pads, are what girls turn to for pain relief. There are little data on the prevalence of absenteeism in girls because of menstrual cramps, or to what extent dysmenorrhea impacts other aspects of a girl's life, such as sports, social activities, school homework, or even sleep.

When menstrual pain gets so debilitating that a daughter will complain to her mother that she needs help, typically mothers bring their daughters to a gynecologist with the assumption that starting oral contraceptive pills (OCPs) will relieve the pain. Many times the pain is indeed lessened with OCPs, but there are also increased risks for headaches, stroke, and blood clots in the lung, among others. Past medical history of any of these problems may preclude the use of OCPs. Non-pharmacological remedies are generally not considered.

We will discuss possible pain-relieving strategies later in this book. However, the point here is that **significant recurrent pain can increase risk for central sensitization and the likelihood for the development or worsening of pain propagated by brain neural circuits.** Also dysmenorrhea, because of hormonal changes associated with menses, can increase other types of pain in some girls, such as migraines, or make IBS or other pain conditions worse. Research about sex differences in chronic pain suggests that **dysmenorrhea**

---

21 *https://andreaportes.wordpress.com/ with permission.*

PAIN IN CHILDREN AND YOUNG ADULTS

may play a role in the higher prevalence of other chronic pain conditions, such as fibromyalgia, migraines and IBS in women. There is also concern about how much testing to carry out to determine if endometriosis is the cause of the dysmenorrhea.

We asked Dr. Andrea Rapkin[22] to discuss dysmenorrhea and the premenstrual syndrome in adolescents and young women.

Dysmenorrhea: Dysmenorrhea describes bothersome menstrual pain located in the lower abdomen. It can be associated with nausea, vomiting, low back pain, diarrhea and headache. Dysmenorrhea is common, affecting 60- 90% of teens; it interferes with participation in daily activities in at least 50%. Primary dysmenorrhea refers to pain with menstrual bleeding in the absence of underlying pelvic disease, whereas secondary dysmenorrhea refers to menstrual pain with pelvic abnormalities.

Most teens with menstrual pain have primary dysmenorrhea. The pain usually begins a few hours before or just after the onset of menstrual bleeding and may last for 1-2 days. The pain can feel like labor pain, with cramping in the lower abdomen, low backache, and pain radiating to the top of the thighs. If the pain begins days to weeks before the bleeding or lingers after the period is over, the diagnosis is more likely to be secondary dysmenorrhea.

Primary dysmenorrhea is caused by an excess of chemicals called prostaglandins that come from the lining of the uterus during the menstrual flow. The symptoms of nausea, vomiting, low back pain, diarrhea and headache are also the result of the prostaglandins reaching the blood stream. The prostaglandins increase uterine contractions and sensitivity that contribute to dysmenorrhea pain.

Symptom Relief: The most effective treatments for dysmenorrhea are non-steroidal anti-inflammatory drugs (NSAIDs) such as ibuprofen or naproxen; they prevent formation of prostaglandins. These are available over the counter and should be taken immediately at the onset of bleeding or mild pain, as they may not be as effective if one waits until the pain is severe. The NSAID should then be continued every 6-8 hours in the dose recommended in the package label for the first day or so of the period. If after 2-3 months there is no significant improvement, options can be discussed with your health care provider. A higher "prescription-level "dose or starting NSAIDs 1-2 days prior to the expected menstrual period or changes in type of NSAID are then recommended. Side effects of NSAIDS are uncommon and generally mild. They can include nausea, heartburn and occasionally fatigue. Medications are better tolerated if taken with food. Girls who are allergic or

---

22 Dr. Andrea Rapkin, UCLA Professor of Obstetrics and Gynecology and expert in pelvic pain.
    www.uclahealth.org/provider/andrea-rapkin-md

CHRONIC PAIN CONDITIONS (B)

hypersensitive to aspirin or have a history of stomach bleeding or ulcers may not be able to take NSAIDs.

Hormonal contraceptives decrease prostaglandin production from the uterus lining. We often recommend them for dysmenorrhea unresponsive to NSAIDS, or for teens who cannot take NSAIDs and who have no medical contraindications to hormonal contraceptives. The latter include birth control pills, patches, rings, shots or implants; all are highly effective. If severe menstrual pain persists on hormones, "extended cycles" of oral contraceptives can be considered to prevent menstrual bleeding.

Heating pads, regular exercise, acupuncture, or transcutaneous electrical nerve stimulation (TENS) have been tried to help dysmenorrhea. How these approaches work is not known. There are no recommended herbal or vitamin treatments for the relief of menstrual pain.

The timing of the onset of the pain with bleeding and the relief with treatment such as NSAIDS or hormonal contraceptives confirm the diagnosis of primary as opposed to secondary dysmenorrhea. The most common cause of secondary dysmenorrhea is endometriosis. Endometriosis is a condition characterized by growths of tissue in the pelvis that come from the uterine lining (endometrium). **Teens with endometriosis usually have very severe menstrual pain that starts up to two weeks before the onset of menstrual bleeding.** *Other symptoms can include deep pain with sexual intercourse, irregular vaginal bleeding and rectal pain with bowel movements. A pelvic examination and/ or pelvic ultrasound can suggest endometriosis but may be normal.*

The initial treatment of dysmenorrhea related to endometriosis is the same as the treatment of primary dysmenorrhea. Confirmation of the diagnosis of endometriosis requires a laparoscopic surgery and is only performed if there is a poor response to treatment or if abnormalities on examination or pelvic ultrasound suggest that this procedure be undertaken. Treatment of endometriosis that is not relieved by NSAIDS or hormonal contraceptives includes removal of or burning off endometriosis tissue inside the abdomen. Medications that temporarily suppress ovarian hormones are also effective.

Premenstrual Syndrome: *If your daughter has bothersome physical and and/or emotional symptoms up to 2 weeks before her monthly menstrual period, she may have 'premenstrual syndrome' (PMS). This is not rare as 20% of adolescents experience pre-menstrual symptoms associated with some difficulty functioning at school, home or work. Severe PMS or PMDD occur in up to 5% of adolescents.*

Premenstrual Dysphoric Disorder (PMDD) *is a much less common form of PMS in which severe emotional symptoms such as depression, irritability, anxiety or mood swings impair functioning at home or at school.* **In the case of both PMS and PMDD,**

symptoms resolve by the time the menstrual bleeding has finished, unlike a purely psychological disorder in which the symptoms do not resolve with menses. The symptom-free interval lasts 1-2 weeks after menstrual bleeding ends, and then the cycle begins again. The typical physical symptoms include abdominal bloating, breast tenderness, sleep disturbances, feeling of tiredness (fatigue), muscle and joint pain, headaches, and food cravings. Sometimes teens will feel that they cannot concentrate or control their behavior during this time. They may have relationship problems, become more argumentative, or withdraw socially.

Exact causes of the symptoms are still unknown. They are not due to hormone imbalance or abnormal levels of hormones, such as estrogen and progesterone. Pre-menstrual symptoms are a result of how changes in these hormones affect brain chemistry.

Diagnosis: A daily calendar documents the severity of symptoms in relation to menstrual bleeding. The easiest way to accomplish this is to list the five worst symptoms down the left hand side of the piece of paper and the days of the month, 1 thru 31 across the top of the paper. At the end of each day, rate the severity of each symptom from 0-3 (0= no symptoms, 1 =mild, 2 =moderate, 3 =severe) and circle the days of menstrual bleeding. After recording a couple of menstrual cycles, the pattern will emerge. If symptoms are moderate to severe and occur during the 2 premenstrual weeks and there are no symptoms or only mild symptoms (0 to 1's) in the week after the end of menstrual bleeding, your teen may have PMS or PMDD. This chart should be brought to the attention of your teen's health care provider. If symptoms are severe, the provider should be consulted sooner, as it may be possible to begin treatment based on the symptom history alone.

Many conditions can be confused with PMS or PMDD and include depression, anxiety, severe stress, substance abuse, and sometimes anemia or thyroid disease. During the first visit, your daughter's primary health care provider should complete a medical history and physical examination to exclude other medical and psychological disorders. Your daughter's PCP may also screen for drug usage, physical, sexual or emotional trauma and eating disorders.

Symptom Relief: Certain lifestyle changes may be helpful for PMS. Firstly, it is important to reassure your teen that changes she is feeling may be related to hormone fluctuations, and that charting will help to both understand the nature of the problem and lead to appropriate treatment. Increased awareness and predictability of symptoms that come from charting can be very beneficial. Also helpful are learning how to better manage stress, practicing a relaxation technique such as meditation or yoga, getting plenty of exercise, improving calcium intake in the diet (dairy products, calcium fortified foods and green leafy vegetables), and avoiding cigarettes. If your

CHRONIC PAIN CONDITIONS (B)

teen cannot tolerate dairy products, administration of a calcium supplement 600 mg twice a day may help to reduce some of the mood and physical symptoms. If there is premenstrual and menstrual pain, over the counter, non-steroidal anti-inflammatory agents (ibuprofen or naproxen) can be tried.

Once the symptom diary has been completed and/or you have visited your provider to rule out other underlying disorders, many treatment approaches are available. Oral contraceptives (birth control pills) may be helpful in decreasing the fluctuation of ovarian hormones, thereby improving symptoms. Sometimes, if the symptoms are very severe such as with PMDD, anti-depressants that increase the neurotransmitter serotonin (SSRI's like fluoxetine, sertraline, paroxetine or citalopram) may be recommended. These medications need not be taken all month, but can be given during the 2 weeks before the period, as long as the symptoms are truly PMDD and not related to premenstrual worsening of an underlying mood disorder. When anti-depressants are prescribed for a teen, joint management with your daughter's physician and a psychiatrist is recommended.

FATIGUE

Fatigue is the overwhelming sense of tiredness and lack of energy that can persist throughout the day. It is a common accompaniment to chronic pain and is linked by common mechanisms and pathways. When pain interferes with sufficient nighttime restorative sleep, fatigue is one outcome. However, in some conditions, no matter how much sleep a child or teen gets, the fatigue persists. When the fatigue is so significant that it is having a major impact on activities of daily living, the condition is called *chronic fatigue syndrome (CFS) and* is now recognized by the Institute of Medicine as a disease in itself, rather than what was previously thought to be a purely "psychological" problem.

Typically, adolescents stay up late either doing homework, texting or talking with friends or other activities; they are tired in the morning and have difficulty getting up to go to school. The school day is not in sync with the adolescent biological clock that is set for late to bed and late to rise. However, there are strategies called "sleep hygiene" that adolescents can carry out that will help with sleep duration and increase the *restorative* type of sleep. We will discuss this more in chapters 11 and 11. Suffice it to say here, that part of the management of chronic pain is to facilitate good and sufficient restorative sleep, with ease of sleep onset (30 minutes or less) and good sleep maintenance (not waking up until morning, after falling asleep).

MITOCHONDRIAL DYSFUNCTION IN CHRONIC PAIN SYNDROMES

There are many theories about the underlying mechanisms of chronic fatigue and pain, one being that it is related to "mitochondrial dysfunction." Mitochondria are the energy generators within each cell in our body. Research suggests that with ongoing stress, either emotional or that related to chronic pain, the mitochondria undergo "oxidative stress." This means that they increase production of "free radicals" which are substances that, as they accumulate in the cell, poison the cell by reducing the efficiency of the mitochondria to work well and produce energy for cells to function. Anti-oxidant" supplements are encouraged to help the mitochondria regain normal function. Foods, such as blueberries, are high in antioxidants. As well, supplements, such as Coenzyme Q10, Acetyl L-Carnitine, and others, work to enhance mitochondrial function (chapter 16). Clearly the best, most economical way is to reduce stressor load and learn how to increase restorative sleep.

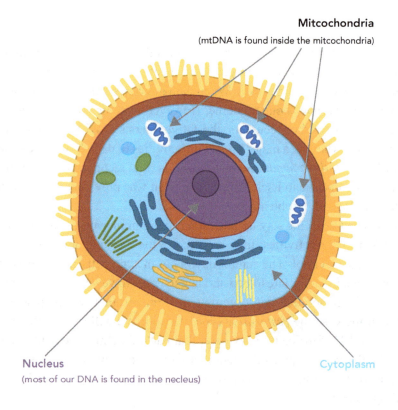

Figure 5.2. Diagram of cell showing place of mitochondria and nucleus.

CHRONIC PAIN CONDITIONS (B)

We asked Dr. Richard Boles[23], a geneticist with detailed knowledge of mitochondrial disorders to shares his thoughts about this new, complicated and sometimes controversial area in pain treatment.

What are Mitochondria? Most cellular energy is made by mitochondria, organelles originally derived from bacteria that live within our cells. In the transition from separate life forms, the vast majority of their genes were lost or transferred to the nucleus. In humans, mitochondria are composed of over 1000 proteins. The vast majority of genes encoding these proteins are located in the nuclear DNA (chromosomes). A few genes remain entirely in the mitochondria and not in the cell nucleus constitute the mtDNA ("mitochondrial DNA" Figure 5.2). The entire mtDNA is active in energy functions. Despite comprising only 37 genes, the compact mt-DNA has a high mutation rate leading both to tremendous genetic diversity from a high number of sequence variants, and to a high rate of pathogenic variants (mutations).

The cytoplasmic-located mt-DNA is inherited only from the mother without recombination, as any sperm mt-DNA that happens to enter the ova is not replicated. In the absence of a recent mutation, a child carries the identical mtDNA sequence to that of his/her mother, full siblings, and maternal half-siblings, aunts, uncles, and grandmother. These "matrilineal" relatives share the same mtDNA sequences and are often affected in families that carry mtDNA mutations[50]

Mitochondrial diseases. Mitochondrial disorders can be caused by mutations on either the mt-DNA or the nuclear DNA. In its "classical" form, mitochondrial disease is often progressive and can be ultimately lethal. Since nerves are electrical and have high-energy requirements, "hard" neurological abnormalities are common: mental retardation, seizures, stroke, ataxia, dystonia retinopathy, sensorineural hearing loss and cardiac conduction defects. Muscle is another tissue with high-energy demands, and clinical manifestations can include cardiomyopathy, muscle weakness, ocular myopathy, and smooth muscle myopathies (gastrointestinal and vascular disease). Far more commonly, "Functional" symptomology manifests as chronic pain, fatigue and gastrointestinal conditions, fibromyalgia and often dominates the clinical presentation in lesser-affected patients, as well as in relatives of more-severely affected index cases. Mitochondrial diseases are more likely to strike at times of stress, due to the high-energy demands. Examples of stressors include fasting, exercise, illness, and psychological stress.

Patients with mitochondrial disorders frequently present with chronic pain, and often meet diagnostic criteria for chronic pain as in functional disorders including migraine,

---

23   Richard G. Boles, M.D., Medical Director, Courtagen Life Sciences, Woburn, MA
     www.mitoaction.org/blog/dr-richard-boles-functional-mitochondrial-disorders

non-specific abdominal pain, complex regional pain syndrome (CRPS), fibromyalgia, tem-poromandibular disorder (TMD). Several other functional conditions include irritable bowel syndrome (IBS), chronic fatigue syndrome (CFS), cyclic vomiting syndrome (CVS), postural orthostatic tachycardia syndrome (POTS), tinnitus, chronic idiopathic nausea, and intersti-tial cystitis (IC), among others. Depression and generalized anxiety disorder are often placed in the same category, or as related conditions[36].

Since the term "functional" varies among medical sub-specialties, and these con-ditions are generally associated with aberrant AUTONOMIC responses[37-40], the term "functional/ autonomic-related" (FAR) disorders can be applied to this group. Diagnosis is dependent upon fulfilling a number of clinical criteria based largely on subjective symptoms without the benefit of confirmatory biomarkers[41]. There is no clear dividing line between those conditions in which pain is a primary or secondary contribution. Patients/ families often have several such conditions, both primary and secondary.

- *44% of patients with IC also have symptoms suggestive of IBS (v. 12% of controls)*
- *59% of CVS met the standardized criteria for generalized anxiety disorder*
- *67% of people with migraines fulfilled criteria for CFS43*
- *75% of patients with CVS are projected to develop migraine by age 185,27,28.*
- *20%-80% of TMD patients suffer from additional chronic pain disorders such as headache, low back pain, fibromyalgia, and IBS .*

These findings suggest that at least some of the genes comprising the familial aggre-gation of the FAR/pain disorders reside on the maternally-inherited mtDNA. Since energy is a requirement for life, all cells require energy for essential every function. Thus, mitochondrial dysfunction usually manifests in more than one tissue, and usu-ally causes more than one sign or symptom. Some common features include:

- *Dysfunction of at least 3 different nerve / muscle tissues (e.g. myalgia, depression and ptosis)*
- *Gastrointestinal dysmotility affecting more than one level of the gut (e.g. GERD and constipation)*
- *Disease that changes over time as being intermittent /or protean manifestations at different times)*
- *Time course in regular cycles, or intermittent episodes triggered by stress (e.g. viral illness, psychological stress)*
- *Severe fatigue with post-exertional malaise*
- *Dysautonomia (e.g. tachycardia, POTS, temperature intolerance)*

CHRONIC PAIN CONDITIONS (B)

- *Occasional multi-system involvement, particularly low blood counts, pancreatitis, liver transaminase elevations, endocrine gland problems.*

- *Protean manifestations in "matrilineal" relatives (related all through women, thus sharing the same basic mtDNA sequence).*

Treatment Approaches. Mitochondrial dysfunction generally involves the production or persistence of increased levels of reactive oxygen species (ROS) and other free radicals. These byproducts of respiration damage macromolecules including DNA (causing further mutation), proteins and lipids. If damage accumulates faster than repair, this leads to disease progression that may be irreversible. Thus, antioxidants are frequently prescribed in these patients. Beyond antioxidants, several natural substances are known to have effects in mitochondrial energy metabolism, including the B vitamins and carnitine. Although antioxidant, vitamin and cofactor therapies are in wide clinical use in chronic pain patients, scientific study has been sparse.

There are a large number of products with reported mitochondrial effects on the market, and no single substance or treating philosophy is best for every patient. Treatment should be individualized. Here are tips which express the opinions and practice of this author:

Coenzyme Q10 is generally a first line therapy. Coenzyme Q10 can be effective in a wide variety of symptoms and clinical manifestations related to chronic pain disorders. In the author's experience, it is generally under-dosed, and many preparations on the market have poor bioavailability. Blood levels can be very helpful in guiding therapy. A level of greater than 3 mg/L is generally required for clinical efficacy and levels over 4 mg/L being ideal. Individuals with severe intestinal failure can be very difficult to reach therapeutic levels. Side effects are rare, and occasional insomnia responds to limiting dosing to earlier in the day.

Vitamin C, Vitamin E and Alpha lipoic acid are frequently used. Since antioxidants prevent future cellular damage, efficacy is delayed by weeks or months, often with full effects only seen after a year. Gastrointestinal side effects are common, except with vitamin C and may necessitate ramping or lower dosing. As very high dosing can have pro-oxidant effects, moderate dosing of multiple antioxidants seems prudent. For children ages 3-5, half dosing is given. Infant and toddler dosing is individualized.

Carnitine deficiency. Operating as "trash trucks of the cell", L-carnitine is often depleted in patients with mitochondrial dysfunction due to the excretion of high volumes of byproducts of defective metabolism. Lesser degrees of carnitine insufficiency can lead to vague functional symptoms (e.g. pain, fatigue, weakness) that can be corrected by L-carnitine supplementation. The free carnitine level is important in gauging supplementation, as that value represents the available carnitine to complex with metabolic byproducts. A common side effect is a foul body odor often referred to as "fishy", which is caused by gut bacteria metabolizing carnitine. This odor often responds to lowering the dosage given, or riboflavin supplementation. Carnitine also can cause GI upset.

***B vitamins** are involved in energy metabolism, and as such are often used to treat mitochondrial disease and FAR/CPS disorders. In particular, riboflavin (vitamin B2), which is a cofactor in multiple mitochondrial enzymes including complexes I, II and III of the respiratory chain, is often used in migraine. However, many other B vitamins and/or their derivatives acts in mitochondrial metabolism including thiamine (B1), niacin and **nicotinic acid** (B3), pantothenic acid (B5), pyridoxine and pyridoxamine (B6), biotin (B7), folate (B9) and the various cobalamins (B12). They are often given together as a "B complex", of which there are many brands. A common preparation is a "B100" or "B50", whereas the number indicates the milligrams of riboflavin per tablet, among other things.*

***Magnesium** is another cofactor in energy metabolism that is often used in migraine prophylaxis. Many other minerals, including selenium, are also needed for proper mitochondrial function.*

***Creatine** serves to store energy, as phosphocreatine, in nerve and muscle. Inborn errors of creatine biosynthesis or transport lead to progressive neurological dysfunction and movement disorder, which generally responds to creatine supplementation.*

Don't forget about diet and exercise.

- *Fresh fruits and vegetables provide many antioxidants not available as supplements.*

- *Post-prandial hypoglycemia and associated symptomatology can be ameliorated by a diet rich in low glycemic index foods and protein, with less processed foods.*

- *A moderate to high protein diet can be helpful in some patients, possibly by providing amino acids to replenish Krebs cycle intermediates. This is especially true in sick and hospitalized patients, whereas parental nutrition may be needed.*

- *Fasting can provoke disease in many patients with mitochondrial dysfunction, and frequent meals and snacks can sometimes be helpful.*

- *Exercise increases mitochondrial size and number, and is often effective in reducing symptomatology if frequent and in moderation. Both the benefits and need for careful moderation are heightened in cases with chronic/post-exertional fatigue.*

Although difficult to treat in many cases, antidepressant drugs are widely used in practice to treat the FAR/CPS disorders. The common response of these conditions to antidepressant drugs suggests shared causative factors. The therapeutic response to antidepressants includes tricyclics, serotonin uptake inhibitors, monoamine oxidase

CHRONIC PAIN CONDITIONS (B)

inhibitors, and atypical agents. Among these conditions, migraine and IBS have been most studied and often have efficacy whether or not the patient has depression.

Psychotropics can often be helpful, possibly due to direct effects on mitochondria. Tricyclics: Amitriptyline is frequently used to treat a range of pain disorders including CVS, migraine, CRPS, fibromyalgia, and IBS. Efficacy may take 1-3 months. Side effects include lethargy and irritability. A slow increase in dosage is important, and if slow enough this drug often is tolerated even in those that failed the drug in the past. Prolongation of the electrical conduction in the heart (QTc) is a rare, but potentially serious, side effect; monitor ECG before/ after therapy.

SSRIs and SNRIs: These drugs have some efficacy against the chronic pain disorders and are prescribed in this setting, especially in cases with co-morbid depression. Among these drugs, Zoloft is often used; it appears to induce less lethargy.

SLEEP PROBLEMS

Children may have trouble falling asleep or staying asleep for many reasons, including pain, anxiety, depression, or just an "active brain that won't turn off." Sleep deprivation is an additional factor that keeps pain active. There are some excellent strategies, not involving medication, that facilitate improved sleep. Dr. Harvey Karp, a well-known developmental pediatrician and author of many books and DVDs on infant and toddler development, behavior, and sleep, describes what he calls the 5 "S's" that he believes activates a neonatal response, the "calming reflex", that can quickly reduce infant crying and promote sleep[24]. His comments and further details appear in Chapter 12.

In the next chapters we will discuss specific diseases that have pain associated with them, like arthritis, intestinal inflammatory conditions, cancer and sickle cell disease among others.

---

24   Harvey Karp, MD, FAAP, Creator DVD/book, *The Happiest Baby on the Block.*
    www.happiestbaby.com/about-dr-karp

This pain is present every day
Unyielding, oppressive, still there.
Why doesn't it take a day off,
Who said, "Life is always fair?"

Inhabited by the unwanted
I feel victimized, possessed.
I ask myself all those questions,
"What did I do? Was I too stressed?"

How much is psychological?
How much is left to chance?
Will it get worse or better?
Should I take a reflective glance?

Depression displaced by anger
I felt helpless, betrayed by fate.
Blaming myself, my parents, my genes
I faced my own Watergate.

I began to count my losses,
Labored through my grief,
My life, my body, my ego
All vandalized by this thief.

For a while I wallowed and floundered.
Kicked by the foot of fate,
Then one day I passed a mirror and said,
"This is your life. It's getting late!"

Suddenly that's when it hit me.
I'd had enough of that pit.
My life was leading me around
Instead of me living it.

I began to look for solutions
If this pain is always to be.
I had to find some hope in my life,
Imprisoned, I longed to be free.

I took a personal inventory
Of all that I have left,
Gradually I stopped asking, "Why?"
And began feeling less bereft.

I've learned to love each day
Even the dark side and strife
For hidden within the heartache
Is a seed of renewal, called life.

—SUE FALKNER WOOD-HTTP://WWW.EVERYDAYHEALTH.COM/COLUMNS/
LIFE-WITH-CHRONIC-PAIN/A-POEM-ABOUT-CHRONIC-PAIN/

CHAPTER 6

DISEASES ASSOCIATED WITH CHRONIC PAIN:
ARTHRITIS, CROHN'S/ULCERATIVE COLITIS, SICKLE CELL AND CANCER

ARTHRITIS

INFLAMMATORY BOWEL DISEASES (IBD)

- Ulcerative Colitis and Crohn's Disease (Regional Ileitis)
- Discussion by the experts

SICKLE CELL DISEASE

- Patient and parent's perspective

CANCER & BONE MARROW TRANSPLANTATION

- Post-Operative Pain
- Bone Pain
- Hospital Resources for Pain Management In Cancer

PAIN IN CHILDREN AND YOUNG ADULTS

ARTHRITIS

For most children with arthritis, chronic pain is not a huge issue... if the arthritis is well managed. Children may have some increased pain during physical therapy but that pain usually resolves after the physical therapy session has ended. Sometimes, however, the inflammatory process is difficult to treat. For example:

> *Jodi is a 9-year-old girl with juvenile idiopathic arthritis (JIA) whose large joints hurt and were inflamed. While her treatment with methotrexate helped initially, after one year the methotrexate was no longer effective. She was to start a biological modifier medication (Enbrel) but that required a weekly injection. However, she had a severe needle phobia and despite pre-medicating her to reduce anxiety prior to the Enbrel injections, she would panic and need to be held down. She developed severe antici- patory anxiety before each injection to the point that parents chose to stop treatment until efforts to reduce her needle phobia could be successful. During the time off treatment for arthritis, her pain and inflammation became worse.*

> *We were consulted and after seeing us, Jodi began working with one of our team psychologists to learn cognitive behavioral therapy (CBT) strategies to reduce her anxiety and desensitization to reduce her needle phobia (see chapter 15 for more on these therapies). After 4-6 weeks, she was able to successfully receive injections by her father without the need for other anxiety-reducing medications. The sense of pride in her accomplishments furthered her ability to receive Enbrel injections; her disease and pain symptoms improved.*

For some children with arthritis, long-term difficulties getting the disease under control lead to ongoing and significant joint pain, which itself sensitizes the central nervous system and sets up increased pain signaling in the brain and through the nerves traveling up and down the spinal column. Thus, even when the disease itself is under good medical control, electrical, nerve signaling components, activated by the prior prolonged period of pain, add to current sensations causing pain, even though the disease is under good control. This pain is not *nociceptive* (related to inflammation), but it is *neuropathic* related to changes in neural signaling. The treatment then needs to be aimed at central neural pain mechanisms rather than "treating the disease" directly by reducing inflammation.

For some children, the time for getting the disease under initial control with effective disease-targeted therapies is challenging and prolonged. In these situations, short-term nociceptive pain-relieving medication may be needed, such as meloxi- cam (a potent anti-inflammatory medication) or opioids, if anti-inflammatory agents are not effective. In this case, reducing pain until the disease itself can be brought under control with disease-targeted medications can also reduce the likelihood of

88

DISEASES ASSOCIATED WITH CHRONIC PAIN (A)

extended nociceptive inflammatory pain triggering central neuropathic pain. After receiving the effective disease-related treatment, the temporary analgesic medication can be weaned off and discontinued.

We asked Laura E. Schanberg, MD[25], and Fellow, Dr. Rebecca Sadun, to discuss arthritis in children.

Arthritis – pain, swelling, and inflammation of one or more joints – can occur in children of any age. In a child under the age 16, arthritis that lasts longer than six weeks is called juvenile idiopathic arthritis (JIA); formerly juvenile rheumatoid arthritis (JRA). In JIA, the child's immune system attacks the lining around joints (synovium). If left untreated, damage will extend to the bones that are part of the inflamed joint. **Diagnosis and treatment is focused both on improving current symptoms and on reducing or eliminating long-term damage** *from ongoing joint inflammation.*

A pediatric rheumatologist will work with your child's other doctors to help diagnose and treat any of the various types of JIA. Great resources describing each type of JIA and the treatments are described in more detail at this website in the footnote.

Types of JIA: *Some JIA attacks one or just a few joints; if < 4 at diagnosis, the child has oligoarticular JIA and is treated with steroid injections into the swollen joints and/or with anti-inflammatory medications like ibuprofen. If they progress to develop involvement of five or more joints, called extended oligoarticular JIA, they need stronger medications. If five or more joints are involved from the beginning, this is called polyarticular JIA. Some of these children have a blood test that shows either rheumatoid factor antibodies (RF), or anti-citrullinated peptide antibodies ("anti-CCP."). Most children with polyarticular JIA, unlike adults, don't have antibodies.*

Another type of JIA, systemic-onset JIA, causes fever, rash, swollen lymph nodes and other symptoms besides arthritis. At diagnosis, kids with systemic JIA are often quite sick and may need multiple medications to control disease and pain. These may include steroids, methotrexate, and other biologic agents including blockers of interleukin-1 (anakinra/Kineret™ or canakinumab/Ilaris) and interleukin-6 (tocilizimab/Actemra™) that are especially effective in treating this type of JIA.

Sources of Pain: *For many children, pain and swelling occurs around the joints rather than in them. When the inflammation is at the attachment of the tendon to the bone, also known as an enthesis, the child's arthritis is called enthesitis-related JIA. Often, these children have pain in the low back, knees, ankles, and feet. The medications already mentioned can be used to treat this type of arthritis; in addition, a medication called sulfasalazine is often helpful.*

---

25 Laura E. Schanberg, MD, Professor of Pediatrics, Co-Chief of Pediatric Rheumatology at Duke University Medical Center. Dr. Rebecca Sadun MD, Fellow, *http://pediatrics.duke.edu/faculty/details/0019107*

PAIN IN CHILDREN AND YOUNG ADULTS

Arthritis in Other Conditions *Children can also get arthritis associated with other conditions like inflammatory Bowel Diseases (IBD), (e.g. Crohn's or ulcerative colitis). The skin condition psoriasis is associated with arthritis; these kids are diagnosed with psoriatic JIA. Both IBD-associated JIA and psoriatic JIA can be controlled with anti-inflammatory medications, but often require sulfasalazine, methotrexate, or a biologic medication to achieve full control.*

Treatments *The goal of treatment is to eliminate swelling completely, as we know that this reduces the chance of long-term joint damage and chronic pain or disability. For many children, remission is possible – after a period of excellent arthritis control, their doctor can gradually reduce the number of or dose of medications, and may eventually stop one or more medications entirely.*

Children with polyarticular JIA, especially those with RF or anti-CCP antibodies, need medications beyond anti-inflammatories and steroid injections to suppress the immune system. The most commonly used medication is methotrexate. In general, children who continue to have symptoms and swelling despite methotrexate will receive a Tumor Necrosis Factor (TNF) inhibitor; the two most common are etanercept/ Enbrel™ and adalimumab /Humira™ and are called biologics. There are new biologics to treat JIA being tested all the time. Some children need to begin a biologic from the time of diagnosis. Even if the IBD or the psoriasis is fully controlled, ongoing joint inflammation leads to pain as well as permanent disability. Therefore, controlling the arthritis is as important as controlling the IBD or the rash.

Preventing Damage *Pediatric rheumatology teams help kids be as active as possible and lead relatively normal lives, but some children will have limitations. They may participate in PE or even in school sports, but their joints may not handle extremely intense athletic training necessary for becoming an elite or professional athlete. Likewise, some sports may be great (swimming) while others are not a good fit (gymnastics). Pediatric rheumatologists encourage children with all types of JIA to stay physically active, but limitations may be set to reduce the risk of further injury.*

Stopping Treatment *While some children go into remission and never have another flare of symptoms, others may need to start back on medications at some point in the future. Coming off medication is best managed by a JIA expert. If the child has pain or swelling during or after the process of weaning medications, it is important to alert the child's doctor right away.*

Unique Features of Pain in Arthritis *Not infrequently, children will experience ongoing pain, even when their arthritis is well controlled. This occurs for several different reasons.*

DISEASES ASSOCIATED WITH CHRONIC PAIN (A)

- *Subtle ongoing inflammation not evident on physical exam; sometimes an MRI is necessary to identify this.*

- *During the period of active arthritis, the muscles around the joint weakened; and this can often improve/ resolve with physical therapy.*

- *Permanent joint damage may have occurred during the period of active arthritis. Physical therapy can be helpful, and occasionally a brace or other device can help support the joint and reduce pain. In rare cases, surgery is needed.*

- *If the child's arthritis is in the knee/ankle, sometimes one leg grows longer than the other, which can lead to pain. Physical therapy and a lift in or on the shoe can be helpful.*

- *A child who had pain during the period of active arthritis may develop central pain (changes in brain connectivity). This results in increased sensitivity and "top-down" pain propagators, rather than having ongoing "bottom-up" inflammation as a cause of the pain. This type responds best to medications aimed at neuropathic pain as well as mind-body interventions.*

Summary *Pain in arthritis can be useful, helping to alert the patient, parents, and doctors that there is inflammation and arthritis requiring treatment. For many children, pain will resolve as the arthritis comes under control. For other children, however, the pain itself can become a problem that requires specific treatment in addition to the treatment of the arthritis itself. Two helpful Duke Websites appear below*[26].

A mother comments

"Julia" a mother of two children with Juvenile Arthritis comments on her journey to find pain relief for her sons.

> *One of the hardest things for a parent to endure is to helplessly watch their child suffer. As a parent of two children with Juvenile Arthritis, this is a feeling that I was well acquainted with, especially after my older son Grant, had a life-threatening flare. In this situation, the first (and correct) instinct is to stop the disease in its tracks, with the hopes that whenever the root of the problem is managed, then the pain issues will also be resolved. We thought that "fixing" the arthritis would also "fix" the pain, but we learned that things are not always so simple.*

> *When the initial shock of dealing with a serious flare is over, and the physical crisis is under control, it would seem as though the pain should subside and return to bearable levels. This isn't always the case, and absolutely was not for my son. Even though his arthritis was active, it was controlled according to physical exams and lab results. This was not what we*

---

26 www.dukemedicine.org/blog/growing-pains and www.arthritis.org/arthritis-facts/disease-center/juvenile-arthritis.php

were seeing at home. Despite the good reports from specialists, his pain levels were out of control and affected every area of his life. Pain awoke him at night; his sleep was fitful and irregular, which negatively affected mood as well as his ability to focus in school. There wasn't a single area of his life that pain did not infiltrate or have a negative effect. Tired and irritable, he would become more hyper focused on his discomfort, which magnified the pain and created a vicious cycle that was heartbreaking to witness. Nothing seemed to help, and despite our best efforts, the situation continued to deteriorate.

Some doctors didn't understand the pain Grant was feeling was real. They encouraged him to "get tough" or even questioned our motivation to get treatment, concerned that we might be drug seekers. The pain he was feeling simply didn't add up with his test results. Out of desperation, we decided to see a specialist in Pain Clinic, hoping that maybe we could find a solution there. This was one of the best decisions we ever made. I knew my son. I knew something was still wrong, and I trusted my maternal instinct to keep pressing for answers. I was unwilling to accept the condition my son was living with every day as an unavoidable side effect of his disease. I knew that something else had to be causing him such agony, but we just didn't know why.

We had no idea what to expect in Pain Clinic, but when we went it was like a breath of fresh air. They believed my son, and reassured him that what he was feeling was real. They recognized a cause for his pain. The relief he felt from being heard and understood was physically visible, and an emotional turning point for us both. Although we did agree to start a regimen that initially included medications, most of the modalities were methods that helped him learn to manage pain, including the use of his mental toughness to reduce or overcome uncomfortable physical sensations. ***Stopping or reducing these sensations before they were out of control stopped the pain cycle.*** *This blended approach not only helped him work through his physical issues, but also helped him work through his emotions and put him back into control. His sleep improved, his moods improved, his physical condition improved, and finally, and his pain improved. When his pain was reduced, his inflammation also decreased, having a positive effect on his underlying illness. When we trusted him and treated him as a whole child, the outcome was greatly enhanced. No child should have to live in pain. I am very grateful that we found help to navigate a course to wellness, and that we didn't give up before my son was able to find not only relief, but the tools to help him manage his disease and pain throughout his entire life.*

INFLAMMATORY BOWEL DISEASE (IBD)

As noted before, resolution of pain and other GI symptoms follows after effective disease-targeted treatment. We won't talk about specific food enzyme deficiencies

DISEASES ASSOCIATED WITH CHRONIC PAIN (A)

and other intolerances here related to sugars, called lactase or fructase deficiencies or celiac disease; these tend to resolve by avoiding foods containing those substances. In the case of lactose intolerance, adding Lactaid™ to digest the lactose can eliminate symptoms with ingestion of milk sugar.

Infectious causes of abdominal pain include ulcer-type pain associated with infection with Helicobacter *Pylori*, and other infections such as Giardia and other parasites, treated effectively with specific antibiotics as targeted treatments. Children taking high doses of non-steroidal anti-inflammatory agents (NSAIDS), such as ibuprofen for extended periods, can develop abdominal pain related to gastritis (irritation with inflammation of the stomach lining). Typically, this condition resolves with stopping the NSAIDS.

In this section, we discuss three inflammatory bowel diseases: Crohn's disease, ulcerative colitis, and the controversial "eosinophilic esophagitis." As with other states, **when the disease is under good control, the abdominal pain and other gastro-esophageal (GI) symptoms should resolve, unless there has been a prior history of ongoing pain during the period of getting the disease under control.** When that happens, central sensitization may occur with continued abdominal pain and GI symptoms. The persistence of pain, even after effective disease treatment, might be the result of top-down neuropathic pain. The effective pain treatment then involves the 'electrician approach' in addition to the intestinal-focused nociceptive (plumbing) approach.

Regional Enteritis, Ulcerative Colitis & Eosinophilic Esophagitis

Inflammatory bowel disease (IBD) is a condition of ongoing or recurrent inflammation within the intestinal tract. (IBD should not be confused with irritable bowel syndrome or IBS, which we discussed in Chapter 5) There are several forms of IBD. Ulcerative colitis is an IBD that is limited to the large intestine (colon). Early signs include left-sided abdominal pain that improves after bowel movements, joint pain, and progressive loosening of the stools that are often bloody. Severe abdominal pain and bloody stools create disabling symptoms for children before the disease is first diagnosed or during times of increased inflammation. Treatment is aimed at reducing inflammation in the colon, usually by specific anti-inflammatory medication. Removal of the colon is an option of last resort.

Crohn's disease is another IBD in which there is patchy inflammation that involves all the layers of the intestine wall. The early signs of Crohn's disease in children are often vague, making diagnosis difficult. Abdominal pain over the navel or on the right side is most common and may appear long before pervasive diarrhea. There also may be joint pain and fever before there are any changes in bowel

PAIN IN CHILDREN AND YOUNG ADULTS

patterns. Decreased appetite and weight loss are often misdiagnosed as symptoms of anorexia nervosa, school anxiety, or psychological problems.

There are effective anti-inflammatory treatments that prevent or reduce the inflammation and this usually resolves the pain issue. Not every child with IBD actually has abdominal pain, even though there may be small areas of intestinal inflammation. However, in children who might be at risk for development of chronic pain, **severe bouts of inflammatory-related abdominal pain or surgery can set off central top-down neuropathic pain.** In this case, the nerves carrying pain signals from the intestines to the brain get "turned on" and the signals become magnified so that the brain perceives just as much pain as if there were active inflammation, even though the intestines may be fine after anti-inflammatory treatment. This condition occurs in rare cases of significant prolonged pain prior to the removal of the entire large intestine in ulcerative colitis. In this example, **the brain region activated during the period of severe disease may remain "turned on" still causing the experience of belly pain**. When abdominal pain continues after successful treatment of intestinal inflammation or colon removal, treatment is aimed at central neuropathic pain.

There are sometimes outside-the-intestine manifestations of IBD, including arthritis or arthralgias (joint pain without inflammation), and skin rashes. However, the hallmark of IBD is inflammation of the intestine and typically abdominal pain.

Discussion by the experts

Dr. Shervin Rabizadeh[27] discusses the current status of mechanisms and treatments for Crohn's disease and ulcerative colitis below.

> *Inflammatory Bowel Disease (IBD) is a condition of chronic intestinal inflammation that impairs the quality of life for hundreds of thousands of children and adults. IBD patients often are classified into 2 diseases, Crohn's disease and ulcerative colitis. Though the exact mechanism is unclear, both diseases occur in people with specific genetic risk factors within the right environmental setting when a person's immune (defense) system attacks his/her own intestinal tract. In Crohn's disease, the inflammation can happen anywhere within the intestinal tract, while in ulcerative colitis, the inflammation is limited to the large intestine (colon). Crohn's patients will present with debilitating abdominal pain, weight loss, and growth failure, anemia, diarrhea and recurrent fevers. Ulcerative colitis patients often present with rectal bleeding, diarrhea, urgency for bowel movements, sensation to have a bowel*

---

27   Dr. Shervin Rabizadeh, a pediatric gastroenterologist specializing in IBD at Cedars-Sinai Medical Center and UCLA Associate Professor of Pediatrics. www.cedars-sinai.edu/Bios---Physician/P-Z/Shervin-Rabizadeh-MD-MBA.aspx

DISEASES ASSOCIATED WITH CHRONIC PAIN (A)

movement but without production, abdominal pain especially prior to bowel movements, and recurrent fevers. Both Crohn's disease and ulcerative colitis patients can have extra-intestinal symptoms such as joint pains and rashes.

The goal of treatment for IBD is remission, which is defined as the patient not having any symptoms. This is often achieved by re-regulating the immune/defense system with medications. Local anti-inflammatory medications, similar to those for the skin, can work for patients with milder forms of ulcerative colitis. However, some ulcerative colitis and Crohn's disease patients require the long term use of stronger medications that will control their immune system by decreasing the number of certain types of cells or certain proteins that act as signals that control the immune reaction. These medications have potential side effects but the risk of active disease and its sequelae far outweigh the potential harm from the medications. Surgery, especially in ulcerative colitis where colon removal is possible, can lead to resolution of the disease.

We also asked Dr. David Ziring[28] to provide his comments on IBD.

Inflammatory bowel disease (IBD) is commonly thought of as being either Crohn's disease or ulcerative colitis based on location and behavior. Roughly 38,000 children in the US currently suffer from Crohn's disease and 23,000 from ulcerative colitis.[1] We now know that there are several conditions that, when combined, lead to IBD. For instance, a child has to have inherited genes that place him/ her at risk of developing IBD (whether or not anyone else in their family has it.) These genes lead to changes in the immune system, changes that affect how our immunity recognizes and responds to the normal bacteria in our intestines. With new testing methods, we have a much better appreciation for the types of bacteria that inhabit the intestines in someone with IBD compared with people without the disease. Lastly, there seems to be an inciting trigger for IBD that can include stress, infection, antibiotics, smoking, and other environmental influences. This does not mean these factors cause IBD, as children affected were going to develop the disease at some point in their lives, but these triggers "unmask" the disease.

Crohn's disease results in inflammation and ulcers anywhere in the GI tract, from mouth to anus. This inflammation, over time, causes swelling of affected parts in the intestine and eventually scarring that can either narrow the intestine or even cause a hole to form. A child with Crohn's often presents with abdominal pain and weight loss. They may have unexplained fevers or bloody diarrhea. Or, they may simply have stopped growing unexpectedly. Everyone's Crohn's disease is different. Medications used to treat Crohn's disease alter the immune system to prevent it from

---

28 Dr. David Ziring, a pediatric gastroenterologist and UCLA Associate Professor of Pediatrics who heads the IBD program at UCLA. www.uclahealth.org/provider/david-ziring-md

causing damage to the intestine when it is attacking the normal bacteria there. These medications are called "immunomodulators" (methotrexate or mercaptopurine) or "biologics" (such as infliximab (Remicade™) or adalimumab (Humira™).

Ulcerative colitis, on the other hand, is inflammation that is confined only to the large intestine (the colon) and is found only in its lining. For most children, the entire colon is affected and the inflammation tends to be more severe than in adults with ulcerative colitis. Children with ulcerative colitis typically first complain of diarrhea, often containing blood, and they occasionally have stomach cramping or urgency to use the restroom. Sometimes they feel a particular sensation as if they are unable to pass the entirety of their bowel movement, or that once they do, they need to return immediately to sit on the toilet.

Mild ulcerative colitis is often treated with anti-inflammatory drugs that coat the lining of the colon. But colitis that is more severe requires aggressive medications, similar to those used to treat Crohn's disease.[5]

Finally, we thought that this section would not be complete without some comments about eosinophilic esophagitis (EE), as this condition is becoming increasingly recognized, although approaches to treatment may differ by institution. Dr. Jorge Vargas[29] discusses this complex condition.

Eosinophilic Esophagitis (EE) is a rare immunologically mediated condition, characterized by a peculiar swelling of the tube that connects the mouth to the stomach, the esophagus, which was recognized as a disease or disorder only since 2005. We do not have a good explanation of how it happens or why it presents the ways it does.

The characteristic symptoms vary according to the degree of swelling of the esophagus, whose function is to propel the different textures of food we swallow to the stomach in a matter of seconds, where big chemical changes will happen to that "bolus" of food in the first steps of digestion. So the period of contact of each bolus, solid or liquid, with the lining of the esophagus is very short and demands a major coordination of movement of this tube-like structure to produce the required action. This process involves opening and closing at the site of connection to the stomach to allow food to enter quickly and to prevent food from backing up into the esophagus. Some backing up into the esophagus occur normally, mainly after a meal, and this is called "reflux". If this happens with excessive frequency, or for prolonged periods, then the stomach contents, which turn acid after we eat, may irritate the lining of the esophagus.

---

29 Dr. Jorge Vargas, Clinical Professor of Pediatrics . A UCLA pediatric gastroenterologist who has significant experience treating EE. www.uclahealth.org/provider/jorge-vargas-md

DISEASES ASSOCIATED WITH CHRONIC PAIN (A)

Diagnosis: Any swelling will have a consequence on the way the esophagus moves or propels the 'bolus.' Thus, food bolus can move quickly or, with major swelling, movement can be slowed to the point of causing an obstruction. The latter is felt as a sensation of difficult swallowing, a bolus being stuck somewhere in the chest behind the breastbone called "dysphagia" [from the Greek: Dys= disordered or bad & Phagus= eat]. This sensation can be painful. (Odynophagia)

If we then think in physical terms, this difficulty will be more apparent with solids than with liquids. Dysphagia will be manifested very differently by age, developmental stages and ability to communicate. The infant manifests this sensation with refusal to eat solids or even some liquids, and the consequence of poor intake at that age may translate into poor growth. As the child grows, dysphagia can be better expressed, with sensation present or first ascribed to solids and then to liquids, to a point when the swelling may be so advanced that it may suddenly cause the impaction of solid food in the esophagus. The classic presentation of esophageal obstruction in a young adolescent is usually happening after eating a hot dog.

Sometimes the problem shows up with cough or wheezing because of increased secretions. Sometimes the child can show skin 'allergies' to different foods or environmental factors such as humidity, temperature, dust or pollen. When combined with the sensation of dysphagia, primary care physicians may diagnose "reflux." Most children will be treated initially with medications that reduce or control acid secretion in the stomach and some may actually have some improvement of symptoms. But a large number, as the symptoms persist, will be referred to a gastroenterologist with the idea that they have severe 'reflux-disease'. These children are then studied in more detail and the characteristic findings of EE may then be confirmed.

Endoscopy is the one test that will reveal the presence of swelling of the esophagus with the appearance of white bumps under the lining of the esophagus. But microscopic appearance through biopsies document that these bumps are made up of bunches of inflammatory cells called eosinophils, which are related to allergic reactions. While eosinophils are also seen in many types of injuries in the esophagus, such as acid-related injury, the number of eosinophils (over 15 per high power field) allows for the diagnosis of EE, specifically also when seen predominantly in the upper part of the esophagus, as opposed to eosinophils seen mostly in the lower part of the esophagus as in acid reflux, where most of the chemical contact with the acid is expected to happen. Rarely some children will also have increased eosinophils in the blood. Motility studies if done will be abnormal, but that is a non-specific finding related to the swollen esophagus. pH and other monitoring for increased acid exposure as in reflux will demonstrate a lack of correlation between pain symptoms and episodes of reflux.

Rather than EE being the result of an "allergy" to specific foods, recent research has documented a more complex situation of a dysfunctional response that may be immune but not specifically to a food item, even if there is a visible clinical response to dietary exclusions and to the use of 'elemental' diets or diets that contain molecular structures small and simple enough not to cause any possible allergic reaction.

Therapy: *There are several therapeutic approaches to treatment. Very strict protein elimination diets and non-palatable elemental diets are difficult to impose on school-age children or adolescents and create stressors that impact mood and function. The other approach is to give the child steroids systemically (swallowed in a pill form) or in a non-absorbable form topically to act locally on the lining of the esophagus. A problem with this latter method is that the response lasts only a short time, but combining the topical steroid with a carbohydrate or sugar (syrup) will make it stay a bit longer in contact with the affected areas to reduce the swelling.*

If the narrowing of the esophagus has caused food impactions, then dilations of the esophagus may be needed, although these are done more frequently in adults than in children. Topical steroids can have immune system side-effects, increasing the likelihood of fungal infections in mouth and esophagus.

Parents may receive conflicting approaches to treatment from otherwise wise and knowledgeable pediatric gastroenterologists. The differing opinions relate to the use of a strict diet with gradual additions of food proteins, with or without repeated endoscopies and biopsies, use of systemic vs topical steroids, or some equivocation about the number of eosinophils to make the diagnosis.

SICKLE CELL DISEASE (SCD)

Sickle Cell Disease (SCD) is an inherited blood disorder that causes continuous destruction of red blood cells, episodes of intense pain, vulnerability to infections, organ damage, and, in some cases, early death. It is most prevalent among African-Americans and Hispanic-Americans. Health experts estimate that one out of every 500 African-American children and one out of every 1,400 Hispanic-American children are born with SCD. Dr. Tom Coates[30] shares his expertise in this section on SCD.

James is a 15-year-old young man with SCD. Over the years, he experienced bouts of pain in his chest, stomach, arms, and legs caused by the blockage of blood flow due to the sickled shape of his blood cells. In the past, James' sickle cell pain or "crises,"

---

30   Thomas D Coates, M.D., Professor of Pediatrics and Pathology, Section Head of Hematology, Head, Sickle Cell and Hemoglobinopathy Center, Children's Center for Cancer and Blood Diseases, Children's Hospital Los Angeles, USC Keck School of Medicine. http://profiles.sc-ctsi.org/thomas.coates

DISEASES ASSOCIATED WITH CHRONIC PAIN (A)

as he called them had occurred once yearly. However, since he turned 13 years, his pain crises occurred more frequently and required more emergency department (ED) visits and hospitalizations. Sometimes the pain was brief, other times it lasted hours, days or weeks. He began to tire more easily and was having problems fighting infections. He tried his best to manage his pain at home, but it was becoming difficult.

James always tried to maintain a sense of humor about his pain and was often upbeat and joking with his doctors and the nurses who treated him. However, in the last two years his mood changed. He became sullener. The doctors began to wonder if James was coming to the hospital "just to get drugs," and James began to mistrust the doctors. His more intense and frequent pain crises forced him to rely increasingly on the ED and the hospital for intravenous (IV) fluids and stronger pain medications. His treatments escalated with repeated blood transfusions, causing iron overload and requiring medications to bind his iron so that it wouldn't poison his organs. His depressed mood, however, was getting in the way of his regularly taking his medications; his body was suffering.

Origin of Pain in SCD People with SCD have red blood cells that contain an abnormal type of the oxygen-carrying part of the red blood cells (hemoglobin). Normal hemoglobin is a liquid and when it releases oxygen, it remains liquid. Sickle hemoglobin transforms from liquid to solid gel when it releases oxygen into the tissues. When the sickle red blood cells release oxygen, they become rigid, take on a sickled or crescent-shape, and have difficulty passing through small blood vessels. When sickle-shaped cells block small blood vessels, less blood reaches that part of the body. Tissues that are starved for oxygen eventually become damaged. If organs or body parts are deprived of oxygen, there is a buildup of chemicals at nerve endings, and pain signals become activated.

Imagine that a blood pressure cuff that keeps getting tighter and tighter until your arm turns blue is squeezing your arm. After a while, your arm will begin to ache and the pain may become unbearable. This is the type of extremity pain experienced by people with SCD. The magnitude of this pain is similar to that which occurs with a bone fracture. It is severe. These episodes of pain usually start in one region of the body such as an arm or leg and increase in intensity over hours. The pain can be so severe that it can require powerful pain medications such as opioids like morphine.

Arthritis medicines like ibuprofen are taken around the clock to suppress the inflammation due to the damage from the sickling. These painful episodes often last from 2 to 7 days. The pain often cannot be managed with oral medications at home; and it becomes necessary to be admitted to the hospital to receive infusions of pain medication directly into the veins.

Children and adolescents with SCD also develop headaches and low back pain from chronic muscle spasm and lack of oxygen in their spine. They experience joint pain,

PAIN IN CHILDREN AND YOUNG ADULTS

especially in the hip, when the head of the large bone in the thigh (femur) is destroyed from a lack of blood and oxygen. This hip condition also can cause a deep, aching "referred" pain in the lower thigh above the knee. Therefore, patients with SCD have two types of pain: one directly from the blood vessel blockage itself and the second because of permanent damage to bone or other organs. We do not know why some children have frequent, repetitive pain episodes while others have a milder, intermittent form. What we do know is that the pain varies wildly depending on the child.

There is a third kind of pain called "nerve pain" that occurs in patients with SCD. Actually, nerve pain (neuropathic pain) can occur in any one secondary to an initial acute pain experience. When nerves have been bombarded with enough signals from the damage secondary to poor blood flow, they start sending off pain signals even when the initial damage has stopped. This secondary nerve pain is difficult to treat and requires different approaches. Typically, opioids do not help this pain and in fact can make it worse. This kind of pain can continue relentlessly for days, weeks or even months after the initial insult. Patients state that they "have pain all over" or that they have "burning of their skin", or "their skin feels like it's on fire". They may complain of pain even with very light touch or other stimuli that usually are not painful. Clinicians who are not familiar with it ("neuropathic pain") often miss the diagnosis of nerve pain. In fact, medical personnel who don't recognize the symptoms may think that the patient is hysterical or making the symptoms up or "drug-seeking."

One of the most difficult things about nerve pain is that the medicines and approaches required to manage it are quite different than medications for pain directly due to blood flow blockage or bone damage. Opioids like morphine or hydromorphone (Dilaudid™) can make nerve pain worse. Non-drug treatments like massage, acupuncture, meditation, and imagery can be very helpful for nerve pain, since the persistence of the nerve pain takes place from messages in the brain. To make matters even worse, sickle patients can have both kinds of pain simultaneously. It is very important that sickle patients be aware of nerve pain because the treatment for it may be to stop or greatly reduce opioid use.

The severity of pain and need for opioids (and especially failure of opioids to help misdiagnosed nerve pain) may cause healthcare providers to conclude that sickle patients are "drug seeking" or addicted. In fact, the incidence of true drug addiction in sickle cell patients is the same as in the general population. This is striking, since sickle cell patients are exposed to a lot more prescribed opioids than most people without SCD. Fighting these misconceptions is a very difficult problem for these individuals. One of the best recommendations we have heard, with respect to this misconception, came from a psychologist who had SCD. When she was out of the hospital, and not in crisis, she dressed in the business attire she wore every day and

DISEASES ASSOCIATED WITH CHRONIC PAIN (A)

made an appointment to meet with the emergency room staff that treated her when she was in crisis so they could see her the way she usually was.

SCD and The Autonomic Nervous System: A New Link *There is new research that provides data about risk factors for increased acute pain crises and even for the development of chronic pain in young people with SCD. We now know that some people are more physiologically sensitive to stress effects in their body so that increased stress impacts their autonomic nervous system (ANS), with higher sympathetic ("fight or flight") nervous system (SNS) activation. These stressed individuals have increased circulation of adrenalin, increased pain signaling volume ("louder pain"), and more stress-related vasospasm (blood vessel narrowing), with increased opportunity for sickling to occur.*

Causes of Crises *Acute pain itself is a trigger for a vaso-occlusive pain crisis through its impact on the ANS (by increasing SNS activity). Thus, it is important to get acute pain crises under rapid control to reduce their continuance and increase in severity. In addition, the sooner those acute pain crises are controlled, the less likely it is that central sensitization will lead to more widespread chronic neuropathic pain. The frequency and severity of sickle cell pain crises can be reduced with regular hydration (drinking lots of liquids), exercise, a healthy diet, and by preventing exposure to low oxygen situations such as mountain-climbing. We also think that activities that reduce stress like yoga, massage, psychological strategies, and meditation can help reduce the frequency and severity of crises. We know for sure that stress and anxiety can greatly increase the magnitude of pain once it starts, so learning to help control stress can help manage pain. We think that the autonomic nervous system that is involved in stress and pain responses is hypersensitive because of the SCD itself, so learning stress control is particularly important for people with SCD.*

For most people with SCD, stress, anxiety control and hydration alone will not prevent all pain episodes. Management of painful crises begins with having a treatment plan and medicines set up in advance of the pain. Hydroxyurea is a medicine that is scientifically proven to reduce frequency and duration of pain crises by 50% in sickle cell patients. It also reduces the death rate significantly from SCD as well as reducing many long-term complications. All patients with SS type SCD should take this medicine daily. A nutritional supplement called L-Glutamine can also reduce SCD pain crises.

The Future *The outlook for SCD is increasingly hopeful. Regular management of complications, stress reduction, Hydroxyurea and now L-glutamine can make a significant impact in the day-to-day quality of life of SCD patients. Bone marrow transplantation offers the possibility of cure of SCD, though this cannot be done in all patients because of lack of suitable donors. Perhaps even more importantly, the*

PAIN IN CHILDREN AND YOUNG ADULTS

long awaited promise of gene therapy is finally about to be realized. Gene therapy means that bone marrow cells from patients with SCD can have their gene defect corrected in the laboratory, and the 'corrected marrow' is given back to the patient. The first sickle cell patient received this novel therapy in late 2014 and this experimental therapy is now open to new patients.

All individuals with SCD should be seen regularly by health care providers with special expertise in SCD to help them manage their disease and to keep them up to date on the latest developments. SCD is rare, and most physicians, including hematologists, have not managed many SCD patients so it can It can be hard to find individuals with significant experience. However, it is important for each affected individual to find a sickle cell center of excellence. The rarity of the disorder makes is especially important for all people with SCD to learn about the disorder and its management.

Patients and Parents Speak

Dr. Coates and I have had the pleasure of knowing Brianna, a lovely and bright young woman who is now 19 years of age and has SCD.

Brianna tells her story with recommendations for teens with SCD on how to get the best care.

My memories as a young child revolved around pain in my legs and the hospital. The pain was so intense it felt like a million knives and needles stabbing and pricking my legs twenty-four hours a day. Just to have a sheet, blanket, or even clothes touching my legs would make it worse. Once I hit middle school, it had gotten so bad that it affected my ability to walk; and I was ordered a walker. Going up stairs was impossible, and I would fall down while trying to walk from class to class. My mother and I were looking for answers from our healthcare team, but all they offered us was more pain medications at higher and higher doses. Eventually, we received a home healthcare nurse who gave me high doses of narcotics since the school nurse was not comfortable giving me those medications, especially at such high doses. After a while, the doctors began telling me that I would just have to "deal with the pain" and that they had exhausted all options and didn't know what to do anymore. At that point, I started to agree with them. This would just be something I would have to deal with and there was nothing anyone could do about it.

My major frustrations really centered on the doctors. Most people go to the doctor for help when they are sick and expect that their 10 years of medical school will allow them to fix the problem. Yet, for me, I was told 'I was faking' or that I would just have to deal with it. Mom throughout the whole time never gave up and I appreciated her words of encouragement, but at the same time I was getting tired. I didn't really want

DISEASES ASSOCIATED WITH CHRONIC PAIN (A)

to keep going to all these doctors and not see any type of results. Each doctor we saw who didn't know what to do, or told me I was faking, added a layer of depression and frustration with the entire healthcare system.

Then, one day, mom stumbled across this book for parents with children with chronic pain written by Dr. Lonnie Zeltzer. After she finished reading the book, she decided to email her and see if we could possibly get a consult. By some form of grace, she replied pretty quickly and was willing to see us. Mom said we were going to see this new doctor that may be able to help; I'll admit I was skeptical. If every single doctor we had seen in the past couldn't help us, then how could she? But, I still had some hope left inside and was willing to give it a try. I was surprised that after I told her exactly what I was feeling, she told us that she knew what was wrong and could actually fix it! With a little work and different types of therapy we were able to get my chronic pain under control. I went on and finished middle school, high school, and even ran track for about two years.

My advice to teens and young adults with Sickle Cell Disease: Never give up and never stop trying to find answers. There is always an answer. You just have to figure out the pieces that put it all together. There will be times you want to stop looking, and you may even feel hopeless, but if you keep pushing forward things will get better.

Brianna's mother also talks about a mother's journey in this process with advice to other mothers of children with SCD.

What were the major pain challenges for Brianna?

Brianna was born prematurely at 26 weeks weighing 1 pound 8-1/2 ounces and later diagnosed with sickle cell anemia. The combination caused significant issues with her lungs and extremities that kept her in and out of the hospital and ICU on ventilators, antibiotics and central lines and at 14 months of age, in organ failure with double lobe RSV pneumonia and acute chest syndrome. My marriage suffered under the pressure; I eventually joined the ranks of single parenthood. I was on a first name basis with the hospital staff and our pediatrician's number was on speed dial.

What were your major frustrations in that journey…with healthcare docs and nurses?

In order to manage her raging sickle cell disease and prevent any further damage to her lungs, she received monthly blood transfusions to suppress her bone marrow and "turn off her disease" for several years. We decided to wean her off transfusions, understanding that her disease would return but the attempt backfired and landed her in the hospital three times in two months with pain and viral infection.

On the 3rd admission, nurses and doctors said, "the patient could be seen laughing at the nurses' station and did not appear to be in any pain until her parent called to check on her." The attending physician, clearly frustrated after attempting to manage her symptoms, told me he felt that I was causing the problem. Several attempts at a diagnosis of neuropathic pain, chronic pain, Complex Regional Pain Syndrome were made as her condition continued to deteriorate to the point of needing a wheelchair off and on for several years. By this time her pain was running the entire household and it was definitely in charge. Whenever something as light as a sheet was placed on her legs, she would end up screaming and writhing in agony, her pain unresponsive to high doses of narcotics. When I looked at my daughter all I saw was her disease; I could not see her anymore.

Brianna's pain controlled every aspect of our lives, it decided when it wanted to come and go. It was a constant companion; it existed, and so did we. Every decision I made afterward caused me to question if I was doing the right thing. I had no idea; my compass had been broken.

For two years I drove her four hours' round trip every three months to see a doctor who helped both of us develop our coping muscles and introduced us to non-opioid type medications. He mentioned Dr. Zeltzer during one office visit and suggested that Brianna would benefit from seeing her due to her work with alternative therapies in conjunction with traditional medicine. I wrote her an extensive email and received a response from her and by the time we actually met, it felt like we had been around the world.

I remember the day she walked into the exam room. She was a tiny woman who exuded what I can only describe as a serene and calm demeanor. Immediately I felt a sensation of a heavy weight being lifted off my own shoulders after she said she knew what my daughter's problem was and that she could help. She saved my daughter and saved me too.

Mom's advice for parents of children with Sickle Cell Disease:

First, be open-minded. Second, "begin with the end in mind" to ensure the best outcomes for your child. What do you see your child doing in 20 years? What kind of life do you see your child having? College, career, and family? Visualize what you want for your child, figure out what you are going to need to make it happen, work backwards from there and create a plan by setting concrete goals with your team. Pull in all the resources you can to assist and support you. Anything not in alignment with the ultimate goal goes by the wayside.

Believe that you are an integral part of your child's healthcare team and you and your child's voice should always be clearly heard. You should never be made to question your instincts. Trust them. You aren't crazy.

DISEASES ASSOCIATED WITH CHRONIC PAIN (A)

We asked Tiffany, age 25 years, with SS disease to comment for the book.

There's entirely too much I want to say. I have faced issues with not only being an adult with this disease, but also there are issues with being seen by pediatrics.

My advice to parents you know your child and or children best. Don't ever let anyone tell you or them you're wrong. If that means you have to pick up a cell phone and page your doctors yourself, do what it takes for your voice to be heard. I am now recording everything. I have been treated very inappropriately, and to protect myself I am now documenting everything.

To the patients if you don't take anything else away from this I hope you take this. Do not let anyone tell you who you are. Never doubt yourself. You know your body, and you know what works best for you. Be open to suggestions, but don't let anyone talk down to you.

I hope together we can start making changes in the minds of doctors and nurses, but we have to do it together. It's really difficult to be positive. I was extremely disrespected to the point where I felt like I didn't mean anything to those people. No one should go through that ever. And I will not tolerate it ever again.

My advice to parents is that you know your child best. Don't ever let anyone tell you that you're wrong. If that means you have to pick up a cell phone and page your doctors yourself, do what it takes for your voice to be heard.

*My advice to the patients, if you don't take anything else away from this I hope you take this. Do not let anyone tell you who you are. Never doubt yourself. You know your body, and you know what works best for you. **If that means you have to pick up a cell phone and page your doctors yourself, do what it takes for your voice to be heard.** Be open to suggestions, but don't let anyone talk down to you.*

I hope together we can start making changes in the minds of doctors and nurses, but we have to do it together. Best Wishes Tiffany

Her mother commented below:

My name is Lavender and I'm a mother of two: "T" age 25 and "D" age 15;

They both suffer from Sickle Cell Disease. Our family has experience with both the Adult and Pediatric sides of the medical care needed for Sickle cell patients. The challenges that we've had to face were truly unbelievable. From being turned away from hospitals to being labeled as a "drug seeker". The sad reality is that ignorance still exists.

Pain management for Sickle Cell patients is a challenge that needs to be evaluated, educated and changed. The transition from pediatric care to adult care is shocking and overwhelming. The pediatric care is filled with education, compassion and respect. The adult care severely lacks knowledge, compassion and respect for the adult patients. Despite the adult patient life experience with this chronic debilitating illness, physicians continue to ignore, label, stereotype and disrespect patients' concerns about medical care.

To all the individuals that are open minded to CHANGE, may I suggest to the Sickle Cell community: create a binder with your current medical information. Include your Hematologist contact information, latest test, latest lab results and any medication you are currently taking. It's very important to have/or know your history and that it be available during an Emergency Room visit. Most of all, INSIST that the Emergency Room contact your physician that is currently caring for you.

To the Physicians caring for Sickle Cell Patients:

Please listen to the patient and don't dismiss what they are saying. Sickle Cell is not an "all in one" disease; it has to be treated individually. What's good for one patient may not work for another. Contact the treating Hematologist or their Pain Management Specialist. Most of all consider the discomfort, frustration and pain that Sickle Cell patients feel.

My continued Prayers for a cure and change with the care for Sickle Cell Patients. Lavender

Late Breaking news note

Because of patients like Brianna, Dr. Coates launched a research program with several other specialists, including myself (LZ), to understand the relationships between pain and reduced blood flow in sickle cell disease, with the goal of preventing pain crises before they begin. The research team is examining ways to identify those individuals, whose nervous system is more biologically reactive to stress and to pain, resulting in more frequent and severe episodes of vaso-occlusive pain crises. This research is examining mechanisms for how this stress-pain-reduced blood flow link happens and ways to alter the pathways leading to pain crises in these individuals. Other research efforts, led by Dr. Donald Kohn at UCLA, are studying gene therapy with attempts at curing sickle cell disease. Unfortunately, there are still many doctors who believe that patients with sickle cell disease are "drug-seeking" when rather they are seeking help for pain crises that have not been adequately treated. It is hoped that the future will bring better pain care for these individuals and better understanding of the disease to be able to prevent pain and ultimately find a cure.

DISEASES ASSOCIATED WITH CHRONIC PAIN (A)

CANCER PAIN, BONE MARROW TRANSPLANTATION (BMT) & OTHER CANCER CONDITIONS

> *I thought pain was part of having cancer... I had to get through it. Now I know you don't have to just get through it; I don't have to be a macho man. I have cancer and I deserve not to be in pain...It was nice to just lie in bed with my mucositis pain, not having to talk, but knowing that I wasn't alone; my family and friends in the room got me through the hardest times.*
>
> *M.B., a 16-year-old adolescent with leukemia, reflected on his journey through chemotherapy and bone marrow transplantation.*

Most children with cancer do not have ongoing chronic pain. However, certain situations related to disease and treatment can be associated with pain; the most common causes relate to procedures. Pain can be associated with needles for blood tests, IV placement, lumbar punctures, injections, and other distressing procedures, such as nasogastric tube placement through the nose (Table 6.1).

Table 6.1   Strategies to Reduce Pain & Distress with Procedures
1   Topical patches/ creams applied to skin to numb area for appropriate time before the procedure or needle stick (e.g. topical lidocaine)
2   Minimize number of times the child must be poked; cluster lab tests together;
3   Take medications by mouth as much as possible
4   Use breathing, distraction, guided-imagery or hypnosis techniques during procedures
5   Group time periods when child needs to be sedated to do more than one test.
6   Light sedation (such as nitrous oxide or midazolam (Versed) during procedures,
7   Invasive procedures (bone marrow biopsies) require deeper sedation/anesthesia using propofol plus lidocaine analgesia under anesthesiologist-monitored conditions
8   Preparing for the procedure in advance, often with the help of a child life specialist

Bone marrow/ Stem cell transplantation (BMT)

BMT has its own set of unique pains

Mucositis: Chemotherapy and radiation cause irritation of cells lining the digestive tract (mucositis); this includes areas from the mouth down to the rectum.

PAIN IN CHILDREN AND YOUNG ADULTS

Mucositis is a typically expected pain problem that occurs after BMT and lasts 10-14 days.

Mucositis also is a common side effect of chemotherapies including methotrexate and Adriamycin. It can make eating and swallowing difficult, cause abdominal pain and difficulty with passing a bowel movement, or even cause painful urination, another organ lined with mucosa. Treatments for mucositis pain include the following:

- *Continuous* (a "drip" or around-the-clock) opioid pain medication during periods of severe irritation (rather than on an "as needed" basis)

- Topical numbing medications before taking oral medications or eating

- Extra pain medication immediately before taking oral medications or eating

- Distraction and other psychological therapies, such as breathing techniques and imagery can also be helpful

Radiation therapy (XRT) can be part of the conditioning for BMT

XRT uses high-energy rays that cause heat and swelling (inflammation) in the mouth, throat or intestines. Sometimes chest or other area XRT can cause skin irritation and pain. Local anesthetics like lidocaine syrup, "gut rest" (no food by mouth with nutrition through IVs), and topical creams and anesthetics can be helpful. Also, as with all pain, psychological and behavioral strategies can alter suffering associated with the pain as well as reducing the pain itself.

Post-operative pain

Post-surgical pain is acute pain that occurs after surgery or tumor removal or other treatment-related reasons. Good post-operative pain management is imperative to reduce the risk for continued chronic pain. Strategies for post-operative pain management include (See also Table 6.1):

- Continuous opioid or non-opioid pain medication (i.e. a "drip" or around the clock) for a period of time after the surgery (e.g. 1-2 days) rather than "as needed" dosing

- long acting numbing agents at the end of the surgical procedure

- Acetaminophen around the clock, as a way to decrease opiate use

- Psychological, behavioral, complementary (e.g. massage, hypnotherapy, acupuncture, music) therapies

DISEASES ASSOCIATED WITH CHRONIC PAIN (A)

Bone pain

Bone pain can be related to bone marrow infiltration with tumor cells (e.g. leukemia or lymphoma), or with bone cancers, such as osteogenic sarcoma, Ewing's sarcoma, or in metastatic disease with spread of cancer into the bones. Treatment is typically with long-acting opioids, with short-acting opioids for "breakthrough" pain to avoid pain spikes. If there are nerve impingements by tumors, then treatment aimed at neuropathic pain will be a useful addition. With osteoporosis (thinning of the insides of the bones), medications aimed at osteoporosis as well as vitamin D and calcitonin can be helpful.

Hospital Resources for Pain Management in Cancer

For any type of cancer-related pain, there should be effective treatments and, as parents, you can and should be advocates for applying optimal pain relief for your child.

- Ask if there is a pain management or palliative care service in the hospital to help your child's primary team with other pain treatment ideas if your oncology team is doing its best, but your child is still suffering.

- Remember that during hospitalizations, your physical presence with your child is invaluable as a support, distractor, and guide.

- Provide opportunities for your child to discuss fears, distress, and anger.

- Help your child cope with distractions, stories, interactive games, as well as massage. These are all helpful for your child to get through this experience.

- If social work support is available to you, take advantage of this opportunity.

- If child life specialists and child psychologists are available for your child, take advantage of those supportive staff as well.

- For your child's sake, it is important that you also take care of yourself and muster the support of family and friends as best as possible.

(See chapter by Michaela Nalamliang, nurse practitioner and clinical coordinator of the Mattel Children's Hospital UCLA's pain and palliative care program[6]

Dr. Jacqueline Casillas[31] provides some guidance for parents in this process. Her bottom line: For your child's sake, **it is important that you also take care of yourself and muster the support of family and friends as best as possible.**

---

31 Dr. Jacqueline Casillas, Associate Professor of Pediatrics, UCLA, Pediatric Hematologist-Oncologist, Associate director of the UCLA-LIVESTRONG™ Survivorship Center of Excellence www.cancer.ucla.edu/Index.aspx?page=384

PAIN IN CHILDREN AND YOUNG ADULTS

Most children being treated for cancer have not been seriously ill prior to their diagnosis, and so have not had the experience of chronic, recurrent, or acute pain episodes from multiple needle sticks in a short of time period. Nor have they had the experience of large teams of doctors and nurses coming into a room to care for them. This results in additional stress as children have mainly experienced doctors' visits as well-child checks with brief pain associated with immunizations or minor injuries. So when a child is diagnosed with cancer, she can become anxious, fearful and overwhelmed due to the fast pace of painful procedures including multiple blood sticks, sedation for scans and procedures and surgical management.

The child is not psychologically prepared to cope with the invasive nature of treatment for a life threatening pediatric cancer diagnosis. In addition, the pain experienced with the first medical procedure at the time of diagnosis sets the expectations of pain to be experienced by the child for all future procedures. ***If the pain is not well managed initially for the child, there can be post-traumatic stress symptoms (PTSD) experienced by the child due to memory recall of invasive procedures during treatment.*** *These painful memories continue beyond the treatment into the survivorship period.*[7]

What can you do to support your child to minimize the traumatic experiences associated with both the acute and chronic pain they may experience during their cancer journey?

Keep A Journal That Records The Pain Experience - What Helps… And What Hurts: (see Chapter 10). *If putting a numbing cream on the skin prior to starting an IV helped to minimize the pain for your child, make sure the nurses are aware of this so they can plan ahead to get the order for the anesthetic cream and to place it 20 minutes prior to the needle stick.*

If there have been times when your child is going to have a procedure (e.g. a CT scan) with sedation or he needs to have his central line (i.e. Port-A-Cath) accessed, which can be traumatic, ask the anesthesia team who will be completing the sedation for the scan if they can access the port when the child is being put to sleep. ***Being proactive with your healthcare team about the specific needs for your child will provide better care for him/ her.***

Discuss *with your oncology team what will be expected for the diagnostic and treatment plans and how this accords with the developmental level of your child. For the school aged child or adolescent, pain assessment and plans for management of upcoming painful procedures should occur early on, where there is family support in a non-threatening environment. But, if the child is in the ER and will be admitted for ongoing care, the family can ask for a nurse from the oncology floor who is a favorite for the child to come to the ER to access the line, if this results in less trauma/pain for*

DISEASES ASSOCIATED WITH CHRONIC PAIN (A)

the child. Child Life Services serve as another resource to help provide personalized, targeted developmental support for painful procedures and treatment regimens.

Child Life Services can also advocate and interface with the treating team to explain methods that should be used to minimize pain (for example, clear descriptions of what will be occurring prior to the procedure will help a pre-teen be less anxious going into the procedure, or obtaining and listening to music via headphones for the adolescent can also help calm them).

Self-Care for the Caregiver– *Given the key role that parents and family play in the care of the child going through cancer treatment, it is critical to recognize that there are other factors that impact pain perception. Parental fear or anxiety or tiredness, also impact the pain experience for the child cancer patient. The cancer care journey is very long and often has bursts of intensities of treatment, whether it be prolonged hospitalizations or lengthy recovery time from procedures such as surgery or bone marrow transplantation.*

*During this time, the parent may not be able to get restful, restorative sleep if they are in the hospital for days or weeks. There may be other caregiver demands like children at home; or commuting at a distance from the treatment center. This can all result in mental exhaustion and fatigue. However, a parent who is able to get rest and take care of his/her own health will be that much stronger caring for their child. **So, take others up on the offers given by family and friends so you can get a night's sleep away from the hospital.** When someone else takes a "shift" with the child in hospital, it allows the parent to step away for a period of time. In this way parents can maintain better physical and mental health. Then you will be in the best possible state to alleviate anxiety and fear for your child as he/ she goes through treatment.*

In the next chapter, 7, we will discuss how pain can become persistent in select groups of children because of electrical circuit issues.

CHAPTER 7

DISEASES ASSOCIATED WITH CHRONIC PAIN:
AUTISM, COMMUNICATION RELATED DISORDERS, CEREBRAL PALSY & RARE CONDITIONS

AUTISM, AUTISM SPECTRUM DISORDERS AND PAIN

- Expert and parent commentary

CEREBRAL PALSY (CP), DEVELOPMENTAL AND COMMUNICATION DISORDERS

RARE CONDITIONS

- Ehlers-Danlos Syndrome
- Syringomyelia/Chiari Malformation
- Fabry Disease

In this chapter, we review how and why pain is such a perplexing problem with children having features of the Autism Spectrum. The amount and frequency of pain that a child experiences with them varies. Some have little, while other children have significant distress. The differences relate to the extent and type of disease, ease of controlling the underlying disease-related factors causing pain, and whether there are other contributors such as anxiety, learning disabilities, developmental factors, depression, and coping issues that increase or decrease the pain signals.

You will see how this works in the cases that follow.

AUTISM AND PAIN

Autism spectrum disorder (ASD) is a (neuro)-developmental condition with varying degrees of problems in communication and social interaction. That is, there is a "spectrum" of severity of symptoms. Some children have high levels of communication but minimal *empathy* (being able to understand, appreciate what another person is feeling) and difficulty with social connectedness. They may have more difficulty "reading" non-verbal cues from others and may be seen by peers as "odd, nerdy, and different." However, peer relationships can evolve around common interests, such as with computer games. Children with ASD have broad levels of intelligence despite communication and social difficulties. They can be extremely smart, with special expertise in focused interest areas, or their intelligence may vary.

Children with ASD often have habits that constitute obsessive-compulsive behaviors with repetitive movements or perseverative needs and wants. **In relation to pain, their perseveration may focus narrowly on the pain, such as with a headache or stomachache in ways that make distraction and other coping strategies very difficult.** Because of communication difficulties, some children with ASD appear to be oblivious to pain. But, in fact, they may be expressing pain in non-traditional ways such as head banging or other self-injurious behaviors. Often, the behaviors are treated without determining their underlying reasons, such as anxiety and/or pain.

> *Arnie, a 10 year-old with ASD, kept banging on his chest and hitting his chin. It was thought, after consultation with the Autism Think Tank NJ that he might be suffering from gastroesophageal acid reflux (GERD).), He was placed on a three-month trial of a proton-pump inhibitor (to reduce acid in his stomach); the behaviors went away.* **(www.autismthinktanknj.com)**

Experts and parents give advice

Dr. Ricki Robinson[32], a national expert in childhood autism, discusses her views on ASD.

> *What Is Autism? Autism is a developmental disorder that affects a child's ability to communicate and relate. No longer considered rare, recent studies show that 1 of every 68 children in the US is living with autism. While no two children with autism have the exact same symptoms, they do have several features in common that include:*

---

32 Dr. Ricki Robinson, a Los Angeles pediatrician and well-known expert in childhood autism, *Autism Solutions: How To Create a Healthy And Meaningful Life For Your Child* Ricki G. Robinson, M.D., M.P.H. www.amazon.com/Autism-Solutions-Create-Healthy-Meaningful/dp/0373892098 www.drrickirobinson.com/index.html

DISEASES ASSOCIATED WITH CHRONIC PAIN (B)

- Delay in understanding (receptive) and use (expressive – gestural/ spoken) of language,
- Difficulty with social interactions,
- Resistance to change and repetitive behaviors,
- Unusual responses to sensory input (sound, touch, pain) frequently associated with overly dramatic body movements or behaviors

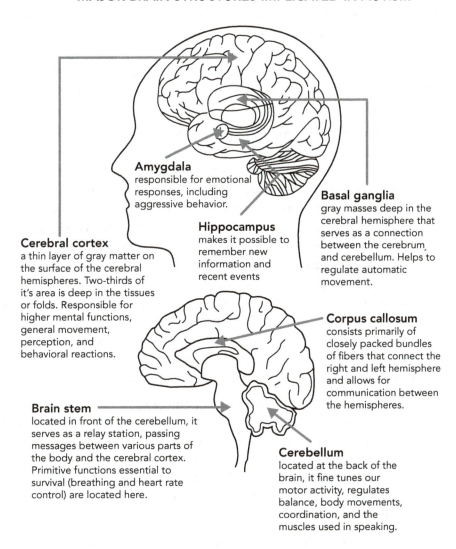

Figure 7.1. *Major Brain Structures Implicated in Autism.*

The degree of challenge in each symptom category can vary from mild to severe, with the variation in symptoms leading to the overarching diagnostic term, Autism Spectrum Disorders (ASDs). While all the causes of ASD have not been identified, research suggests that each affected child may have a genetic predisposition initiated through environmental exposures. This gene/environment interplay influences a child's developing brain by producing less nerve cell-to-nerve cell (neuron) transmission of information. The "under-connectivity" in key brain areas then results in the child's difficulty in processing sensory information (including pain), learning, communicating and relating as well as producing some of the typical behaviors seen in ASD. See figure above.

Anxiety In Autism *Anxiety affects over 80% of children and adolescents with ASD; they demonstrate anxiety or nervousness in many of the same situations as typical children. Children with ASD especially experience generalized "free floating" anxiety (everyday worry associated with tension, irritability, sleeping difficulties and stomachaches), separation anxiety (leads to dependence on adults) and social phobias (leads to social isolation and few peer friendships).*

If your child suffers from anxiety, he may experience strong internal sensations of tension that include a racing heart, breathing quickly, muscle tensions, sweating and stomachaches. The difference for a child with ASD compared with their counterparts is that the intensity of these symptoms is present throughout the day at greater levels and at much greater intensity for longer periods of time than for typical children. When a sensory stimulus is given to children with ASD, their responses are greater than typical children and it takes them up to 20 times longer to return to their baseline. Thus, it stands to reason that children with ASD are experiencing stressful body changes throughout the day. This may be due to the under-connectivity in the areas of the brain (amygdala, hippocampus) where we understand and react to stressful situations based on previous experiences. Children with ASD have great difficulty learning from sensory experiences - both those coming from the environment and from their own bodies. For example, routine situations for a typical child such as the fire alarm test in school can be overwhelming, painful and frightening for a child with ASD.

Pain Perception Is Unusual In ASD *Children may be under-responsive to pain and not realize, for example, that they have been burned when touching a boiling pot on the stove. A child who is over-responsive may find a simple soft touch extremely painful and upsetting. The same is true for pain originating within the body. Since many children with ASD don't comprehend the signals from within their body, this poor body comprehension may make it difficult for them to localize the site of pain or what the sensation even means.*

Children With ASD May Not Understand Environmental Or Body Cues *We all take in environmental cues through our sensory systems, both external (e.g. sight,*

DISEASES ASSOCIATED WITH CHRONIC PAIN (B)

sound, touch, taste, smell), and internal (e.g. balance, pain, body regulation –e.g., sleep, hunger). From this we learn about our bodies and our world. Experiences, paired with shared meaning, gives us the framework to respond appropriately, enter into relationships and to think and be creative. Children with ASD, however, may not understand their environmental or body cues as might be expected, and therefore their responses can be unusual… and definitely not as expected. I often feel that most children with ASD are doing whatever it takes to get through a day in an environment that is extremely frightening and anxiety-provoking for them. Not only are they living in this frightening world but they are often aware that they're not interpreting their surroundings like other peers or siblings. This heightens their anxiety even further.

The individual learning profiles of these children are often characterized by uneven and poor comprehension of what people say, with delays in processing that information. Weak visual-spatial processing and/or poor motor planning further exacerbates their processing and comprehension challenges. If a child falls apart, it may be that he is scared, worried or in pain, or because he realizes his body doesn't respond as he would like it to. A child with ASD is likely to have increased anxiety when he has an idea but he can't convey or act upon it.

Given the sensory challenges that children with ASD experience, it is not surprising that their inner world is often confusing, frightening and painful. Without a means of clear communication, they have limited ability to influence what is happening to them. This lack of control further adds to their anxiety and the "fight or flight" response, that we all understand in anxious and frightening situations. Your child's behaviors in these situations are likely described as "just part of his "autism" or "difficult behavior". However, these behaviors are predictable by knowing your child's individual profile of sensory and motor challenges. If, for example, he is over-responsive to sensory input, he may become aggressive, explosive and/or increase his repetitive behaviors. If your child is under-responsive, he may become more self-absorbed or run away (even bolt) from the situation. The same is true when your child is experiencing painful body sensations. For example, children with ASD experiencing ear infections or gastrointestinal symptoms such as stomach acid reflux or constipation may be irritable, aggressive and even, if the pain is extreme, self-injurious - which may resolve when the medical concern is treated. During these highly anxious/painful times, even if your child has communication abilities, he may be unable to access his language as he becomes more and more upset - especially as the situation escalates for him. Reducing anxiety and relieving pain can significantly improve your child's wellbeing. When the debilitating symptom and underlying causes are treated, progress can resume.

What Can You Do to Help? *If you are a parent of a child with ASD it is important to consider your child's behavior as his means of communicating. This is especially true*

PAIN IN CHILDREN AND YOUNG ADULTS

if there is an escalation of his typical behaviors, in which case he may be experiencing increasing anxiety/pain issues. Determining the source of his changed behavior generally takes much thought, and may take the help of your treatment team members and especially your doctor if you suspect medical issues play a role. If you suspect your child is experiencing anxiety/pain:

1 *Recognize his individual pattern of responses in these situations (they often repeat under these circumstances and can be an identifiable "signal" for you).*

2 *Examine and control your responses to his behavioral pattern - during these highly upsetting times parents, caregivers, treatment team members can "add fuel to the fire", escalating your child's anxiety.*

3 *Determine the cause (such as medical, environmental changes, or undiagnosed processing difficulties that may be adding to his confusion).*

4 *Help your child understand what is happening, and assure him as best you can (using nonverbal as well as verbal communication) that you and the team will try to help him feel better.*

5 *Treat or eliminate specific problems (e.g. medical, modulating the offending environmental stimuli, decreasing the academic challenge).*

6 *Target his anxiety in the short term by using calming, interactive sensory motor techniques that you know work for your child (create a "sensory rescue kit" to keep at home, school and car to be available when needed).*

7 *Help your child in the long term by solidifying his developmental capacities that support comprehension and help him achieve mastery of his world - this can eventually decrease his fears, help to normalize his responses and allow him to be more comfortable and less reactive in his environment.*

When anxiety/ pain is excessive and/ or becomes chronic in nature, anti-anxiety medication may give additional support to your child (see chapter 17) - your medical team will be a useful resource.

But always remember, if your child has ASD, addressing and treating his anxiety and pain issues will not only help him feel better both in his body and mind, but will also support his developmental growth and be a step along his journey to achieving his full potential.

Paul Abend, D.O.[33] founded the Autism Think Tank NJ bringing in a group of experts on different aspects of care for a child with autism. The ATTNJ consists

---

33   Paul Abend, D.O., Clinical Assistant Professor, Department of Physical Medicine and Rehabilitation (PM&R), Kessler Institute, UMDNJ-New Jersey Medical School, Medical Director of Rehabilitation Services, Robert Wood Johnson University Hospital at Rahway. www.autismthinktank.org

DISEASES ASSOCIATED WITH CHRONIC PAIN (B)

of Drs. Tim Buie (pediatric gastroenterologist), Margaret Bauman (child neurologist), Charles Henry (child psychiatrist), Ralph Ankenmann (child psychiatrist), Raffi Tachdjian (pediatric allergist), Talin Babikian (child neuropsychologist), and Lonnie Zeltzer (Pain Medicine) . We meet as a team by webcam with the doctor and parents of a child with ASD to help with specific problems. On site a social worker harmonizes recommendations from the team and coordinator, Sheri Haiken.

Dr. Abend is the father of a son with autism. We asked him to discuss autism from the perspective a father. He does this in a frank, direct and honest way.

Autism is like no other medical disorder... there is a beginning but no end. It is totally "unpredictable." Lives are shattered and destroyed (mother's, father's, siblings, grandparents) ...Financially, physically, and mentally abused. ... drowning daily with little to no help. This rare disease many years ago has now become an epidemic in the 90's and it is more recently a pandemic (in a very short time), spiraling out of control, on track to "bankrupt" the medical system of care. Time is not a luxury for parents of medically complex autistic children.

What Were the Major Ways Your Son Was Having Pain Or Distress? *Dropping suddenly to the floor, "posturing," crying out while playing quietly, suddenly becoming "self-injurious" (biting his hand, smacking his head) and then attacking anyone that would come to his aid, striking his head against a nearby wall (breaking the sheetrock) or smacking into a TV screen or window.*

When we would drive up to his school (very strict ABA environment) where he knew intuitively they would be placing demands on him (despite being in pain), it would become stressful and/or anxious for him. He would start "tantrums" (when we left, he would be instantly calm and playful).

Various foods and medications would suddenly cause him to scream out or hurt himself (later we would find out that it was the side effects of the medication): Zantac, preparations with peppermint, Depakote, and others.

What Did You and Your Wife Do to Get Help? What Didn't Work? *Reading, Internet, Medical Conferences (we are both physicians), speak with colleagues and speak with parents. It didn't help.*

After many years of very, very "dark times," no one to turn to for help, medical staff at hospitals, horrified to see him screaming and writhing in pain on the ground, prescribed Tylenol with Codeine then OxyContin (for breakthrough) and finally the suggestion by gastrointestinal physician of trying an immunosuppressive drug (Humira) that we had said it was enough.

PAIN IN CHILDREN AND YOUNG ADULTS

Traditional medical care (e.g. gastroenterologists doing endoscopies, colonoscopies, etc.) provided limited medication with no confirmatory diagnosis (lymphoid hyperplasia, enterocolitis, aphthous ulcers, mild gastritis). Non-traditional medical care (e.g. "DAN" doctors and thousands of dollars) for treatment for "dysbiosis" (Flagyl and dietary changes, chelation for heavy metal, IV, patches, and ointments), vitamin therapy injections (B12, etc.), gluten, casein free diets.

What Worked? We found a nationally recognized pediatric gastroenterologist, Dr. Tim Buie, who specializes in autism. Over the phone, we reviewed our story, our diagnostic procedures, blood work, many consultative reports, etc. and immediately came up with a confirmatory diagnosis of gastro-intestinal reflux, brought upon by stress and medication, common in autistic children and very commonly missed by gastroenterologists on exam.

Our son was treated with a very high dose of Prevacid (proton pump inhibitor). We had to take full prescribing responsibility at the pharmacy, since then pharmacist initially would not fill the prescription. We also changed the preparation of his compounded medication (as he does not swallow pills) as well as his other medications with known gastrointestinal side effects that were missed by physicians and pharmacies.

After six long years and being thrown out of two schools and the recommendation by a well-known psychiatrist to have our son placed in an institution, his pain was essentially all but gone and he became actually more agreeable and functioned better, as did we.

What Advice Can You Give to Parents And Children With ASD? Use "tertiary medical experts" with longstanding reputations at excellent academic institutions who have published in medically credible journals and/or written textbooks. Ensure they have a very strong background in specific medical complexities of autism (50% have GI problems and 30% have seizures). Find specialists who know about hormonal imbalance-testosterone in boys and pubertal hormones in girls, since psychotic behavior and rages can occur at puberty. Use their numerous years of experience with children and their ability and willingness to think "outside the box" when necessary (every child is different). Strongly avoid charlatans "trying to profit from these times of misfortune." These families are already financially, physically, and mentally drained but still are desperate for hope and do not want to give up. The goal is to set up "collaboration of these tertiary medical experts" to ensure successful outcome.

These are the stories parents tell about their children: Unpredictability (calm and quiet, explosive and raging). Self-injurious to himself/herself (banging their hands against floors, walls, furniture, TV screen and windows, punching and biting themselves so their hands and face are bloody). Attacking anyone coming to their aid (eyes

DISEASES ASSOCIATED WITH CHRONIC PAIN (B)

wide open and crazed), staring right through you, sweating profusely, heart racing, breathing heavily, high pitched screaming, and writhing in pain on the ground, kicking, punching, biting (through the skin of themselves, their aide or family member). Broken bones (usually facial on self, family members, or aides). Abruptly stopping all behaviors (like a light switch) and returning to a sensitive calm (psychotic amnesia). Aide, family members with bite marks, bleeding, broken bones, bruises, swelling, sheetrock walls, broken glass and furniture, hair pulled out and clothes ripped). Everyone's heart racing, breathing heavy, blood pressure elevated, perspiring, exhausted and wounded, waiting anxiously for the next unpredictable "moment," always on guard, never relaxed. Wondering which episode will take their loved one or themselves to the hospital.

Autism Think Tank Of New Jersey These experiences and stories from other parents lead us to create the "Autism ThinkTank of New Jersey," with tertiary medical experts collaborating without bureaucratic politics of hospital systems. The ThinkTank has provided the light for parents after their experiences of years with minimal help and essentially no one to call. We and other parents live in a dark and horrible abyss of recurrent nightmares and helplessness, feeling the constant danger of a loved one, yourself, and others. This is the world that most of us live in and that needs to be changed.

Gastrointestinal Symptoms and Abdominal Pain in Children with Autism

The most common symptoms in children with ASD are abdominal pain and constipation. Dr. Timothy Buie is a pediatric gastroenterologist in the Harvard Ladders Program in Boston, and an expert on GI problems in children with autism and a member of the New Jersey Autism Think Tank (NJATT). Here he and Nurse Katherine Murray[34] discuss highlights some of the secrets of these GI related issues that parents should understand to be effective advocates for their child with ASD.

In Autism, behaviors, not words are the secret to understanding gastrointestinal symptoms. Children with autism often "tell" us that they are having pain or distress, but too frequently we do not understand the "language of behavior" they are speaking. We have learned that many children with autism communicate discomfort by means of their behaviors. The child may point to a spot of pain on her belly, but due to other autism-related factors, such pointing may, or may not, be reliable. However, if a child is consistently tapping on his/her chest or belly, parents and doctors should think hard about whether this is an actual expression of pain.

---

34   Timothy Buie MD, Director of Gastroenterology and Nutrition, Lurie Center for Autism at Massachusetts General Hospital for Children; Assistant Professor of Pediatrics at Harvard Medical School; and Katherine F. Murray, BSN, RN; Research Nurse, Gastroenterology and Nutrition, Massachusetts General Hospital for Children

Think about your own threshold for temper. If you have an underlying headache or pain, you are much more likely to get annoyed or angry about little things that would not usually set you off. If you see behaviors set off that way in a child who previously tolerated transitions or requests, you should think about medical factors or new anxiety that might account for change.

New behaviors and new body positions (such as twisting the neck or arching the back, contorting the face and mouth, or arms outstretched in unusual ways) may be posturing from distress. We certainly consider underlying medical factors when we see this. If a parent/caregiver sees strange behaviors, taking a video of these events to share with the healthcare provider can be very helpful to sort things out.

Eat to treat. *If we look at odd or sometimes difficult, problem behaviors as signs of pain or distress, not just unwanted behaviors, then we often find the hidden medical problem that explains the behaviors. For instance, the child may press on an area of distress or bring a parent's hand to that spot, not solely for sensory input, to use it as a tool to apply pressure when seeking relief. If one can't grab for the antacid, then eating frequently or constantly drinking cool liquids may be the only way a child can help themselves with heartburn - this is what I call "eat to treat." Some children even put ice cubes on their chest or seek ice to chew as a marker of heartburn. These actions make sense if you think about it, but initially they look strange only if you consider them as behaviors.*

Those who have little language skill often have behaviors, such as aggression, when in pain. Self-biting or other self-injury (such as head banging) is another common behavior meaning pain. There are many reasons these behaviors may occur, including anger at transition requests or frustration with attempts to communicate. But by using functional behavior evaluations we often find that there are not obvious "functions" to some behaviors. We should look hard at those unexpected or unexplained behaviors as a marker for pain. Frequent aggression or self-injury often can have a medical trigger.

Empirical treatment is one approach. *Take acid reflux or constipation for example. Not all children need testing to prove that acid reflux or constipation is a problem. The idea for the treatment comes from particular symptoms or the evaluation of behaviors. If these issues are suspected, we often suggest a trial of antacid or constipation management. This treatment can be guided by your pediatrician or family physician. We advocate that your healthcare provider chooses a regular dosing schedule as a therapeutic treatment trial and then evaluates your child for any response to that treatment. If there are improvements in target behaviors, this supports that behaviors are occurring because of the treated medical issue. A lack of response to a treatment trial does not always exclude an underlying medical condition. In that circumstance,*

DISEASES ASSOCIATED WITH CHRONIC PAIN (B)

we pursue a medical work-up in children who have suspicious symptoms or behaviors that have not been responsive to treatment trials.

We are doing better cataloging some of the behaviors that communicate pain, but many heath care workers haven't learned this language yet. Be patient and you will teach the medical community how to listen better.

Dr. Margaret Bauman[35] has extensive expertise in childhood autism and is also a member of the NJATT. She discusses the neurodevelopmental problems and communication difficulties that often get in the way of recognition of pain in children with ASD and thus effective treatment. She offers advice on managing sensory sensitivity and integration problems that these children often have as well as how to facilitate communication.

Biology of Autism Approximately 50% of ASD individuals are non-verbal or significantly hypo-verbal. Although there is an increasing effort to provide these children a "voice", it remains difficult for them to express pain and discomfort even with the use of sign language and gesture, picture communication systems (PECS), a variety of technological devices or voice output systems. Although we do not fully understand why correctly communicating or localizing discomfort is challenging, a phenomenon that can also be seen in some verbal and "high-functioning" individuals, it is likely that neurobiological inaccuracy in the processing of sensory information plays a role. Compounding this situation is the fact that it can often be very difficult for parents and caretakers to know if and how the ASD individual is experiencing pain or discomfort, given that the signs and symptoms of even fairly routine illnesses and disorders may be expressed very differently in autism as compared to neurotypical persons.

Illness and Behavior Interactions Research has documented an association between physical illness and problem behaviors in this ASD population: disorders such as constipation, allergies, and premenstrual syndrome, as well as urinary tract and ear infections are frequent. The causal relationship between behavior and physical illness has been supported by the fact that when these disorders are effectively treated, the behaviors in question improve or disappear. It has been proposed that it is not physical illness itself that results in problem behaviors but the pain and discomfort that accompanies the specific illness. Problem behaviors can include the following

- *Self-injury, pinching and aggression,*
- *Sensory seeking behaviors: pressure on the abdomen, head, or chest,*

---

35 Dr. Margaret Bauman, Clinical Child Neurologist in the Integrated Center for Child Development; Associate Professor of Anatomy and Laboratory Medicine, Boston University School of Medicine. www.iccdpartners. org/ABOUT/Staff/MargaretLBauman.html

PAIN IN CHILDREN AND YOUNG ADULTS

- *Repetitive hitting of the head or other body parts,*
- *Screaming, tantrums,*
- *Running, pacing,*
- *Gulping, facial grimacing, biting, chewing on non-edibles,*
- *Sleep disturbances.*

Any unexplained behavior or new disruptive behavior should be investigated for a possible associated underlying medical condition. Causative medical conditions may be difficult to localize and identify, especially in non-verbal or cognitively impaired individuals. Signs and symptoms usually recognized by most medical professionals or caregivers are often absent, making the search for potential causes challenging.

Common physical illnesses *These include ear infections, sinusitis, sore throat, dental pain (cavities, impacted wisdom teeth), gastrointestinal disorders (gastritis, esophagitis, ulcers, reflux, celiac disease, inflammatory bowel disease, constipation, diarrhea, Crohn's disease), urinary or bladder disorders, injuries, fractures, menstrual irregularities, allergies, and infections among others. All of these physical disorders have been associated with disruptive behaviors in individuals with developmental disabilities including ASD. Thus it is imperative that any ASD individual, whether a child or adolescent who presents with disruptive behaviors and/or new problem behaviors, should be evaluated for a potential underlying medical condition before these behaviors are assumed to be the result of emotional or psychiatric conditions.*

It is becoming increasingly apparent that ASD individuals can and often do experience added medical conditions that are often associated with problem behaviors. Often these physical illnesses have been missed or ignored due in part to difficulties in obtaining a meaningful medical history and the challenge of conducting a thorough physical examination in a non-verbal patient whose behavior may interfere with performance of a detailed assessment. However, the identification of potential physical illnesses is of critical importance; many are treatable, often resulting in reduced discomfort and improved overall health, reduced problem behaviors and better quality of life.

In spite of great progress, there still are many unknowns in how to relieve symptoms in children with Autism. We frankly don't know why one will work on some children and not on others. Here Hillary Bedell discusses her experience with one boy with ASD using Energy Therapies and CranioSacral methods.

J.R. is a ten-year-old mostly nonverbal severely Autistic boy who was referred to me because of gastrointestinal problems, including pain, constipation and self- injurious behavior that comes with the pain.

124

DISEASES ASSOCIATED WITH CHRONIC PAIN (B)

I felt the most important thing for an Autistic child would be to make him feel at ease with me. To that effect I work out of my home. The first times I saw J.R. I didn't put my massage table up. I had asked his parents what he likes before they came to see me and they said music. I brought out my guitar and put it on the living room floor. When the family came into my living room, I asked his mother to sit on the floor with J.R. and me. J and I strummed the guitar a little and he smiled lot. He made what I later learned were his happy sounds "Bah-bah-bah" I copied him and soon we were rubbing heads together and laughing. Then I asked his mother to sit back with J. between her legs. I proceeded to send energy up his legs. It made him very quiet and calm right away. After completing the energy healing I asked his parents if he would like to lie down on the couch because I wanted to do craniosacral therapy. His parents said he loves the couch. I put my hand on his neck and his sacrum and felt into the craniosacral flow.

The second time he came his parents said he was having a bad morning and was in a lot of pain. I tried the guitar and he hit it. His parents who saw how calm he got with the energy healing said, "he doesn't need the guitar he just needs you." He was pacing back and forth and hitting himself. I then asked his mother to sit on the floor with him between her legs and I gave him some energy healing. He calmed down right away. His parents were shocked. They said the pain usually lasts a very long time and never ends like that.

I used a craniosacral position called the Transverse Facial Membrane Release on his sacrum and his diaphragm because I thought it would be good for constipation. After the session he had a bowel movement. The next day his mother emailed me and wrote "Guess who had the best day?"

Energy Healing is effective on Autistic children and because they are so sensitive, they feel it immediately. I also use it to pull their energy down from their head and so they can be more in their bodies. With JR I did a lot of "clearing and filling" in his abdomen and sacrum area to help out with his constipation. When he is very agitated I put my hands on either side of his heart and send energy in and it calms him down. (If you want to try this just pretend the energy is like a hose sending water from the center of your hand into the heart.)

As JR's gastrointestinal problems improved I began using more CranioSacral therapy on him to help with his behavior. Dr. John Upledger, an Osteopath and CranioSacral pioneer, spent three years at the Center for Autism in Michigan researching CranioSacral Therapy on Autistic children. When he noticed so many of the children had Temporal lobe compression he developed a technique called the Ear Pull. (No pulling involved, CranioSacral Therapy uses only light pressure to achieve its goals, about 5 grams) When I tried this technique on JR he cried inconsolably. Then I used

PAIN IN CHILDREN AND YOUNG ADULTS

an alternate technique for Temporal Compression that uses light compression on the Mastoid Process alternating from side to side. When I do this he gets very quiet and seemingly blissful and we can stay in this position for several minutes.

I used many techniques to free up the structures of the brain and to enhance the craniosacral flow, from massaging the sutures to compressing and decompressing the sphenoid and the parietal bones. I also use a cranial lift with the tips of my fingers where the occiput meets the neck, which is very freeing on the structure and the fluid in the system.

After some time working with JR his parents wrote "we noticed a significant reduction in visceral sensitivity, less self-injurious behavior, improved relaxation and a return to his more playful self."

Pain in Cerebral Palsy (CP), developmental and communication disorders

Children with CP typically have ongoing muscle spasms that are the most common cause of their pain. They have difficulty communicating pain if their motor involvement impacts ability to speak so that others can understand them. If confined to a wheelchair they may develop backaches or other chronic pains from sitting for long periods of time. If they have tight heel cords, their gait may be further affected besides the impact of difficult voluntary motor ability; this in turn causes other muscle adjustments to complex walking patterns.

We asked William L. Oppenheim, M.D[36] and UCLA pediatric orthopedic Fellow, Jennifer J. Beck, MD, to comment on pain and its treatment in children with cerebral palsy.

Cerebral palsy (CP) is the most common cause of childhood disability affecting 3 per 1000 children in the United States. It is a group of chronic conditions caused by damage to one or more areas of the brain, with impairment in movement and muscle coordination. The damage takes place before, during, or after birth when the brain is still developing. Half of patients with CP will have other neurologic abnormalities, including sensory and cognitive impairments, seizures, balance and coordination issues, and difficulty eating, swallowing and communicating.

Spastic CP *is the most common form of CP at 80%. It is characterized by inappropriate opposing co-contractions of muscles in response to improper brain signals.*

---

36   William L. Oppenheim, MD, Margaret Holden Jones Kanaar Professor, Emeritus Chief, Pediatric Orthopedics, Director, OIC / UCLA Center for Cerebral Palsy David Geffen School of Medicine at UCLA; and b. Jennifer J Beck MD, Pediatric Orthopedic Surgery, Sports Medicine, Assistant Clinical Professor, Department of Orthopedic Surgery, Associate Director, Orthopedic Institute for Children's Center for Sports Medicine, David Geffen School of Medicine at UCLA

DISEASES ASSOCIATED WITH CHRONIC PAIN (B)

This results in a feeling of stiffness that can affect the trunk and extremities leading to contractures, joint dislocations, curvature of the spine (scoliosis), foot and other deformities. These conditions frequently interfere with the patients' quality of life by restricting mobility, interfering with sitting/positioning, and compromising the ability to perform daily activities and hygiene.

Chronic pain *It is a feature in 65% of children and adults with CP. Pain may be difficult to interpret in non-verbal children but is usually manifested by crying, grimacing, writhing, acting out, increasing tone, and difficulty in dressing. It may be overlooked in children who routinely grimace or make alarming sounds. Parents and caretakers can usually perceive changes in behavior in daily care activities, but often find that they cannot localize or quantitate the pain with any consistency. Nevertheless, caretakers and parents are in the best position to monitor children for pain as well as the response to pain treatments. Their observations should always be taken into consideration in any medical evaluation.*

Pain Assessment *In an attempt to improve pain assessment in children with CP, caretaker and patient questionnaires and other measures have been developed. These include observations such as activity level, vocal communication of pain, eye movements, facial expressions, interest in food, and the quality of social interactions. However, their interpretations leave them open to controversy causing them to be largely used in research at the present time.*

Like any painful condition, the first line of treatment depends on identifying a pain source and addressing it directly. Health care providers and surgeons, in particular, must be certain of the source of pain in children and not overlook non-orthopedic causes such as urinary tract infections, upper respiratory tract infections, gastrointestinal motility issues and GERD (gastro-esophageal reflux disease). The causes of pain in children with CP differ from that of adults with CP and commonly relate to spasticity or contractures that cause an inability to position properly, dress comfortably, or sit for an extended length of time. In addition, braces and other equipment can be ill-fitting and generate local discomfort. In teens and adults, pain is often a result of degenerative arthritis from affected joints.

Although movement of stiff joints may cause pain, lack of movement can cause skin breakdown and wounds that may be painful. Many children with cerebral palsy have less soft tissue to protect their boney areas leading to pressure pain and even progressing to skin ulcers. Careful fitting, modification and renewal of seating systems and walking aids can help prevent pressure pain and sores. Attention to nutritional requirements, possibly leading to the surgical placement of a feeding tube, may result in the child being more comfortable in general while reducing the incidence of fractures, infections, and other confounding events. Hidden fractures may disguise themselves as infection and occur due to poor bone quality and difficulty with and during positioning. These are easily overlooked or misdiagnosed unless considered during a careful examination. Seizure and spasticity control are also important in preventing fractures and other musculoskeletal injuries.

Pain Prevention *The emphasis of treatment in children is often directed toward the prevention of pain, for example by keeping the hips located and the spine straight. X-ray evidence of joint malposition does not in itself suggest a painful condition. The child and parent should be questioned about pain during every medical examination. Most minor musculoskeletal pains seem to respond well to physical therapy, occupational therapy, or serial casting. In addition, pain from spasticity can be treated with a variety of medications including Baclofen, Klonopin, Diazepam, and Botulinum toxin (Botox). Baclofen can be taken orally but is most effective when delivered directly to the spinal cord region by a subcutaneous pump and a catheter placed within the spinal canal. Chronic use of pain medication is possible but often problematic due to the development of tolerance and decrease in efficacy over time. Selective posterior rhizotomy, a neurosurgical procedure, is another popular method of ameliorating spasticity and its associated pain.*

Over time, spasticity can cause large, rigid deformities that may become true contractures. These deformities include hip dislocations, scoliosis, and knee and foot deformities. Though these are rarely painful in childhood, they can evolve to painful conditions in adulthood so they are frequently addressed surgically in childhood. When several levels such as hips, knees, and ankles are addressed in a single surgical session, it is referred to as SEML (single event multilevel) surgery. Although usually transient, pain from surgery is something children with cerebral palsy frequently encounter. A variety of anesthetic techniques are now available to make surgery more tolerable for these children. These include pain blocks, epidural anesthesia, and muscle relaxants. Pain pumps have also been useful in SEML surgery.

Summary *There are many non-operative and operative modalities available to children with CP to prevent and treat pain. While it is relatively easy to talk in general about characterizing pain in of a group of disabled patients, in practice it can be very challenging to determine the source and the solution on an individual basis. Pain prevention and treatment plans must be individually developed, ideally by a health care team specializing in CP, together with the family.*

RARE DISEASES

Here, we will discuss three rare diseases for which pain can be prominent: Ehlers-Danlos Syndrome, Chiari-Syringomyelia, and Fabry's disease. Dr. Shahram

DISEASES ASSOCIATED WITH CHRONIC PAIN (B)

Yazdani[37] gives an overview of these conditions and the problems these children may have that are associated with pain. Dr. Yazdani edited a textbook on rare diseases of childhood to inform pediatricians[38].

Ehlers-Danlos Syndrome (EDS)

Ehlers-Danlos syndrome is a rare genetic connective tissue disorder that may cause generalized or focal pain from one or several conditions such as increased joint mobility, "doughy" over-extensible and fragile skin, easy bruising, and poor wound healing.

There are 6 major classifications and two additional rare forms of this disease described in the literature. EDS is categorized based on symptoms, genetic cause and inheritance pattern. Subtypes of EDS are inherited as an "autosomal dominant" or "autosomal recessive" disorder. Autosomal dominant has the presence of one abnormal strand of DNA to cause the disease, while "autosomal recessive" diseases require two strands of the abnormal DNA to manifest. Autosomal recessive diseases typically require both parents to carry the abnormal gene and pass them onto their offspring. However, autosomal dominant diseases require only one affected parent or new (de novo) mutation to cause disease.

__Clinical Presentation__ In the classic form of EDS, patients experience fatigue, recurrent hernias, various cardiac and vascular disorders, lung disease, gastrointestinal and urinary bladder complications in addition to their joint and skin disorders. Other sub-types of EDS can additionally present with retinal detachment, dysautonomia such as postural orthostatic tachycardia syndrome (POTS), decreased muscle tone, frequent fractures, tendon rupture and recurrent dislocations.

__Diagnosis__ Individuals who are experiencing excessive joint mobility or dislocation, translucent skin with poor wound healing and unusual scars or easy bruising should discuss the possibility of this disease. Although genetic testing is available to identify most types of EDS, diagnosis of this disease is based on the clinical criteria.

Upon suspicion of EDS, referral to a geneticist is highly recommended. Furthermore, upon the identification of the disease subtype, referral and follow-up by cardiology, ophthalmology, pulmonology, and orthopedist are indicated. The overall clinical presentation of EDS may mimic other conditions such as Marfan syndrome, Larsen syndrome, osteogenesis imperfecta, or cutis laxa. Affected Individuals who plan to get

---

37 Dr. Shahram Yazdani, Clinical Professor in Pediatrics, UCLA. Pediatric expert on rare diseases,

38 *__Chronic Complex Diseases of Childhood: A Practical Guide for Clinicians__* by Shahram Yazdani ,Sean A. McGhee, E. Richard Stiehm Brown Walker Press, 2011. www.amazon.com/ Chronic-Complex-Diseases-Childhood-Clinicians/dp/1599425351

pregnant should discuss the possible complications of pregnancy with their physician. Also, those who are known carriers of EDS gene should discuss the odds of having affected children with a clinical geneticist based on the inheritance pattern of their EDS gene and their partner/donor's genetic status.

Treatment *Patients with EDS generally suffer from a variety of chronic and acute pains that may mimic fibromyalgia, various types of arthritis, or irritable bowel syndrome. Treatment of the pain component of EDS should begin with education regarding life-style changes and low impact exercises that improve muscle strength and stamina, while avoiding heavy lifting and isometric exercises that could lead to injury. Thus implementation of physical therapy by an expert therapist in collaboration with the managing physician is essential for optimal outcome. Cognitive behavioral therapy seems to be of some value in treating pain, while medications are most useful in treating the side effects of pain such as insomnia, dysautonomia, anxiety, and depression.*

Medications such as amitriptyline, duloxetine, pregabalin, and milnacipran are reported to be of benefit, as monotherapy or combination therapy in treating the pain of EDS. Generally, platelet-inhibiting analgesics such as ibuprofen and aspirin should be avoided, as they may lead to increased bruising and prolonged bleeding.

Case History *A 14-year-old teenager was seen for the complaint of shoulder and back pain after daily swimming practice. His history was significant for unusual hyper-flexibility of his joints and absence of morning stiffness, fever or other symptoms. Family history was also significant for joint hyper-flexibility in his father. Further examination indicated unusually stretchable facial skin. Genetic testing confirmed the suspicion of EDS.*

He was subsequently referred to cardiology to rule out aortic dissection and further monitoring. To treat his pain, he was advised to continue with moderate water exercises or even competition, as tolerated. He was also recommended to use rest, alternating warm-and-cold compresses, and over the counter pain reducers for mild to moderate pain. For the more severe acute pains, he was advised to use tramadol. Fortunately, he continued to have good use of all his joints with no progression to chronic pain or joint damage.

Fabry Disease

Introduction *This rare condition is characterized by pain in the hands and feet with red spots on the skin that are dilated blood vessels covered with a thick protective layer of keratin (angiokeratomas). Fabry disease is caused by the deficiency of the enzyme alpha-galactosidase A (α-gal A) one of a category of conditions known as*

DISEASES ASSOCIATED WITH CHRONIC PAIN (B)

"lysosomal storage diseases". Affected individuals are predominantly male. Although female carriers of the X chromosome mutation are typically "asymptomatic carriers", they may have manifestations of this condition too.

***Clinical Presentation** The earliest reported manifestations of Fabry disease in boys and girls have been gastrointestinal issues (age 1-4 years) followed by tingling sensation of toes and fingers/neuropathic pain (age 2-4 years). The clinical presentation can be non-specific, including decreased perspiration, heart or kidney disease, heat/cold intolerance, (eye) corneal and retinal abnormalities. The neurological manifestations of this condition include pain crises and also numbness, tingling, intermittent or constant pain in the arms and legs, gastrointestinal discomfort. These sensations can be triggered by stress, fatigue, severe exercise or heat. Other neurologic manifestations of Fabry disease typically appear during adulthood and stem from the vascular changes in the brain that lead to stroke, sudden blindness, and abnormally dilated arteries and veins (aneurism).*

***Diagnosis** Since males typically have a more pronounced presentation of this condition, symptoms and family history along with laboratory testing of the enzyme activity levels provide a more definitive result and shorter diagnostic odyssey. However, female carriers with milder symptoms typically require genetic testing. This is due to the fact that 50% of affected female carriers have normal enzyme activity levels. Prenatal and newborn screening for Fabry disease are of limited value due to poor correlation between the genetic findings and severity of the symptoms. However, such testing can prevent incorrect or delayed diagnosis of this disease.*

Patients with the suspected family history and symptoms of Fabry disease should be promptly referred to a geneticist for further testing and discussion of treatment options, if confirmed. Depending on the constellation of symptoms, other subspecialties such as, audiology, ophthalmology, cardiology, pulmonology, gastroenterology, pain-management, and child development may need to be involved. In severe instances, psychiatric support is needed to help patients and their families deal with the emotional burden of this disease.

***Treatment** Enzyme replacement therapy (ERT) should be considered in severely symptomatic cases, or when there is evidence of organ damage. Early treatment may prevent some of the manifestations of Fabry disease. Other supportive measures include blood-pressure control to protect the heart and the kidneys and to prevent stroke. Antiplatelet therapy using aspirin or dipyridamole is also used as adjunct pharmacotherapy to prevent strokes in high-risk patients.*

Neuropathic pain is a common presentation of Fabry disease that has been reported in up to 80% and 60% of affected boys and girls, respectively. Although ERT may improve neuropathic pain in the long run, it is not a cure, and patients often need to resort to preventive measures such as avoidance of heat and exhaustion. It is note-worthy that some patients with severe nerve damage may feel no pain prior to ERT, while subsequently experience pain for a short period of time due to the functional improvement of their small nerve fibers. However, in severe cases medications such as carbamazepine, gabapentin, and amitriptyline may be of benefit. In adults, use of antidepressants and anxiety reducing medications may also prove beneficial. Non-steroidal anti-inflammatory medications such as ibuprofen should be avoided due to their burden on the kidneys.

We asked "Marina", a mother of a child "J" with Fabry Disease, to reflect on her journey to find answers for successful pain treatment for her son.

My son's pain is like any long voyage: providing me with some sense of accomplishment over successfully navigating unforeseen hurdles. It has been an intense and multi-faceted trip with frustration, helplessness, guilt, and fear overwhelming me for what appeared to be an endless journey.

J's pain began when he was ten years old, but he was 15 before he was diagnosed with neuropathy, one of the cardinal symptoms of Fabry disease. I often asked myself what I missed and whether or not I asked the right questions at the doctors' offices we visited while searching for help. I got frustrated not knowing what the cause of my son's pain was, and felt helpless when I could not ease it. As he got older, and his pain intensified with greater frequency, I felt fear that he would suffer lifelong pain. Guilt was always with me when I gave him opioid painkillers, which turned him into a zombie in order to stop him from and crying and screaming. I had to hope that he would not become an addict to these powerful medications. Worse of all, I discovered that I had the first genetic mutation of Fabry's in my family and thus, have passed on this genetic disease to him.

Thanks to caring doctors, healthcare professionals, and the Fabry community, my son can live a normal life: his pediatrician, who never gave up searching; his genet-icist /Fabry specialist who understood and recognized his needs; his neurologist who accepted that he needed a pain specialist and referred him to Dr. Zeltzer; and several healthcare professionals who guided us through treatment while also steering us through the insurance maze; and the Fabry community which provided us with a wealth of information as well as moral support.

While my son's younger years were filled with uncontrollable pain, he has since learned to manage his pain by using the various techniques recommended by Dr. Zeltzer and her team. These techniques include biofeedback, visual relaxation and maintaining regular daily and bi-monthly doses of medication. Most importantly, my son can identify and recognize his own pain triggers. By learning how to avoid them, he reduces the frequency and intensity of his pain.

DISEASES ASSOCIATED WITH CHRONIC PAIN (B)

Ten years into this journey, I am very proud for what J has accomplished and how he has learned to cope with an inherited genetic disease. He is now living the typical life of a post-teenaged youth, asserting his independence from his parents while attending a University of California institution as a mathematic-computer science major.

Syringomyelia

The word Syringomyelia means "flute-like" spinal cord and refers to disorders that involve fluid-filled cavitation of the spinal cord that commonly extends through the neck and chest area. There are four anatomically distinct sub-types of Syringomyelia. This condition affects both genders equally and is found in all racial and ethnic groups. Syringomyelia is typically associated with another congenital malformation of the cranium and brain, called Chiari malformation type I. Rarely it can be caused by trauma or toxins and has been associated with increased cerebrospinal fluid within the brain and spinal cord. There is no clear consensus on the mechanism of syringomyelia formation in children.

Clinical Presentation: Syringomyelia can present with multiple neurosensory abnormalities including head and neck pain, numbness and tingling of the arms and legs, and severe pain with non-painful stimulation of the skin by light touch or wind. Headache and neck pain often resemble migraine or tension headaches. The type and severity of the pain also depends on the location of the syringomyelia and the duration of time that it has been left untreated. Individuals with syringomyelia may also develop abnormal curvature of the spine (scoliosis) over time.

Diagnosis: If this condition is suspected, a detailed history and physical along with a referral to an expert neurologist or neurosurgeon is warranted. Magnetic resonance imaging (MRI) of the entire spine is often confirmatory and can shorten the diagnostic odyssey. In cases of suspected vertebral anomaly, a plain X-ray or computed tomography (CT) of the spine is helpful. In symptomatic patients with increased pressure of the spinal fluid, or compression of the brain and spinal cord, a neurosurgeon should be consulted.

Treatment: The symptoms associated with syringomyelia are best treated medically, as surgical intervention does not significantly relieve pain, scoliosis and loss of sensitivity associated with this condition. The pain associated with syringomyelia is considered to be neuropathic pain, which classically does not respond well to pharmacologic analgesic interventions. Additionally, the low incidence of this condition has made clinical trials of pharmacologic or non-pharmacologic treatments challenging. Hence, while there is little evidence for medication efficacy, there is no evidence for non-pharmacologic treatments such as peripheral and spinal electrical stimulation in children.

PAIN IN CHILDREN AND YOUNG ADULTS

The medications that have been used with limited efficacy include opiates such as tramadol, morphine, oxycodone, dextropropoxyphene, buprenorphine, fentanyl and methadone, anticonvulsants such as carbamazepine, gabapentin, pregabalin, and topiramate, antidepressants such as amitriptyline, duloxetine, venlafaxine, and local analgesics such as lidocaine, and mexiletine.

The main focus of pain management in syringomyelia should be regaining function through targeted rehabilitation, physical-, occupational-, and speech therapy. Facilitating restful sleep through relaxation techniques, exercise, and in some cases medication is essential for successful pain management. Additionally, the psychological and socioeconomic impact of this condition should be fully addressed.

Case History: *A 19-year old college student was seen for weakness, tingling and occasional pain of his right arm and shoulder. Further examination confirmed decreased sensation, strength and tendon reflexes in the affected arm. The rest of his physical exam, including neurologic testing, was normal. Neuroimaging of the brain and spine indicated syringomyelia with no evidence of Chiari malformation. The extent of the syringomyelia correlated well with his physical exam.*

Patient was advised to receive physical therapy with poor compliance due to his busy college schedule. After two years of worsening symptoms, his physical exam and imaging plateaued. More diligent physical therapy and tincture of time seems to have reversed his symptoms to the point that he eventually regained full function of his right arm with residual numbness. Ironically, he pursued medicine and specialized in surgery.

You now know the basics. In the next section you will learn how to take defined actions to help your child feel better.

SECTION B

START TO TAKE ACTION

"If you can't go back to your mother's womb, you'd better learn to be a good fighter."[39]

—ANCHEE MIN, RED AZALEA

39 www.goodreads.com/work/quotes/89610-red-azalea

The medical practitioners limited their efforts toward ruling out plumbing issues and prescribing traditional migraine medication. Candidly it was the incredibly myopic approach to the problem by our PCP and subspecialists that we take issue with.

—'LIFE: SUBJECT TO CHANGE WITHOUT NOTICE'.
ALEX, PARENT TO MELANIE, 2013

CHAPTER 8

HOW DO I START THE PAIN TREATMENT JOURNEY?

WHERE DO I START?

WHAT DO I ASK MY PEDIATRICIAN?

- The Pediatrician's Dilemma-caring for the child in pain
- Working to identify first-line treatment before referral to a sub-specialist

HOW DO I ASSESS MY CURRENT TEAM?

- When and from whom do I ask for a 2nd opinion?
- Do I need a Pediatric Pain expert?
- How do I find a Pediatric Pain expert or treatment center?
- What questions to ask before seeking a 2nd opinion?
- What are hidden costs in getting a second opinion?

HOW DO I OBTAIN A SECOND OPINION WITHIN MY CURRENT HEALTHCARE SYSTEM?

- How do I get expert care from my prepaid health plan or HMO?
- Obtaining 2nd opinions in an HMO or Kaiser Plan?
- What if my child's physician discourages me from a 2nd opinion?

WHERE DO I START GETTING HELP FOR MY CHILD?

You have known that your child is in pain. After reading Chapters 1- 6 you are sure it isn't a trivial problem. The pain has been present for months now, is not improving, and it is affecting your child's life as well as your family's. What to do?

The professional who probably knows the most about your child and can help initially is your child's pediatrician, family practice doctor, or other Primary Care Provider (PCP) such as a nurse practitioner (NP) or physician's assistant (PA). After listening to your story and performing an appropriate physical examination and targeted tests on your child, he or she may conclude that the pain does not represent a disease and thus may start treatment before referral to a pediatric subspecialist. Such treatment may consist of any combination of physical therapy (PT), psychological intervention, dietary recommendations, sleep education, or a medication. If your child has back pain, then alternatives to carrying a heavy backpack as well as physical therapy would be prescribed. These approaches should be given about a month before assuming that they are "not working."

How do I help my child's PCP develop the best treatment plan for my child?

You now know about the different types of pain that your child might have and the different symptoms related to these pain conditions. You, together with your child, can give your child's PCP a detailed description of the pain and discomfort, and how it has affected your child's life. With this detailed information, your child's PCP can make more precise recommendations to address the problem.

It is thus up to you as the parent to be very clear on describing the problem, how long it has gone on, and why you are concerned... even your worst fears. Perhaps your parent, friend, or sibling had similar symptoms and it had a bad outcome, like cancer or other serious illness. Your physician needs to know this to put your child's treatment plan into perspective.

Be sure to ask questions if you do not understand your PCP's recommendations or do not appreciate how they will address your child's pain. *It is also fine to ask him/her for a reasonable period as to when you should notice improvement.* Remember, some physicians have different experience and comfort levels in handling chronic pain, or even recognizing it as a problem. It is also fair to ask three important questions:

1 "Have you seen this type of problem before?"

2 "What was your experience with it?"

3 "Would you be more comfortable referring my child to a specialist for this problem?"

HOW DO I START THE PAIN TREATMENT JOURNEY?

PEDIATRICIAN'S DILEMMA: CARING FOR THE CHILD IN PAIN

We asked many experienced pediatricians how they thought about chronic pain in their patients. Dr. Lorraine Stern[40] offers some commentary on her 40 years of pediatric experience (side note disclosure: PZ was Dr. Stern's resident and Dr. Stern was LZ's resident at UCLA during our pediatric training!):

The most common persistent complaints that I have had to deal with are headaches and stomach aches... not the isolated, acute bellyache or headache which lends itself to accurate diagnosis most of the time. The child who is missing many school days or frequently has to be picked up early because of pain. This is worrisome to parents and was often times frustrating to me. My first task was to take a detailed history. Some kinds of pain are worrisome: the headache that is severe upon awakening or the abdominal pain that wakes a child at night, weight loss or a slowdown in growth. These are signs that testing is imperative; there might be a serious cause. Most cases are not that clear. Abdominal pain comes and goes, sometimes after eating, sometimes with excessive gas (boys more often than girls, of course). Headaches are worse sometimes in the heat or when a child is hungry or has not been drinking enough water.

A thorough physical exam is an important step, including height, weight and blood pressure. People think that visual problems cause headaches but that is rare. What can contribute is poor body mechanics when sitting at the computer for hours on end. Constipation is a common cause of abdominal pain. Does the child eat enough fiber? The usual chicken nuggets, mac and cheese and French fries diet of the picky eater can be the culprit.

I always ask is whether there is something stressful going on – parental divorce or disagreement, a job loss, a pending move, a death, a friend moving away or bullying at school. Parents are not always forthcoming about that. Several patients with chronic pain had parents who denied problems; but when they came back a few months later the parents were separated or divorced. One of my psychologist friends said, "Feelings are more contagious than viruses." If you are having trouble at home, there is no way your child is not being affected.

One of my patients complained of joint pains severe enough that she could not sit cross legged at school. She had no signs in her blood testing of any kind of arthritic problem but she persisted in complaining. Her mother was understandably worried, when I suggested that perhaps the hostile divorce that the parents were going through might be contributing; she vehemently denied that it could be. After multiple consultations

---

40   Pediatrician Dr. Lorraine Stern, Santa Clarita, CA. http://valpeds.com

with university specialists and many more tests it was determined that this was 'psychological'. Much testing and stress could have been avoided if the possibility had been acknowledged and the child received counseling.

If the child is otherwise well, gaining weight and growing normally, I order some baseline testing that can uncover issues not obvious at first. For example, celiac disease or gluten sensitivity is more common that we used to think; and the symptoms may be vague. Some issues can be easily diagnosed: lactose intolerance needs only a milk free diet for a couple of weeks.

If simple testing and history are not revealing, and I cannot offer a solution, the next step is referral to a specialist. Depending on where you live, pediatric specialists may not be conveniently located but someone who cares for adult stomachs or headaches is not qualified to take care of children. Be sure you are referred to someone who specializes in children. When you go to a specialist, make sure that you take the relevant records with you. Any lab tests, growth charts and X-ray reports should be available to the specialist. Do not trust faxing. I always have a patient hand-carry the material even if I faxed; machines are not fool proof.

HOW DO I ASSESS MY CURRENT TEAM?

We thought long and hard about where to put this section. It could have been placed in the latter part of the book, but we decided to place it closer to the beginning, because at this point you may feel like the situation is getting out of hand. This section will help you decide if you need a second opinion, show you how to find an expert, and prepare you for the actual meeting. It will also explain how to quickly assess your current doctors for their strengths and weaknesses.

See Table 8.1 for the 'rate your current team' checklist. If the NO column has more checks than you are comfortable with (we would be concerned with four or more), then perhaps you should consider a second or even third opinion. This does not mean that you are deserting your current doctor or team. It means you are uncovering all possible avenues for healing. In this way, you'll be more prepared to make strategic choices in the treatment process.

HOW DO I START THE PAIN TREATMENT JOURNEY?

Table 8.1 Assessing My Child's Team — 12-Point Checklist		
Question:	**Yes**	**No**
1 Do I know which doctor is in charge of my child's care?		
2 Does the team communicate with me in a way that satisfies me?		
3 Do my child's doctors take time to answer all my questions?		
4 Do my child's doctors communicate well with each other, so I don't need to be the "go-between" or fill in my own gaps of understanding?		
5 Am I comfortable with and have confidence in my child's doctors?		
Diagnosis:	**Yes**	**No**
6 Have I been told the names of my child's condition and why he has the specific symptoms?		
7 How sure is the doctor of my child's diagnosis?		
8 If I ask for a second opinion, will my doctor refer or recommend me to an unbiased outside doctor?		
Treatment:	**Yes**	**No**
9 How many patients with my child's pain problem does the specialist personally treat each year?		
10 Have the reasons behind each part of the recommended treatment been explained to me to my satisfaction?		
11 Have I been informed about how to get my child functioning again, like back to school, sports, and social activities?		
12 If the doctor doesn't have answers, has he/she referred me to a clinician who can help with the treatment plan?		
13 Is my child's care being given or directed by an expert in pediatric pain management? Do we need that? Will my child's doctor discuss that question with me?		

When do I ask for a second opinion? Do I need a specialist?

Let's just say you have gone through the steps in the sections above. Your child has not improved. What are the alternatives? It is at this point that most parents might ask the PCP if it is time to see another physician, such as a pediatric specialist for the type of pain and other symptoms that your child has.

In many group pediatric or primary care practices, the clinicians may each have special strengths and training, and your child's own PCP may refer you to one with skills in behavioral medicine, tummy pains, or sports injuries. Alternatively, your child's PCP may decide that it is time to see an outside pediatric specialist, whether to a child neurologist for headaches, pediatric gastroenterologist for stomach pain or diarrhea/ constipation, or a pediatric rheumatologist, sports medicine physician, or pediatric orthopedist for a joint or bone problem. The PCP may refer your child to a psychologist for help with behavioral issues, such as school avoidance.

FINDING A PEDIATRIC PAIN EXPERT/ TREATMENT CENTER?

Resources for finding Centers

Ten years ago, it was difficult to find out who and where the experts were located. Economics and the Internet have combined to change this in the consumer's favor. How? Hospitals and experts need to pay their bills in an increasingly competitive environment. They have become "consumer friendly" and advertise in magazines and on the Internet to expand their clientele. Many helpful Internet sites contain advertising from major centers; one click and you are there! For an extensive listing of pain centers in the USA, Canada and Australia, see Appendix A. Pain Center Locator at the end of this book.

There may not be a special pediatric pain center near you and not all children with chronic pain need to be evaluated and treated at a major pediatric pain center. Seeking out such a center or being referred by your child's PCP should take place after primary and condition-specific pediatric specialty care has not resolved your child's pain problem. Some children just need an evaluation by the specialized pediatric pain center with a comprehensive report being sent back from the center to your child's PCP or specialty physician.

It is always important to ask the pediatric pain center if they would be available after the evaluation to answer questions and communicate with your child's primary care physician (PCP) and disease specialist. Some children may require ongoing pain management care from the center and some may require attending a specialized pediatric pain rehabilitation program (Chapter 13).

HOW DO I START THE PAIN TREATMENT JOURNEY?

WHAT PREPARATIONS DO I MAKE BEFORE SEEKING A SECOND OPINION?

It pays to be prepared. In chapter 10, we will describe how to get organized for getting the maximum efficiency from visits to your child's PCP and specialists, including a pediatric pain expert.

What are the hidden costs in getting a second opinion?

There may be several costs in getting a second opinion. The actual doctor's fee is only one of these. For example, a consultation at a university or large clinic might include a "facility fee." This is a charge that the Center administers to pay for their space and operating expenses; it often comes as a surprise to those seeking a consultation and so it is helpful to ask prior to the visit.

What if my physician discourages me from obtaining a second opinion?

This should not happen. You may want to consider changing physicians unless you have no alternatives.

HOW DO I GET EXPERT CARE FROM MY PREPAID HEALTH PLAN OR HEALTH MAINTENANCE ORGANIZATION (HMO)?

An HMO gives you access to certain doctors and hospitals within its network. A network is made up of providers that have agreed to lower their rates for plan members and also meet quality standards. But unlike other insurance plan types, **care is covered only if you see a provider within that HMO's network**. From our experience, few HMOs or health plans offer well-coordinated, well-supported, or high-level expertise in the treatment of complex conditions. They manage common diseases, like diabetes and heart disease, immunizations and well-child care much better than chronic pain. Frankly, they may lack the motivation to provide expertise in narrow specialty areas, such as pediatric pain that costs money and resources. However, larger healthcare HMOs, like Kaiser Permanente for example, are increasing the pediatric pain training of their interested pediatricians.

However, there are often dedicated and skilled healthcare professionals in these groups who get little attention or notice for their expertise. It is your challenge to seek them out and tell them how much you appreciate their service. How do you find them? See Table 8.2.

PAIN IN CHILDREN AND YOUNG ADULTS

Table 8.2   Finding The Right Specialist
1 Ask your child's PCP which physicians in the HMO have the most experience with children's pain/behavioral issues.
2 Ask for a specific referral.
3 After you meet with the "specialist" tell him/her why you chose him/her.
4 Ask your primary doctor to serve as Team Leader to consolidate treatment and interpret what the specialists are saying.
5 Collect, organize your child's medical information. (See Chap.9: Getting Organized)
6 Share the results of your own research with the experts. Ask them to comment on what is applicable to your child. (See Chapter 9)
For Denial of Care, ask why?
• Is the treatment's effectiveness unproven?
• Is the cost too prohibitive to be justified?
• If it is the latter, then you have a strong argument against the denial of your child's care.

Can I Obtain a Second Opinion from my HMO or Kaiser Plan?

The answer is yes... and no. Yes, because usually the plan will allow you to see another physician in the same department as your current physician. Will you get a *different* opinion? Our experience with patients who have come from these plans is that the answer is more than likely, "No." Do doctors not want to disagree? Are they succumbing to financial pressures? Are physicians of similar mind and training? Your guess is as good as ours.

In a prepaid health plan, like an HMO, the contract between you and the organization is that you will use only physicians in their "network." However, *expertise* you *need* may not be in their network. What do you do then? (See Health Care Benefits section in the contract from your HMO/Insurance Company.[8] , Table 8.3, Chapter 18)

What are your alternatives? We have had several patients who have written letters, discussed the complexity of their case with an *ombudsman* and have been persistent "squeaky wheels." They have had their plan pay for an outside consultation at a specialty center, often at a university hospital. You can use the five-point outline below for your challenge letter (Table 8.3). Your plan will not tell you this is possible, but you have nothing to lose (and everything to gain). See also Chapter 18 on handling denials of service.

144

HOW DO I START THE PAIN TREATMENT JOURNEY?

Table 8.3   5-Point Letter Challenging Denials For 2nd Opinion
1 Write a detailed letter to the highest administrative official in the network. Explain the dire straits of the situation your child faces, pain and suffering and change from normal.
2 Let the official know the urgent time frame you face. Request an answer in 7-10 days.
3 Detail reasons that you want the consultation (e.g. results of your web, newspaper or magazine research that indicates a consultation is necessary; informal consultations; that the expertise required is not available in your network).
4 Explain consequences of expertise being unavailable/ not meeting your child's needs.
5 If #1-4 is not successful, you may be better off going outside your network. Pay the cost of the consultation. Argue about it later, based on info you get from consultation.

CONCLUSIONS

No one said that this process was going to be easy. Our desire is that your efforts to get a needed second opinion are successful, and that it leads you to understanding the options with a Therapy Plan in place.

In the next chapters, you'll learn more about the following:

1 Using your skills to surf the Internet and find detailed information about your child's pain,

2 How to get organized to get the most effective care for your child,

3 The biopsychosocial model of pain: which factors can influence your child's pain?

4 The integrative model: needed components of care for childhood chronic pain.

"There is no future in dwelling on the past."

—PAUL ZELTZER, 1998

CHAPTER 9

THE WEB AND INTERNET FOR CHRONIC PAIN INFORMATION

I AM OVERWHELMED BY TOO MUCH INFORMATION

CHAT ROOMS AND GROUPS: ARE THEY HELPFUL?

EVALUATING TRUTHFULNESS OF DIFFERENT WEBSITES

FIVE QUESTIONS TO ASK ABOUT PAIN INFORMATION WEBSITES

TIP-OFFS TO RIP-OFFS

BRINGING INFORMATION BACK TO YOUR PRIMARY CARE PROVIDER

TALKING WITH MY CHILD'S DOCTOR ABOUT MY RESEARCH

PAIN IN CHILDREN AND YOUNG ADULTS

I AM OVERWHELMED BY TOO MUCH INFORMATION

Do these suggestions from relatives and friends sound familiar?

- Use only "holistic" medicine doctors
- Find an expert or major center to get your child's treatment
- Give your child St John's Wort; it "cured" my child's headache
- Fibromyalgia is a life-long condition
- There is a doctor in Texas that cures fibromyalgia
- The Jimson Pain Center has a special machine that cures headaches
- CRPS is a life-long condition
- You should bring your child to my father's anesthesiologist; he is the best pain doc in the state!

On the one hand, information is power. On the other hand, you may find yourself frozen by the overwhelming amount of medical information on the Internet. You are going to read many articles. You are going to meet people who have miracles to sell for the small price of your house or your first-born child. How do you remain sane and use what is important to answer questions about your own child's specific problem? How do you distinguish between good and bad advice? How do you manage all the information on this journey and then bring it to your doctor?

Remember, our purpose for this book is to empower and equip you with relevant, critical knowledge about options. As part of your decision-making process, many parents seek answers to important questions on the Internet, especially if they are unsuccessful in obtaining information from their child's physicians. After you find these answers, you must then resolve this next series of questions:

- How do I evaluate the information I find?
- How do I present it to my doctor?
- Will my doctor be upset with me for sharing this information and wanting to try this new treatment?

You may have some concerns about doing an Internet search. For instance, **many people are worried about offending their doctor by doing so.** To this, we respond that there is no reason to feel awkward; it does not negate your current treatment program and you can inform your doctor that you are "leaving no stone unturned." It also means that you and the "medical professionals" are starting to work as a *team*. **You are now asking your physician for help in *understanding* material, rather than blindly *following* recommendations.**

148

THE WEB AND INTERNET FOR CHRONIC PAIN INFORMATION

CHAT ROOMS AND GROUPS: ARE THEY HELPFUL?

Chat rooms allow you to communicate with people in real time, just like talking to a group of people at a party. You enter a "room" and every time you write a message, everyone in the room sees it instantly. Chatting online allows you to meet and speak with other individuals who have interests similar to yours. Below is an example of such a string:

    To find a chat room or group:

- While logged on to the web, type in your browser's URL *http://answers.yahoo.com* in the entry field. This will take you to *Yahoo!* Many people also use Google, since it is designed to give results which are prioritized on the basis of popularity.

- First click on the left-hand listing> "More" and this takes you to the "Health" site.

- Then Enter "IBS" or "chest pain" and answers may come up while you can click and see what is being discussed. *A commercial site sponsored by a medication comes up first.*

- Ideally you want sites on "IBS in children" or "chest pain in children" as examples

- Or go to "Health and Wellness" or type in your specific condition or diagnosis and see if there are groups for your condition of interest. Add the word "children" or "adolescents"

- For Google try > "Google chat group pediatric pain" and see the results.

- In using listservs, many people find that using a non-identifying "signature" is helpful to avoid having to type it each time To do this:

  - If you use Outlook, under <Tools> then <Options> then <Mail Format>, you can set up one or more signatures to include your relevant information. Many folks on the listservs can help you.

- *Remember*: People on line are often dissatisfied and may be undiagnosed. Thus you must be careful in taking advice or even believing what is said in these anonymous "rooms."

- Explore chat rooms and use them for support, advice, and coping. Be prepared for the raw stuff in the beginning. You will be exposed to many successful outcomes… and some not-so-successful ones. Many people's stories may echo similarities to your situation, but keep your focus.

- You must be wise and realize that not all the questionable or negative outcomes will happen to your child.

PAIN IN CHILDREN AND YOUNG ADULTS

Table 9.1	Chat Room & LISTSERVs & Group Sites on the WEB
Pediatric Pain Listserv	*http://neurosurgery.mgh.harvard.edu/pedi/ pedipain.htm*
Pediatric Pain Program Listings	*http://pediatric-pain.ca/ pediatric-pain-mailing-list*
Child Needle Phobia	*http://pediatric-pain.ca/for-families*
Needle pain	*http://www.ncbi.nlm.nih.gov/pmc/articles/ PMC2528903*
Brain anatomy/function for kids/ adults	*http://faculty.washington.edu/chudler/introb. html#bb*
Pain Chat	*http://www.medhelp.org/health_chats/ archive/30*

- Explore these chat rooms and use them for support, advice, and coping. Be prepared for the raw stuff in the beginning, though. You will be exposed to many successful outcomes… and some not-so-successful ones. Many people's stories may echo similarities to your situation, but keep your focus.

- You must be wise and realize that not all the questionable or negative outcomes will happen to your child.

Table 9.2	Medical Decision-making and the Internet
1	Read best approaches to your child's condition: Internet sites & written resources.
2	Friends, family, and advocates can help you to conduct Internet searches.
3	Evaluate web pages critically. Question the source. Be on the lookout for exaggerated claims and aggressive advertising.
4	Recognize the difference between commercial/ personal web pages and governmental/educational centers of excellence.
5	Get your doctor's opinion on the options that sound best to you.
6	Always ask the doctor what she or he would do in your circumstance.

EVALUATING TRUTHFULNESS OF DIFFERENT WEBSITES

There Are Two Dark Sides to The Internet in Any Chat Room:

- There is always a chance someone in the room is not telling the truth.
- Motives for what people say in the rooms may be questionable.

THE WEB AND INTERNET FOR CHRONIC PAIN INFORMATION

- It is not uncommon for someone who needs investors to try the chat rooms to drum up business. Never give out your full name, address, or phone number to someone in the chat room.

- Discuss your Internet findings with your doctor before taking action. You handle this as you would with any health information that you obtain from more traditional sources (newspapers, magazines, television, etc.).

- Once you start looking for information and open the door, you will be deluged. This wealth of information is a double-edged sword. Much of it is meant for medical professionals, some is purely subjective, a portion is unreliable; some is plain dangerous. Furthermore, reading about a therapy that was a "cure" for one person and "hazard" for another can be confusing.

If you see something interesting, discuss it on one of the lists. You may learn of new options, better treatments, and clinical trials through these chat rooms. However, just to be sure, you should discuss the advice that you obtain here with your healthcare team.

Unfortunately, there is no surefire way to control false or misleading claims on health-related Internet sites, so be cautious about using the Internet to diagnose or treat your child.

FOUR QUESTIONS TO ASK ABOUT PAIN INFORMATION WEBSITES[9]:

1 Which entity is responsible for the site?

   a Government agencies (web addresses that end with ".gov"), universities (".edu"), and reputable organizations (".org") usually contain more reliable information.

   b Is it a commercial (".com") site? Many commercial sites are hyping a product or designed to sell you something, although some commercial, pharmaceutical sites do provide useful information.

   c Try to distinguish between promotion, advertising, and serious content within any commercial site. This can be difficult as an increasing number of legitimate organizations include ads on behalf of their sponsors.

   d Remember that many sites have paid to be listed near the top of a search, so that commercial sites will be prominently placed above governmental, educational, or organizational sites.

151

PAIN IN CHILDREN AND YOUNG ADULTS

For example, on page 1 of a Yahoo! search for "child pain," there are two "sponsored" (paid) commercial sites appear at the top: Guess what they are hyping?

> *Children's Advil® Relief | Childrens.Advil.com*
> *Childrens.Advil.com/Pain*
> *Relieve Your Child's Aches & Pains With Children's*
> *Advil®. Visit Site!*
> *Children's Pain Relief www.MOTRIN.com*
> *For The Nights When It's More Than Just A Bad*
> *Dream. BE READY.*

2 What are the credentials of the individual(s) posting the information?

    a Is it posted by someone with medical expertise? Are persons with science or medical expertise consultants or advisors to the site? Are information sources listed? Is the site kept up-to-date?

    b Does the site feature outlandish claims and testimonials?

3 If a product or treatment seems too good to be true, it probably is.

4 Can you contact the site for more information?

Reputable sites provide an e-mail address for a person who is responsible for the site. The response that you receive will provide a clue as to the site's reliability.

TIP-OFFS TO RIP-OFFS

New health frauds pop up all the time, but the promoters use the same old tricks to gain your trust and get your money. According to the Food and Drug Administration, here are some red flags:

1 Claims that the product works by a secret formula. (Legitimate scientists share their knowledge so peers can review their data.)

2 Advertising for this product can only be found in the back pages of magazines, as newspaper advertisements in the format of news stories, by telemarketing or direct mail, or 30-minute "infomercials" done in talk show format. (Bona fide treatments are reported first in medical journals.)

3 Claims that the product is an amazing or miraculous breakthrough. (Real medical breakthroughs are few and far between.)

THE WEB AND INTERNET FOR CHRONIC PAIN INFORMATION

4 Promises of a quick, painless, guaranteed cure. (Anything that has the words "guarantee" or "cure" requires skepticism)

5 Testimonials from satisfied customers. (These "customers" may never have had the disease that the product is supposed to cure; they may have been paid advocates, or they may never even have existed!)

Table 9.3 Helpful Pain Websites	
American Pain Society: General Pain Information	*http://americanpainsociety.org/education/enduring-materials*
American Academy Pediatrics:	*www.aap.org /*
Society for Developmental and Behavioral Pediatrics:	*www.sdbp.org /*
Children's Cancer Pain Network:	*www.childcancerpain.org*
National Childhood Cancer Foundation	*www.nccf.org/*
Concussions	*www.aan.com/concussion www.cdc.gov/headsup* *www.neurosurgery.ucla.edu/concussion*
Client & family resources about pain, including infographics about chronic pain	*www.hollandbloorview.ca/toolbox http://hollandbloorview.ca/ClientFamilyResources/FamilyResourceCentre/MychildhasAtoZ/Pain*
Finding a Treatment Program	*www.americanpainsociety.org/uploads/pediatric_chronic_pain_clinic_list_12_2013.pdf*
General on pediatric pain:	*www.uichildrens.org/pain-control*
General on pediatric conditions:	*www.keepkidshealthy.com* *www.pediatricnetwork.org/index.htm* *www.kidshealth.org*
General on medical conditions:	*www.healingwell.com*
National Council for Headache Education	*www.achenet.org*
Meditation	*www.innerkidz.org; www.insightla.org; and www.braveheart.org*

TALKING WITH YOUR DOCTOR ABOUT YOUR RESEARCH

Gather your family, friends, and advocates to brainstorm and think critically about the sources and their authenticity. Choose the treatments that you are interested in discussing further with your child's medical team. Then ask your child's PCP or other team members what they would advise for your child's case. Together, develop an action plan. See Table 9.2.

We are all biased by our experiences, education, and cultural attitudes – doctors included. Sometimes, those biases are valuable. Other times they can be limiting. Ask.

Now it's on to the next chapter, Getting Organized, so that you will have "handles" and "drawers" for the knowledge you are gaining.

CHAPTER 10
GETTING ORGANIZED:
THE KEY TO REGAINING CONTROL

*And the day came when the risk to remain tight in a bud
was more painful than the risk it took to blossom.*

—ANAIS NIN. FRENCH-AMERICAN POET: 1903-1977

CREATING THE MEDICAL NOTEBOOK

- Materials I need to get started
- Why I need a notebook
- What I put in my notebook
- How to use my notebook
- Sample questions to ask the expert
- A Medical Dictionary

SEPARATE FILE FOR ALL MEDICAL/ INSURANCE BILLS/ CORRESPONDENCE

PLANNING NOT TO GET OVERWHELMED

155

KEY PREPARATIONS FOR GETTING HELP

It pays to be organized whether you are fixing a leaky faucet, meeting with your tax accountant, or getting your automobile's transmission repaired. The principle is the same for overcoming and getting control over any illness. ***Organization of your child's information is the key.*** Through our experience with thousands of children and families with chronic pain, and observing more successful ones, we have found three activities that are essential:

1 Creating a notebook;

2 Keeping medical-related bills and insurance papers in one place; and

3 Planning to *not* get overwhelmed.

STEP 1: CREATING YOUR MEDICAL RESOURCE NOTEBOOK

Organizing your child's medical information is the first step in regaining control of a situation that might seem out of balance right now. It may sound silly but we suggest you follow the steps in making a **medical notebook.** Later, you can decide if it was good or bad advice. Having these data at your fingertips saves significant time and aggravation, because medical records, blood tests, scans etc. are lost or not available when you most need them (like at midnight in the emergency department).

Materials you need to get started.

Obtain the following and assemble your notebook as soon as possible:

- Three-ring, loose-leaf binder
- 10 dividers, labeled as they appear in Sections 1-10 below (Table 10.1).
- Lined Notepad or loose-leaf paper, lined, three-hole-punched (for Section 6)
- Two types of plastic storage sleeves 8 ½" x 11", three-hole-punched
  - One holds business cards (baseball trading card size) with 5 x 2 = 10 slots/page.
  - These can be found in office supply or drug stores in packages of 10 (e.g., Wilson-Jones #21471 "Business Card binder pages") (Section 1)
  - The other is to hold several CD-DVD disks. (Section 4)

GETTING ORGANIZED: THE KEY TO REGAINING CONTROL

Table 10.1   Content of My Medical Notebook
Section 1. Business Cards or "Who's who?"
Section 2. My chronological summary of my child's chronic pain journey
Section 3. Blood, Urine, and Stool Tests
Section 4. Imaging: MRIs, CT/other Scans, X-ray's, Ultrasound Reports
Section 5. ECG, EEG, other tests, pathology reports, procedure reports, surgery reports
Section 6. Hospital discharge summaries, emergency department visit reports, consultation reports and follow-up notes
Section 7. Medications: A Summary of past/present meds & doses
Section 8. Questions and Answers at Doctor Visits
Section 9. Resources and References
Section 10. Calendar

Using my notebook

Section 1 – Business cards or "Who's who"?

Business cards of doctors, consultants, health professionals, social workers, insurance companies, and case managers are easy to find in the 5 x 2 plastic slots. When you meet with a new professional, write the name and contact information in this section. If you obtain a business card, place it in the sleeve or case—no more searching under couches, through drawers, and in handbags for a name or phone number. Your time is too valuable for that. Pop it in your smartphone too.

Section 2 – Chronological summary- my child's chronic pain journey

This is helpful information to send to the consultant your child will be seeing for the first time. It provides the big picture and story of your child's journey with pain. While your child's doctor will still obtain a verbal history from you and your child, having this outline will help keep dates and sequences of events clear.

Section 3 – Blood, Urine, and Stool Tests

Why are you collecting these reports? Isn't the hospital or doctor supposed to do this for you? As if you don't already know, it isn't a perfect world. Having these records immediately available saves a lot of time in delays and mix-ups caused by tests that may be done in different hospitals or laboratories. You should always ask for copies of your child's test results for your chart. Immediate access to this information within our patients' personal notebooks has spared

PAIN IN CHILDREN AND YOUNG ADULTS

countless hours of waiting to have test results faxed or emailed over and also reduces need for repeat testing when test results cannot be located. When we prescribe medications and calculate dosages for your child, especially if your child has been on medications for a long time, it is helpful to review your child's blood chemistry profiles to ensure that all organs are functioning normally and can handle the medication. Without this availability, there may be a delay while waiting to receive a FAX copy of the report from the testing laboratory. Worse yet, there may be some liver impairment from certain drugs that your child has been on for a long time without this being recognized. Clearly we would want to take your child off the offending medication and not prescribe any other medication that could affect the liver.

Section 4 – Imaging: MRIs, CT other Scans, X-ray, & Ultrasound Reports

Each time your child has an imaging study, it is helpful to obtain both printed copies of the imaging reports as well as the actual images (CD-DVD) before you leave your doctor's office or the imaging center. The CD-DVDs are inserted into plastic sleeves in this section of your notebook with the dictated reports. Most centers will provide a CD-ROM that includes a software program called eFilm™ to enable you to view images on computer with Microsoft Photoshop or similar program.

Rosa, a 15-year-old girl who played competitive softball had arm and shoulder pain and numbness that had stumped 10 doctors before us. Dad, an engineer, had the CD-ROMs in his notebook. He told us that "all the MRIs and scans" had been done. We looked at her CD-ROM and noticed that a regular chest X-ray had never been taken. We ordered a chest X-ray and made the diagnosis of congenital extra cervical rib that was compressing the nerves to her arm from the brachial plexus on the affected side. This was after she had two years of ineffective medications and interventional procedures because all the MRI's and scans had been "normal." She needed to have surgical removal of the extra rib to get relief.

- What if doctors question your record keeping? It's your right to have this information, even if a few medical personnel are skeptical about your request. Don't let any doctor, nurse, or assistant intimidate you.

- You can get these documents from the doctor who ordered the test or the radiologist who interpreted it. Your physician should not be upset by this. Speak up! Ask for your copies. Place the written reports in your notebook in the chronological order.

GETTING ORGANIZED: THE KEY TO REGAINING CONTROL

Section 5 – ECG, EEG, other tests, and pathology, procedure, and surgery reports

Many medications impact the heart's electrical activity and rhythm as identified by the electrocardiogram (e.g. prolonged "QTc"). If your child has had a fairly recent ECG, review of the QTc on the ECG would be useful to be able to prescribe that medication at the time of the visit. History of different procedures and surgeries are best reviewed with the direct reports from those events.

Section 6 – Hospital Discharge Summaries, Emergency Department Visits, Consultation Reports & Follow-Up Notes

This is where you can keep your child's time-sequenced history of hospitalizations, emergency department visits, and doctors' visits, as they occurred. You can use this section when your child meets a new physician. When we see a new patient, it may take us 5-10 minutes to review a summary like this, but it saves us hours of going through the full medical records that might be sent since there may be more information than is needed and in that pertinent information may be missing.

Section 7 – Medications: Past and present meds and doses

Knowing which medications and dosages your child is taking, and when they started or stopped, allows your doctor or future consultants to sort out any side effects your child might be having, and knowing what worked or didn't work for your child in the past. For example, you may tell us that your child had a certain medication in the past that "didn't work." Yet in reviewing this medication history, we might find that the reason that the medication "didn't work" was because the doses given were sub-therapeutic (far too low to be effective). **Know your child's medications and doses.**

> *Mark, an 11-year-old mature preteen, had chronic daily headaches for three months. His grades started to slip from all "A"s to "C"s and he could not play sports because of the headaches. During our two-hour interview we got a list of medications that had been tried. We noticed that he had developed acne at a young age and asked if he had been taking anything for it? Mark's dad volunteered that Mark had started daily minocycline that the dermatologist prescribed but could not remember how long ago. When we looked at the medication log in the medical file that they brought to the visit with them, we found that the minocycline (a tetracycline-type antibiotic) started two months before the headaches began.*
>
> *On exam when I (PZ) looked at his eyes (retina) with an ophthalmoscope, I found that he had signs of increased cerebrospinal fluid pressure in his head. We knew that tetracycline can cause increased intracranial pressure so we asked him to stop his*

10

159

PAIN IN CHILDREN AND YOUNG ADULTS

minocycline, ordered a brain imaging study to confirm our diagnosis, and gave him a medication to reduce the increased pressure. Five weeks later, the headaches went away and have not returned in two years. We were easily able to make the correct diagnosis because the family had the records at their fingertips.

See Table 10.2 in the Appendix for template charts to record medication, doses, who prescribed it.

Section 8 – Questions and Answers

This is your journal section to record *content* of medical or other healthcare visits, conferences or meetings.

1 Put a ledger pad or lined notebook paper in this section.

2 Enter questions you would like to ask your child's doctor, so you are prepared at the next opportunity. Check them off as the meeting progresses. If your doctor is irritated, it is his problem, not yours.

3 Under each question, write the answers that the doctor is giving while the conversations take place. You might have to elaborate on and complete those answers immediately following the conversation, once you have more time to sit and digest all that was exchanged.

4 You will have clear and comprehensive notes to refer to and review whenever you need them. During medical appointments, the information flows so quickly that it's hard to remember it all. You may want to tape record the meetings, if your doctor allows it.

5 It's easy to forget to ask critical questions during appointments with the doctor, particularly when you are nervous about these visits or your doctors are hurried.

Section 9 – Resources and References

On this journey to more knowledge, you will collect handouts, articles, phone numbers, websites and other useful resources. This section stores such information in one place.

Section 10 – Calendar

A small calendar in the medical notebook (not just on your smart phone) makes things technically easier. You can look back to when the last scan was done and write in when the next appointment is scheduled. It's also helpful for detailing when an insurance claim is being questioned, as companies often put the date, but not the reason for the claim. Your smartphone may also hold this information.

160

GETTING ORGANIZED: THE KEY TO REGAINING CONTROL

Okay, the hard part about organizing the notebook is over with Sections 1-10. Now on to getting this "pain thing" more under control.

STEP 2: MEDICAL DICTIONARY AND OTHER BOOKS

Christine, mother of 20-year-old Gene with pain from Fabry's disease, reminded me that a medical dictionary is a must. Dorland's is a classic. Used editions can be purchased on Amazon.com ($11-32) or go to this website *http://download.refer-enceboss.com/index.jhtml*

STEP 3: SEPARATE FILE FOR ALL MEDICAL/ INSURANCE BILLS AND CORRESPONDENCE

Dealing with the health insurance can be overwhelming. For now, file this information and you will learn more about bills, denials and appeals, and insurance later in Chapter 18: Managing Costs, Benefits and Your Healthcare with Insurance. You can use Medical Bill (See Table 10.3 in the Appendix) and Insurance Tracking Forms (Table 10.4 in Appendix) to organize what is paid or owed.

STEP 4: PLANNING *NOT* TO GET OVERWHELMED

Consider bringing someone with you to your child's initial medical appointment

You may not be able to integrate what your doctor says or remember what to ask, especially if you or your child are stressed. Also, doctors are not always aware when they use medical terms or technical language that can confuse. Your "buddy" (your child's other parent or other relative or friend) can help in several ways:

- Discuss and compare with you, after the appointment, what you heard the doctors say (and help you record good notes).
- Offer emotional support, if you need it.
- Ensure that all predetermined questions are asked…and answered to your satisfaction.
- Ask additional questions or ask for clarifications.

So I started doing a status sheet of each of Stevie's symptoms. It's still two pages long. But we cover each of the problems he is experiencing and it lets the doctors know

PAIN IN CHILDREN AND YOUNG ADULTS

everything that is happening. They kind of made fun of me at first, but now it has elim-
inated that initial visit with the nurse asking about symptoms. And it eliminates that
problem that we were experiencing where the doctor comes in the room and asks, "How
are things going?" It's sort of like having an agenda for a meeting instead of a free for
all. And the doctors now all have mentioned that they appreciate it. Marsha, Seattle, WA

Is there a Child Group or Group for Parents?

- Groups provide comfort and understanding. They are a great source of information on treatments, nutrition, costs of care, newer therapies, things your doctor
  does not tell you, etc. They help you know that you are not alone.

- Groups take many forms, from formal meetings near home to informal chats
  on the Internet.

- Many major Child Pain Centers offer group participation in yoga, discussion,
  meditation etc. Some may even have clinical trials in which your child's and
  your participation will be free.

- Ask the pain team at your nearest center what groups are organized for your
  child's type of chronic pain.

- Many local hospitals run support groups. There may even be a chronic pain
  support group for you or your child in your area.

With Internet access and an e-mail account, you can be in continual dialogue with
a community of tens to hundreds from around the world who understand what you
are experiencing with your child. (See Chapter 9)

> *Just knowing you all are out there and that you are on*
> *the other side of this fog we are walking through makes*
> *it more possible to take things one step at a time.*
>
> —JANE, MORGANTOWN, WV.

Ask About Clinical Trials

- For some types of chronic pain, there are experimental studies for new treatments
  for children and adolescents.

- Some may be complementary therapies like yoga or meditation, while others
  may be newer medications.

GETTING ORGANIZED: THE KEY TO REGAINING CONTROL

- Clinical trials are the best way for you to get the latest, state-of-the-art treatments, and typically without cost. To learn more about clinical trials, or to find one look at *www.clinicaltrials.gov*)

Take It One Day at a Time

- Think in terms of taking your own and your child's life one day at a time, until things begin to turn around.
- Don't worry about what your son or daughter will be doing next month or even next week. Okay, so your daughter is out of school, angry, isolated and seems to have "shut down." That's for now... it is not likely to be the future.
- Concentrate on what first steps your team is emphasizing now on the pathway to your child getting better.
- Take a breather and listen to what Melinda, someone who has "been there," has to say.
- Keep a journal or diary.
- Find something to rejoice and be glad about every day.

Ask Your Friends for Help

Following is advice from one dad:

> *As far as trying to manage everything: Can you ask friends to help? People want to help. I have swallowed my pride, as a single parent, and asked for help – friends pick up my other daughter from school and take her to her soccer practice when I have to go bring Julie to the gastroenterologist, the psychologist or the pain doctor; Neighbors even help out with some meals prepared for us; Try to delegate so you can stay strong! You will have your time in life to give back to those that give to you. Take care.*

—SCOTT, FATHER OF JULIE,

A 10-YEAR-OLD WITH CROHN'S DISEASE, ORANGE COUNTY, CA.

Now you know the *why* and *how* of getting organized. The next section is called *My Child Is Being Treated... But Not Getting Better.* In Chapter 11 you'll discover exactly how our own emotions and those around us can have profound effects on pain.

SECTION C

MY CHILD IS BEING TREATED... BUT NOT GETTING BETTER

I stand here naked
Looking in the mirror Sad because
My body is not what it used to be
It was once so tough
A dancer's body both soft and strong
Now it has been weakened by this
It is not the body I know
Legs that won't hold me up
Shape I wish I did not see
But it has survived
I am still alive
And one day I pray It will be my art again [41]

—STACEY YOUNT 2008

---

41   Submitted by: Stacey Yount 2008- http://www.butyoudontlooksick.com/articles/poetry/poetry-i-stand-here-naked/#sthash.binmYXpD.dpuf

CHAPTER 11

EMOTIONS AND CHRONIC PAIN:
EFFECTS ON MOOD AND LEARNING

PAIN TRANSMISSION—PAIN CONTROL

HOW DO WE ASSESS THE "WHOLE CHILD?"

PAIN PERCEPTION: IT'S DIFFERENT IN BOYS AND GIRLS

ANXIETY AFFECTS CHRONIC PAIN: RELATIONSHIP TO THE ANS

HOW ANXIETY GETS EXPRESSED: GENERALIZED, PANIC, OCD, PTSD, PHOBIAS
- Treatments for anxiety

AUTISM: COMMUNICATION/FEELING PROBLEMS
- Social Skills Deficits Training & Autism Spectrum

DEPRESSION, PAIN AND BRAIN CHEMICALS

FOCUS OF ATTENTION

MEMORY AND PAIN

CHILDREN MODEL THEMSELVES AFTER THEIR PARENTS

COPING ABILITY AND STYLE AND PARENT BEHAVIORS

AGE AND DEVELOPMENTAL LEVEL

HIDDEN LEARNING DISABILITIES

HOW ARE LEARNING DISABILITIES RECOGNIZED, ESPECIALLY IN BRIGHT CHILDREN?

PAIN IN CHILDREN AND YOUNG ADULTS

In this chapter we present principles on how the environment and psyche affect pain and vice-versa in the real world. To understand chronic pain, such as Carly's below, it helps to appreciate the various factors that create increased risk for its development as well as those that magnify the pain and maintain it. (See also Chapters 12 & 13)

History Carly, a 12-year-old girl, was referred to me (LZ) by a colleague. She had been in a wheelchair for several months with severe leg and back pain, as well as 'migraines' and abdominal pain. By the time I saw her, she had undergone months of evaluations by orthopedists, rheumatologists, neurologists, and gastroenterologists, with numerous lab and X-ray tests, endoscopies, colonoscopies, and other procedures to find out what was causing the pain. After costly and lengthy testing, the specialists couldn't find anything wrong and didn't know what else to do to help her.

Evaluation My evaluation found that most of Carly's pain was myofascial (musculo-skeletal), which was most likely the result of sitting or lying around for too long following a viral gastroenteritis that left her with ongoing belly pain (that had evolved into IBS). She also had severe anxiety and depression. The anxiety was causing her more pain. The depression was keeping her from feeling motivated enough to cope. Importantly, it was also interfering with her sleep.

Treatment Plan I started Carly on an SSRI (Citalopram) to help her anxiety and depression and to help her sleep. In the meantime, I prescribed a faster acting medication (a "neuroleptic") that would calm her central nervous system since the SSRI would take about four weeks to take effect. I also recommended physical therapy, psychotherapy, biofeedback, and Iyengar yoga. Carly's mom would call me daily to tell me that her daughter was still in pain. We made some adjustments to her medications and I told her that things would not improve much until Carly began at least one of the non-drug therapies I had recommended.

Finally, Carly's parents signed her up for physical therapy and around the same time, the medications began to take effect. Carly's mood improved almost immediately. She began sleeping better and exercising daily, swimming three days a week.

Mom called to tell me that Carly was no longer using a wheelchair. However, mom was upset that Carly's belly pain had not gone away. I wanted to say, "Carly is improving... even faster than I expected... she is walking, sleeping, and exercising! Aren't you excited? I am!" But I didn't. Instead, I bridled my enthusiasm, reviewed her daughter's progress with her. I emphasized that Carly was making progress and that I was sure her pain would improve. I reminded her that medication alone will not be the primary solution and that Carly would need to learn coping skills as well. Again, I reiterated that Carly start psychotherapy for her anxiety and depression. Carly's mom was still holding out for a "quick fix."

168

EMOTIONS AND CHRONIC PAIN

> *Family Dynamics I began to realize that mom's reaction was related to her own anxiety about her daughter. She was especially upset about Carly's refusal to eat when her belly hurt; she viewed the belly pain as much more worrisome than the body pain that had kept Carly in a wheelchair. The more that Carly's mom focused on how little Carly was eating and pushed her to eat more, the more anxious Carly became about eating, and this increased anxiety produced more belly pain and food refusal.*
>
> *After talking with Carly and her mom about the food, fear of eating, anxiety, and belly pain connection, I worked with Carly's mom on a strategy to help her daughter learn how to relax. During one appointment, I suggested to her mom that she needed to take care of herself too, in order to provide a good role model for her daughter. Carly's mom informed me that her primary concern was her daughter and that she had no time to relax. Only after her daughter was cured would she take time for herself.*

To understand chronic pain, such as Carly's, it was not obvious initially how much mom's own fears and lack of self-care were affecting Carly. Indeed these were the factors that magnified and maintained Carly's pain problem. More on this case later.

PAIN TRANSMISSION—PAIN CONTROL

The body's pain system is dynamic—that is, it is active and constantly changing. Remember, there are really two systems working together—pain *transmission* and pain *control*. In the transmission phase, pain signals move from the site of the pain *up* to the brain. In the pain control system, the brain sends messages *down* the nerves to the site of the pain to turn off or reduce the pain signals. **The "outside" factors—like anxiety, parental nagging or questioning, exam time—can all worsen pain by increasing transmission, reducing the efficiency of the pain control system, or by increasing pain perception in the brain,** a phenomenon that relates to the strength and location of intra-brain neural connectivity, i.e., connections of one brain part to another.

Each child needs to be individually evaluated so that as many factors as possible can be, untangled, identified and treated or managed. This is in contrast to the common belief that there is one way to treat migraines, another to treat belly pain, another to treat back pain, tension headaches (myofascial pain).

This is why such simplistic treatment approaches often fail for the group of children with multiple contributing influences on their pain (these are the children that we see in the UCLA and Whole Child LA pediatric pain clinics and who are seen at other pediatric pain clinics nationally). These are the children with "migraines," for example, who fail to get better using the migraine medications that are typically prescribed by neurologists for pediatric migraine.

HOW DO WE ASSESS THE "WHOLE CHILD?"

First, we view the mind and the body as a whole: a continuum. In our patient evaluations, we assess multiple factors in pain perception that are unique to each patient, including: anxiety, depression, focus of attention, memory, gender, parental role models, coping ability and coping style, age and cognitive level, exposure to the pain of others, past pain experiences, expectations, perception of control, and learning disabilities.

Here are a few examples of personalization. Understanding this important principle will affect potential treatment choices. Some children have *"alexithymia,"* that is, **they have a difficult time understanding and then labeling what type of emotion they are experiencing.** They may feel the physical symptoms of anxiety (e.g. rapid heartbeat, fast breathing, and feeling out of breath, sweaty palms, hot/cold flashes, or dizziness) but not feel anxious (at least they do not understand what it means to "feel anxious"). The physical symptoms are worrisome and even scary and are accompanied by dread, a feeling that "something bad is going to happen." But they are not anxious by their own report.

Children also differ in their basic temperament and thus how they respond to pain and even to symptoms of anxiety. Some children are more sensitive to pain and more reactive to it, while others have a higher pain threshold. Some children notice their heart beating faster or dizziness sooner than other children, even at the same heart rate.

Children also differ in the amount of worry that they experience. One caveat, as we mentioned before, is that children with *alexithymia* may have many physical symptoms but not report feeling anxious, yet they still have an anxiety disorder. These are all factors that need to be personalized when recommendations are made.

Let's first explore the factors that, in our experience, most significantly affect pain perception: arousal/anxiety, memory, and attention.

PAIN PERCEPTION: IT'S DIFFERENT IN BOYS AND GIRLS

In the years we have been working with children having chronic pain, it has become clear to us that there are important gender-related differences in pain perception and expression. These differences begin to appear during adolescence, although it is unclear whether these differences are related to age, puberty, or other factors, such as male and female brain differences.

There was an animated cartoon that came across the internet a few years ago. It first showed a pinball machine with hundreds of different balls oscillating at the

EMOTIONS AND CHRONIC PAIN

same time and staying in the machine. That picture was called "the female brain." Then came the picture of two large balls that just dropped. That was labeled "the male brain." Clearly these are caricatures, often of what busy mothers feel are male/female brain differences. However, recent research shows that there are different pathways in response to stress in male vs female brains.

Many types of pain such as abdominal pain, headaches, fibromyalgia, and CRPS-1 are more prevalent in late-adolescent girls than in boys of the same age. This gender difference is negligible in pre-adolescent children. In general, girls also demonstrate more pain behavior. For example, they may show more distress or less tolerance of pain than boys and report higher levels of pain relative to boys.

There also may be psychological factors linked to sex differences that include the ways that boys and girls experience and express emotions, think, and behave. For example, in Western culture, stereotypical behaviors that are considered masculine emphasize showing that you have the ability to withstand pain ("machoism"), while being very sensitive to pain is stereotypical of femininity. Such socialized gender role expectations can influence pain behaviors. Thus, boys' and girls' behaviors may differ because of what they have learned are the "right" ways for boys and girls to behave when they hurt. These differences are learned rather than biological. When LZ first began doing research on male/female differences in pain, she studied elementary school girls' and boys' responses to putting their arm in cold water. When the water was 15°C, boys showed much more tolerance of the water than did girls. But when we lowered the water temperature to a colder 12°C, the "macho-ism" disappeared and boys' and girls' pain tolerance was no longer different.

ANXIETY AFFECTS CHRONIC PAIN: RELATIONSHIP TO THE AUTONOMIC NERVOUS SYSTEM

When the worry is excessive, gets in the way of functioning, and is accompanied by irrational fear and dread, the child has an anxiety disorder. About 75% of the children who come to our pediatric chronic pain clinics have an underlying anxiety disorder or increased anxiety symptoms. This means that their nervous system is predisposed to being aroused or "turned on." They tend to be worriers, perfectionists, sensitive to the behaviors and emotions of others, and become anxious easily. Think of the person as having **a nervous system that is "wound a bit too tightly"; that is, their threshold for anxiety and, therefore for pain, is low.** Children with anxiety are more prone to developing chronic or recurrent pain. Anxiety doesn't cause the pain but it does contribute to, maintain or feed it, and it affects the child's ability to cope. How does that work?

PAIN IN CHILDREN AND YOUNG ADULTS

The autonomic nervous system (ANS) is the part of the nervous system that regulates the body's homeostasis or balance. The ANS consists of two parts: the sympathetic nervous system (SNS) and the parasympathetic nervous system (PNS). (We discussed this in more detail in Chapter 2.)

The PNS is responsible for restorative functions, like digestion. The SNS protects the body as the first response system to threat (actual or perceived). It readies the body for what is called the "fight or flight" response, which is activated when a person feels that she is in danger. When this occurs, the heart starts beating rapidly, breathing speeds up, palms become sweaty, muscles get increased blood flow, digestion shuts down, feelings of stress are intensified, and the body is prepared for either running away or staying put and fighting. To do this, the muscles must have enough oxygen and nutrients, so SNS diverts blood away from the intestines and other internal organs and directs it to the muscles. To increase the oxygen and blood flow in the muscles, the SNS causes the heart to beat faster and breathing rate to speed up. If left unchecked, these symptoms can cause dizziness and shortness of breath.

Anxiety can produce the same body sensations or symptoms, because anxiety is typically accompanied by an increase in SNS activity. Also, SNS nerves connect with sensory nerves that carry information about pain and other physical symptoms to the brain. **During times of anxiety, the entire nervous system gets revved up and causes a child to have nausea, diarrhea or constipation, as well as belly pain.**

Some children are aware of their anxiety because they are aware of thoughts and emotions that are creating the anxiety or worry. However, when sensations, such as nausea, abdominal pain, or headaches, come on suddenly, the child may not connect these physical symptoms to his thoughts or emotions. In this case, you and your child may see the pain as the major problem. And for the moment it is. This is because the child fears the pain and the pain causes more anxiety, which in turn keeps the pain going. Usually, however, there is something underlying this pain/anxiety cycle.

For example, something that has just happened or is about to happen (going to school in the morning) that is anxiety-provoking for your child. **He may not even be aware that school makes him anxious.** However, being bullied by other children, being behind in classes, or having a hidden learning disability or social problems keep a child's nervous system aroused ("turned on") and causes an increase in the volume of the pain signals and, therefore, more pain.

Although an anxiety disorder diagnosis is most often made on the basis of intense worry, physical symptoms are almost always present, such as fatigue, headaches, muscle tension, muscle aches, difficulty swallowing, trembling, twitching, irritability, sweating, hot flashes, dizziness, feeling out of breath, nausea, or diarrhea. Some children with milder anxiety can function well even though they are

EMOTIONS AND CHRONIC PAIN

distressed by their symptoms, while more severe symptoms in other children disrupt function. **Anxiety of any type will make pain worse.** Below we describe the most common types of anxiety disorders (some children will have more than one type).

ANXIETY GETS EXPRESSED: GENERALIZED ANXIETY, PANIC, OCD, PTSD, PHOBIAS

Generalized Anxiety Disorder (GAD)

GAD is a condition that fills the day with exaggerated worry and tension, even though there is little or nothing to provoke it. **Children with chronic pain not only worry about their pain but their worries may be widespread: their family's safety, their own safety, doing well in school even if they are getting As.** They overhear their parents' worries about family's finances or work and take these on as well. These worries are accompanied by physical symptoms, like fatigue, headaches, muscle tension, difficulty swallowing, trembling, twitching, irritability, sweating, hot flashes, dizziness, shortness of breath, or nausea. For children with pain problems, the increase in generalized anxiety-related nerve signals further increase the pain signals anywhere in the body.

Panic Disorder

Panic is an anxiety condition where a child feels terror that comes on without warning. Accompanying symptoms can include heart palpitations (heart pounding and beating fast), sweating, weakness, and feeling faint or dizzy. The child's hands may tingle or feel numb; she might feel flushed or chilled. She may have nausea, chest pain, or feel that she is choking and can't breathe. She might have fears of impending doom, feelings of loss of control, even feeling she is on the verge of death. Sometimes children with recurrent, episodic pain feel panic during the pain episode. The pain brings on an actual panic attack; the panic brings on more pain.

Obsessive-Compulsive Disorder (OCD)

OCD reflects anxious thoughts or rituals that the child feels he can't control. He knows the rituals do not make sense but feels compelled to carry them out; that is, he is too anxious not to do them. For example, he will wash his hands compulsively throughout the day or check the locks on the door multiple times at night. He might feel the need to have everything even (such as touching the alarm clock three more times after he has touched it once) or having to "undo" one thought with another. Some children have OCD characteristics that don't get in the way of their

PAIN IN CHILDREN AND YOUNG ADULTS

daily activities. Others have a severe version where the whole day may be devoted to these behaviors and thoughts. **For the child with OCD, there is no pleasure in carrying out these rituals or thoughts... only temporary relief from the anxiety.** Children with some "OCD symptoms" that do not get in the way of function do not have OCD. Rather, OCD is a disorder only when these symptoms cause disruption of daily activities and thoughts.

Post-traumatic Stress Disorder (PTSD)

PTSD is a debilitating condition that may develop following a terrifying event. The event may have happened directly to the child, such as a car accident, sexual or physical abuse, or even a frightening hospitalization. Or the event may simply have been witnessed by her, such as seeing someone being shot or attacked. **Typically she will have recurring intrusive thoughts and memories of the experience, yet may feel emotionally numb.** She may have sleep problems, flashbacks where she sees the event in her mind over and over, and may avoid the activity or place where the trauma occurred. **Her body may be on hyper-alert so that little things can easily startle her.** In PTSD, the autonomic nervous system resets itself to a lower threshold, so that the sympathetic nervous system gets turned on easily—and little pains become big pains, and little stresses become big stresses.

Social Phobia, often called Social Anxiety Disorder (SAD)

SAD is characterized by anxiety and self-consciousness in everyday social situations. **A child has a persistent and intense fear of being watched and judged by others and may be embarrassed or humiliated by things she does or says.** The fear impedes going to school and engaging in peer-related activities. Children with social anxiety often appear shy and have a difficult time making friends. They worry way in advance of some dreaded situation, such as having to give a talk in front of the class. This condition might also interfere with going to public places such as restaurants, shopping malls, or parks. Physical symptoms include blushing, sweating, trembling, nausea, and difficulty talking. A child may be afraid of being with people other than her family.

Specific Phobias

Specific phobias are intense fears of something that poses little or no actual danger. Some of the more common specific phobias focus on closed-in places, heights, escalators, water, dogs, and injuries involving blood (e.g. needle phobia). Fear of clowns, spiders, and snakes are common specific phobias in children.

EMOTIONS AND CHRONIC PAIN

What is the bottom line here? For children with chronic pain, **the anxiety and its underlying cause(s) must be addressed and treated for the pain problem to resolve**. If children have an anxiety disorder or are chronic worriers, even if they don't meet criteria for a major diagnosable anxiety disorder, they have more difficulty coping with pain and functioning.

It is important for you to know if your child has an anxiety disorder that may be contributing to his pain. And, since anxiety disorders tend to run in families, you might explore whether you or your child's other parent have symptoms of anxiety.

TREATMENTS FOR ANXIETY

These often include medication called selective serotonin reuptake inhibitors (SSRIs) such as sertraline 'Zoloft' or Citalopram 'Celexa' *and* cognitive skill-building tools; but medication is not always necessary. However, in cases where the symptoms are overwhelming the child, it is our experience that medication is the quickest way to calm the anxiety, at least initially and to help the child engage in psychological approaches to treat the anxiety. **These medications also help a child better cope with daily events that cause stress by raising the nervous system arousal set point** (in a sense, like changing the thermostat on the nervous system so that it takes a bigger stressor to "turn it on" and create anxiety).

In the longer term, **mental skill-building tools called cognitive behavioral therapy (CBT) can reduce the thoughts and feelings that spiral into anxiety and then pain**. For example, a child can be taught specific calming and mastery thoughts to replace catastrophic (out of control) thinking as well as breathing and other relaxation techniques. Using hypnotherapy, a child can learn to use his imagination to alter anxiety and pain signals. (See Chapter 14 for a discussion of CBT and child and family therapy for reducing anxiety, and Chapter 15 for more on hypnotherapy.)

ADDRESSING UNRESOLVED GRIEF OR TRAUMA

Children who have suffered a loss, a family member, friend, or even a pet, will go through a normal mourning period. However, with some children, this grief continues beyond what might be considered normal. It interferes with functioning or leads to profound feelings of sadness. Here, psychotherapy can be useful in helping the child to weather the mourning process and feel better.

Children who have experienced or witnessed a trauma (earthquake, shooting, physical or sexual abuse, medical procedures) can suffer from post-traumatic stress

PAIN IN CHILDREN AND YOUNG ADULTS

disorder (PTSD) and have sleep disturbances, flashbacks of the event, intrusive thoughts, be emotional numb, and may startle easily. PTSD will invariably make pain worse and harder to treat and will interfere with a child's life in many ways. Children with PTSD ideally should see a therapist trained in modern methods of PTSD treatment, since recent advances have made our treatment of this condition more effective.

> *Carolyn is a 14-year-old who has had a successful heart transplant. However, she had many post-operative problems, especially with a catheter that carried blood in and out of her body. It had to be replaced once, and she had other painful surgical manipulations in that area of her body. When she was last in the hospital, before we first saw her, the catheter fell out while she was in the bathroom alone; she started bleeding and became panicked. Her anxiety rose quickly and the pain circuits relating to her catheter site became "turned on." She immediately developed severe lower belly pain near the area where her catheter had been. The catheter was replaced successfully, but the pain continued.*

> *None of the cardiologists or surgeons could figure out what was causing the pain even after many tests. Because they couldn't find a "fixable" cause, the physicians didn't know what to do to reduce her pain. When they gave her typical opioid pain medicines, she would just go to sleep, but awakening, still in pain. Fortunately for Carolyn, these doctors understood their own limitations in pain treatment and referred her to our program.*

> *__Diagnosis__ We diagnosed Carolyn with post-traumatic stress disorder (PTSD) resulting from her surgical procedures and the bleeding episode in the bathroom. The PTSD had changed her neural arousal system so that even low levels of pain were hard for her to bear. She had flashbacks of the bleeding episode, trouble sleeping, and intrusive thoughts about her hospital experiences. The sensory nerves from her catheter site kept sending pain signals to her brain creating a memory circuit in her brain that kept the pain going.*

> *__Resolution and Plan__ We used one medication to calm her heightened nervous system and PTSD symptoms and another aimed at her nerve hyper-excitability. We then referred Carolyn to a psychologist trained in PTSD therapy to help her to talk about her stressful hospital experience and to face her fears. She learned CBT skills to overcome the anxiety she felt when she thought about that experience and, over time, she was able to revisit the hospital ward and feel Ok there. Currently Carolyn is off almost all pain and anxiety-related medications. She is going to school, has friends, and is physically active. She no longer constantly worries about her heart or being hospitalized.*

EMOTIONS AND CHRONIC PAIN

IDENTIFYING COMMUNICATION/FEELING PROBLEMS

Children with the condition *alexithymia* have difficulty identifying and labeling their own emotions. They are unsure whether they are feeling sad, anxious, or angry. For these children, negative emotions that remain unidentified, unexpressed and, therefore, untreated, aggravate the pain problem. In this case, therapy teaches children what emotions feel like. The ability to understand your own emotional state is important in both seeking support and in engaging with others in general. A common example is when a child has a panic attack but denies feeling panic or anxiety—*"I wasn't anxious. Just my heart was racing and I felt like I was choking and I was breathing really fast."*

Another kind of communication dysfunction that benefits from therapy is effective *verbal expression*. Some children know what they mean and want to say but have difficulty expressing themselves and finding the right words to say what they mean. This communication difficulty creates great stress for the child and magnifies any existing pain problem.

Social Skills Deficits Training & Autism Spectrum

As we discussed in Chapter 7, some children like Glenn (see his story below) with autism spectrum disorder, have a difficult time "reading" facial expressions and nonverbal behavior of others. To Glenn, social interaction skills did not come naturally. He couldn't figure out what "personal space" was, such as standing by another person at least an arm's distance away. The part of Glenn's brain that interprets the meaning of behavior and understands social etiquette does not work well.

Glenn avoided school because he felt uncomfortable there and had trouble making friends. Peers tended to avoid him because of his behaviors. For example, he was unaware that he was making others uncomfortable by standing too close. He said hurtful things without even realizing it.

> *Glenn is a 14-year-old complaining of headaches that were causing him to sleep poorly so that he said he was always tired during the day. Sometimes he refused to go to school because he just "couldn't get out of bed."*
>
> *Glenn began missing more and more school. When he did go, he had two "sort of" friends, the computer geek and the math whiz. However, school was stressful, because he had difficulty relating to other kids, whom he thought were all "too dumb."*
>
> ***Diagnosis*** *Our evaluation of Glenn indicated symptoms of high functioning autism spectrum disorder (what used to be called Asperger Syndrome). He was very smart, excelled in math and computer science, and there were signs for this diagnosis. He*

11

PAIN IN CHILDREN AND YOUNG ADULTS

was very logical and could be very argumentative, often not "giving up" in an argument at home until he drove his parents crazy. We realized that for Glenn the most stressful part of school was social interaction rather than academic work.

The Plan *He was referred for social skills training in a group format so that he would learn some of the social skills that didn't come naturally to him. For example, he had to learn how to let others children "be right" some of the time and not argue them to death. He had to learn how to make eye contact and smile more, especially if other children smiled at him. He was able to practice these skills with other kids similar to him and they all learned together.*

To return to school full time we developed an incremental plan. Meanwhile he learned biofeedback to control the muscle tension contributing to his headaches. With the combination of biofeedback, social skills training, and a school re-entry plan, Glenn was able to fall asleep better on school nights, awaken more easily in the mornings, and eventually attend school full time.

In the group therapy component, he also learned how to participate in school in ways that took advantage of what he was good at—he joined the debate team and set up "mind-game puzzles" on the computer for the school newspaper. (Typically, only he and his two other friends could figure out the answers, and he loved that!)

Glenn above illustrates how some children need to learn how to interact with other kids. But learning skills (therapy) mitigated some of the isolation that he had been feeling and helped Glenn to incorporate peer-interactional skills such that he began to feel more included at school and to develop friendships.

Like Glenn, Judith had a difficult time at school more because of social settings rather than academics. She was shy, did not know what to do in new social situations, and thus she avoided them. For example, when Judith was on the playground at school and saw a group of kids from her class talking together, Judith would worry that the other kids were talking about her and so she avoided the group, and came home feeling rejected. Her outgoing sister, however, saw the same group of kids and, unlike Judith, her sister approached them, smiling, and asked them what they were doing and if she could join in. Same situation... experienced in two very different ways. Judith had social anxiety, rather than high functioning autism, and needed help with her anxiety and skills and practice to help her cope with social situations.

Social skills training is most effectively taught in the peer group setting so that children like Glenn and Judith can get direct feedback from other children about their behaviors and responses.

EMOTIONS AND CHRONIC PAIN

DEPRESSION, PAIN AND BRAIN CHEMICALS

While depression is most certainly a factor for chronic pain in children, depression typically *follows* the development of chronic pain rather than *causes* it. **Pain and depression share many of the same neural pathways, the same circuitry**. Serotonin is one of the neurotransmitters that makes sure the brain is healthy and functioning properly and is also one of the main chemicals that modulate depression. Chronic pain uses up serotonin like a car uses gas, and when the tank is empty, the car runs less efficiently. Depression occurs when the energy (fuel) of the body starts running low, and the body is not running resourcefully. Brain scans reveal similar disturbances in brain chemistry in both chronic pain and depression, and some of the same medications are used by physicians to treat depression and pain.[42]

Depression and pain problems also can develop simultaneously and be related to other factors, bullying for example. A report published in the *Journal of Pediatrics* in 2004[43] discussed the findings in 2766 elementary school children ages 9 -12 years who reported being bullied at school. These children reported significantly more headaches, sleeping problems, abdominal pain, bed-wetting, feeling tired, and depression, compared with those who identified themselves as bullies or who denied being victims of bullying.

Whether depression occurs as a result of, or independent of pain, it influences pain by leaving the child with low energy reserves and little motivation to be physically active or do other things to help. **Depression disrupts sleep and impairs thinking and concentration**, both of which add to pain. Depressed children may cut back on daily physical and social activities, leaving them with fewer distractions and more time to focus on their pain. Their depression then spirals into feelings of loneliness, guilt and unworthiness, with less and less ability to cope with pain. And pain worsens.

FOCUS OF ATTENTION

Think of the last time that you had a headache (or menstrual cramps if you are a woman). If you just sat and focused on it, the pain probably got worse. The more it hurt, the more you focused on it, and the more it hurt. We know that pain perception takes place in the conscious brain. If the mind is occupied with other thoughts or planning for activities, then there is less room, so to speak, for pain-related brain activities.

Some children in pain have a difficult time shifting their focus of attention. If they focus on the pain, they have a clear pathway for negative thoughts, feelings

---

42   www.health.harvard.edu/mind-and-mood/depression_and_pain
43   http://www.jpeds.com/article/S0022-3476%2803%2900610-3/abstract

179

PAIN IN CHILDREN AND YOUNG ADULTS

of loss of control, fear of the pain, and physical arousal that builds up until they feel overwhelmed.

Distraction (filling the child's attention with other things besides pain), if only for a few seconds, can be very useful in actually reducing pain and the negative feelings that accompany it. **This is why we ask parents *not* to ask their child how she is feeling or if she is in pain.** Such questions only pull your child's attention back to her body and her pain. The best way to reduce a pain problem is to help your child learn ways to function (such as participating in school, doing homework and chores, and engaging in physical and social activities) even while she is in pain. Then she will feel in control and this feeling can and will reduce your child's nervous system arousal, and, thus, the actual amount of pain. **You are not being an evil parent if you push your child to function and have expectations that he can.** These are positive and important aspects of chronic pain treatment.

HOW MEMORY AFFECTS PAIN

Each experience of our lives is laid down in a neural network called a "memory." This happens whether we are conscious of the event or not. For example, there are *biological* memories of painful circumcisions (performed without appropriate pain control), and that these memories may become reactivated during other acute pain events, such as immunizations (see research by Anna Taddio[10]); or that early pain experiences, such as those in the newborn period, may actually alter developing pain pathways for later in life (see research by Maria Fitzgerald and others [11], [12]).

Another example of this kind of "memory" is "phantom pain." For example, if a person's leg is amputated after a bad accident or as a result of a bone tumor, the individual will have phantom sensation for about a year after the amputation. He will feel his ankles flex, his toes wiggle, and his skin may feel warm or cold, even though the leg is no longer there. This is because the areas of his brain that received signals (body position, temperature, sensation) from his leg are present and activated as if the leg were still there. If there was significant pain in the leg before amputation, the neural network that transmitted pain signals would remain active after amputation. This phantom pain can occur in the body even without the removal of a body part.

We have seen many children who have had surgery associated with significant pain before and especially after the operation. For some **the pain remains even after the organ or body part has long healed.** Because the memory of the pain remains in the brain, the nervous system keeps the pain going. This is one reason

180

EMOTIONS AND CHRONIC PAIN

why acute pain needs to be well treated in all children, since there is no way to know which children will develop pain memories. In general, the more psychologically traumatic the pain-related event is, the more likely it is that the memory will be laid down (encoded) in the brain and remain as a pain memory.

Emotionally painful memories can also affect the way and degree to which a child experiences pain. Emotionally traumatic life experiences—such as witnessing someone being hurt or being in an accident—can be embedded in a child's memory. As a result, children may develop a lower threshold for anxiety during future events they perceive as stressful. When this happens, what might seem to us to be "no big deal" can become psychologically debilitating for the child and magnify the pain.

CHILDREN MODEL THEMSELVES AFTER THEIR PARENTS

Children learn many things from watching their parents and how their parents respond to them. **Children learn about how to react to pain by watching how their parents react,** not only to the child's pain but also to their own pain. This learning process is called modeling. Children who have parents with chronic pain who do not cope well will learn ineffective ways of coping with their own pain.

For example, if a child notices that his parent tends to stay home and curl up in a ball when she is sick or in pain, **the child learns that if her own stomach hurts, the best thing to do is not go to school, but to stay home in bed and watch TV.** This is the wrong message for a child to receive; for the longer children miss school, the more difficult it is for them to return to school. School absences and catching up on missed schoolwork become added stressors that stimulate the child's nervous system and increase pain.

Instead, **parents should encourage their children to continue with daily activities even when they are in some pain**. We are not suggesting that you tell your child to just "suck it up" and get on with life, but that a child who continues to do what he can when he is in pain will have less pain and get better faster.

You can ensure that your child takes good care of himself by being a role model for him and taking care of yourself. Parents with children who suffer from chronic pain tend to focus all their attention on the child and forget about their own wellbeing. Your wellbeing is just as important as your child's, because without you he probably won't get better. Also, your child learns to cope in part by watching how you cope. (See Chapter 12 for strategies that you can use to help yourself help your child.)

PAIN IN CHILDREN AND YOUNG ADULTS

HOW CAN YOU HELP YOUR CHILD? SIX PRINCIPLES

When it comes to coping with pain, parents should keep in mind the following:

1 Children sense anxiety in their parents, and this can increase the child's own anxiety and magnify the pain.

2 Pain is worse when paying attention to it… and better if you are distracted from it. If you ask your child if she is in pain, she will scan her body looking for the pain, and find it. If she happens to be distracted from the pain at that moment, it is important for that moment to continue. It is perfectly fine for her to complain to you if she feels pain. (It is fine to ask your child about his/her day or other, non-pain-related topics.)

3 Exercise is good for sleep and chronic pain. Non-impact aerobic exercise is good for almost everyone, but especially for the child with pain. Moderate exercise not only improves the immune and cardiovascular systems, it also improves the pain relief response from the brain, and it puts the body and brain in better overall health.

4 Good sleep means less pain. Impaired sleep makes it more difficult to cope with and reduce chronic pain. In addition to exercise, it is helpful to have a regular routine to regulate sleep. Your child should go to bed at roughly the same time each night, get up at the same time each day, and only use the bed for sleeping (not for doing homework or watching TV, and especially not for texting on a smartphone!).

5 For almost all patients, the pain goes away after the child is functioning normally. Your child is improving when you see improvement in day-to-day activity. To use a basketball term, *"watch the feet… not the lips."*

6 Methods of coping, such as deep breathing, meditation, and imagery exercises, reduce pain and give children a sense of control over it.

Explains Carl von Baeyer, Ph.D[44], a leading researcher in pediatric pain,

There are ways to put pain in the background, and to put more interesting and positive thoughts in the foreground. Sometimes that means paying less attention to pain, and more attention to everything else in the child's life: interests, friends, activities, goals and plans.

---

44 Carl von Baeyer, Ph.D., Professor Emeritus of Psychology and Associate Member in Pediatrics, University of Saskatchewan, and Professor of Clinical Health Psychology, Pediatrics, and Child Health, Faculty of Medicine, University of Manitoba, Canada:

EMOTIONS AND CHRONIC PAIN

AGE, DEVELOPMENTAL LEVEL, AND SKILL IN LEARNING TO COPE

Children learn to cope with pain through practice… and by their successes and failures. As children get older, they learn more ways to cope not just with pain but with other stressors, such as problems at school, anxiety over not being liked, and fear about not getting better after an illness. The coping tools they use then become more plentiful and diverse and, usually, more effective as they get older. As a child's mind becomes capable of more complex thoughts, his understanding of pain and how it affects him expand, and he is able to strategize about what to do to feel better. **But in the beginning, children need help to learn effective skills.**

The types of coping that younger children do when they are in pain are different from what older children and adolescents do. For example, younger children are more likely to seek comfort and physical soothing from a parent. As children age, they should be learning a greater array of self-soothing strategies and become more independent of the assistance of their parents.

In a positive way, they may learn that distraction can be effective and find ways to occupy themselves with activities that take their mind off the pain. They also can learn to tell themselves that their pain will get better, not to worry, and to breathe slowly until the pain passes. Children who have difficulty coping on their own may have significant anxiety, developmental delay (for example, they may be 15 years old but act and function at a younger age level), or may have not learned that they have the ability to cope effectively.

HIDDEN LEARNING DISABILITIES – NOT ALWAYS OBVIOUS

Many children's central nervous systems develop unevenly—that is, some parts develop more slowly than other parts, leading to a delay in specific social, motor, verbal, or other skills. A child may be extremely bright but have an uneven IQ. For example, she may score very high on either the verbal or performance part of an IQ test and relatively lower in other areas. This unevenness can create problems, particularly if she is smart and motivated to do well.

There are many theories about why some children have learning disabilities; however, most remain unproven. Learning disabilities tend to run in families and may be inherited. Other contributors may be head trauma, premature birth, early severe central nervous system infections, being born to a substance-abusing mother, and maternal smoking or alcohol use during pregnancy.

A bright child who tends toward perfectionism can hide her weaknesses by working harder. Learning disabilities in these children go unrecognized until the child begins to unravel because she is no longer able to muster the energy required to continue doing well in an area of weakness. When this occurs, her stress level may increase until her sympathetic nervous system (SNS) becomes hyper-aroused which causes the chronic pain condition to develop. The pain causes her to miss school and fall further behind, which then aggravates the pain condition by producing even more stress. Such is the beginning for the downward spiral of pain. **Sometimes a learning disability may be so well compensated for that it takes a dramatic event such as an injury to bring it to the surface.** Follow Sophie's story below. It illustrates the challenges, difficulties and hurdles one family needed to find answers.

History Sophie, an 11-year-old girl, was well until a few months before coming to the pain clinic. During a competitive soccer practice, a fellow player kicked the ball that hit Sophie in the jaw, causing injury and muscle strain. Following the injury, Sophie continued to play and was in a competitive game that weekend; however, she developed headaches afterward.

Sophie's pain began behind her left ear and then spread to her neck, the left side of the face and her forehead until she developed a hypersensitivity to even the lightest touch across her forehead; she needed to cut her bangs so that they would not touch her forehead. She had multiple tender points along the back of her neck and shoulders. Sophie described her headaches as throbbing, stabbing, burning, or aching, and she reported that squeezing the side of her head helped relieve the pain somewhat.

Sophie rated the pain as a range from "7-9" on a "0-10" scale with an average of "8." She was unable to attend school regularly or do homework; she spent most of her day watching TV and playing on her computer to distract herself. She stopped playing soccer and no longer talked with her friends.

Sophie had seen her primary care physician, two neurologists, an ear, nose, and throat specialist, an orthodontist, a chiropractor, an oral surgeon, and an acupuncturist. A small fracture of her jaw was found through dental X-rays. She was fitted with a special bite plate to reduce strain on her jaw. A CT scan of her head and jaw and an MRI were all normal.

Sophie recently started 7th grade in a new school when the family moved. She had always liked science best and was extremely good in math. Sophie's mother said that Sophie always had trouble in reading and comprehension. However, Sophie always made "As" until this year when she received two "incompletes" in social studies and language arts because she had missed so much school due to her soccer injury and headaches.

Sophie often spent hours doing her social studies and reading assignments. She wanted to get all A's, but the work at the new school was much harder and she didn't see how she could catch up.

Assessment We diagnosed Sophie with head trauma that resulted in a central head-ache with secondary complex regional pain syndrome (CRPS) type I of the head. She also had myofascial pain with multiple trigger points and muscle spasm. Based on her history, we also suspected that she had a learning disability (reading disorder) that was contributing to her headaches and pain-related disability.

Sophie had coped with, and therefore masked, the reading disorder by being smart, a perfectionist, and by putting huge amounts of time into her studies. However, the move to the new school, the stress of the difficult and increasing workload, and school absences due to her headaches overwhelmed her. Her stress and pain mounted until she was unable to attend school at all.

Plan Implementation Sophie was given medications aimed at CRPS (amitriptyline and gabapentin), started physical therapy and Iyengar yoga for the muscle pain that was contributing to her headaches, and she was referred for academic and cognitive testing.

Testing confirmed that Sophie had a reading comprehension and written expression learning disorder. An IEP (Individualized Educational Plan) was set up through her school to provide special help in the areas where she was weak. Her school also agreed to reduce the number of written report assignments Sophie had to complete, presenting them instead as tape-recorded oral reports. Sophie was able to catch up on her work. As this happened, her headaches were reduced until she was able to return to school. Eventually, her headaches went away altogether.

HOW ARE LEARNING DISABILITIES RECOGNIZED, ESPECIALLY IN BRIGHT CHILDREN?

Parents need to look for relative areas of weakness. For example, a child may do well in math and science but have some problems in reading, or related skills. Even "A" students can have relative difficulties in one subject, like math for instance, but the teacher may not be aware that this child is getting good grades in math with great effort and much stress. If you suspect your child may have a learning disability, you can request that the school do cognitive and academic testing, which would include an I.Q. test, or you can have neuropsychological testing done privately. (See also Chapter 17.)

Neuropsychological testing is an important tool to consider in any practice of pain treatment for children. It can identify a child's strengths and weaknesses so that stress on the nervous system can be reduced.

PAIN IN CHILDREN AND YOUNG ADULTS

According to Dr. Leah Ellenberg[45], who often evaluates our patients:

Neuropsychological Evaluation This includes an interview with parents detailing the child's birth and development, social and emotional functioning, school history and interests as well as family history of educational and psychological functioning. The child will meet with the neuropsychologist for approximately six hours of individual testing, usually in two to four sessions.

Assessment This includes an IQ test that is multifaceted such as the Wechsler Intelligence Scale for Children, Fifth Edition, which tests: Verbal Comprehension, Perceptual Reasoning, Working Memory and Processing Speed. Depending on the child's age and ability level, various tests are used to assess language functioning, visual spatial analysis, perceptual motor skills, attention, various types of memory, executive functioning, academic skills, and learning style. Other tests assess emotional, behavioral, and social functioning.

Following testing, the neuropsychologist will meet with parents and the child to discuss the findings and recommendations.

Dr. Ellenberg notes, "I prefer meeting with parents alone first and then meeting with the child in the presence of one or both parents so that they can reinforce what I tell the child."

At the End of This Process parents and child should understand the child's individual issues and learning style. Particular problems can then be dealt with. For example, a learning disability may require individual tutoring or educational therapy (work with a learning specialist who can teach strategies for overcoming areas of weakness) as well as accommodations at school (extra time on tests or shortened assignments). A child with an attention problem may need a school setting with smaller classes, individual tutoring, or medication. Emotional or behavior problems may require individual or family psychotherapy."

In this chapter, we have covered emotions, learning, and how age and development can affect pain. Chapter 12 will describe how parents can help their child by establishing better sleep patterns and relaxation techniques..

---

45 Dr. Leah Ellenberg, Child neuropsychologist, Clinical Associate Professor of Pediatrics at UCLA School of Medicine. www.leahellenberg.com

CHAPTER 12

HOW PARENTS CAN HELP THEIR CHILD

Good parents give their children Roots and Wings. Roots to know where home is, wings to fly away and exercise what's been taught them.

—JONAS SALK, PHYSICIAN, DISCOVERED EPONYMOUS VACCINE FOR POLIO

IS YOUR CHILD GETTING ENOUGH SLEEP?

HOW TO HELP YOUR CHILD GET A BETTER NIGHT'S SLEEP

- How to Help Your Child Get a Better Night's Sleep
- Dr. Harvey Karp's "Pearls"
- Implementing your sleep plan-- improving sleep hygiene

RELAXATION TECHNIQUES

- Relaxation Breathing Exercise for Parents
- Muscle Relaxation Techniques
- Muscle Relaxation/Muscle Contraction Exercise

FAVORITE PLACE

MINDFULNESS MEDITATION

PAIN PREVENTION: STRESSES AND WARNING SIGNS

187

In this chapter we are going to give you guidance on how to help your child when their pain flares, gets worse, and your child is having difficulty coping, even what to do in pain emergencies. We will provide step-by-step guidance on several useful pain and stress reducing techniques, such as breathing, muscle relaxation and mindfulness. You will also learn strategies for helping your child get a good night's sleep, lack of which is one of the major contributors that makes pain worse.

Remember, **the goal for the treatment of children with chronic pain is not** *"to get rid of the pain first,"* but rather to *"help him function and then the pain will fade."*

While doctors use medicines and other therapies to calm the nervous system and alter pain circuits in the brain, it's up to you to help your child carry out the tasks of daily living, including getting a good night's sleep, eating well, going to school, doing schoolwork, socializing, exercising, and participating in family activities, including home chores. Most parents want to help their child to function but don't know what to do. This chapter will give you the tools to help your child.

Remember, you are a role model for your child. The more you take care of yourself, the more likely that your child will also begin to practice self-soothing.

IS YOUR CHILD GETTING ENOUGH SLEEP?

One of the frequently missed assessments for children in pain is attention to sleep… and getting enough of it. Being sleep-deprived is a set-up for a bad day, for parent and child.

To answer the question, take note of the answers to the 8 questions below in Table 12.1. If you answer yes to several of these questions, the chances are your child isn't getting enough quality sleep, especially if she has a chronic pain problem.

Table 12.1 Getting enough Sleep?
1 Does your child have trouble falling asleep? What time does she go to bed?
2 Does she have problems *staying* asleep, once she falls asleep?
3 If she wakes up during the night, does she waken several times, and then have difficulty falling back to sleep?
4 Does she have difficulty getting up in the morning?
5 Is she fatigued during the day?
6 Is she on her iPhone™ texting or watching TV in her room before bedtime?
7 Does she nap during the day?
8 Does she take medication for sleep and is not sleeping? Does this medication help with sleep but make her feel groggy the next day?

188

How to Help Your Child Get a Better Night's Sleep

Sleep is a cornerstone of pain relief. Not getting enough restorative (refreshing, healing, deep) sleep is devastating to a child's body. Children typically need more sleep than do adults. Children with chronic pain who are not getting sufficient restorative sleep have more difficulty learning how to cope because their brain does not learn as well when it is sleep deprived. This is especially true for adolescents whose sleep cycle is often at odds with the requirements of the school system. The lack of restorative sleep at night creates a vicious cycle: chronic pain can cause insufficient sleep, and insufficient sleep maintains the pain.

First step in helping your child sleep is to develop a plan together with her to insure a good night's sleep. For example, if Jamie has trouble sleeping at night, the answer isn't, "What one thing can I do to get her to sleep?" or, as we often hear, "Can you just give her something to make her fall asleep!" If Jamie is not falling asleep, let's review the possible reasons why not. (Table 12.2) Once you know the reasons, it is much easier to come up with a treatment plan. Take note of the following:

Table 12.2   Reasons for sleeping difficulties
1   What time is she eating dinner? (If she is eating a heavy meal right before going to sleep, the food may be interfering with her sleep.)
2   Is she consuming caffeine products—such as soda, chocolate, or tea—before bed?
3   What does she do after dinner and at night to get ready for bed? Watch TV or work on computer or play videogames? (The more active she is, especially on the computer or with videogames, the more aroused her nervous system will become, the harder it will be for her to fall asleep.)
4   Do they watch TV, play computer games, etc. while in bed? (The bed should be the place where they can read or listen to soft music and get ready to go to sleep.
5   Does she have a bedtime routine? (Developing routines is helpful, especially for the child who has sleep difficulty.)
6   If she is < 13 years old, do you spend any time with her at bedtime in her room so that bedtime is associated with pleasant parent-related activities? (e.g telling a story; massaging her head, neck, and shoulders; talking about things that happened during the day.)
7   Is it hard to leave her room? Is bedtime dragged out 1+ hr.?
8   Is she sleeping in her bed or your bed? (Goal = to sleep in her own bed.)
9   Does she have a need for a nightlight? (if so, then a small nightlight can help her avoid larger lights that might interfere with sleep.)

PAIN IN CHILDREN AND YOUNG ADULTS

Dr. Harvey Karp's "Pearls"

We asked Dr. Harvey Karp[46], one of the world's foremost Pediatric experts on sleep in infants and young children, to offer some "pearls of wisdom."

Sleep is a wonderful puzzle! We spend a third of our lives in it, yet it seems as foreign as the depths of the ocean. Over the past thirty years, however, we've uncovered fascinating new clues to help us better understand this misty frontier. For example:

Sleep struggles are among the most common challenges new parents face. (Exhaustion is such a stressful experience that the elite Navy SEALs are put through sleep deprivation to train them to endure torture!) And this is not an isolated problem for the parents of babies. One third of toddlers fight bedtime and half still get up once a night (one in ten wakes twice... or more!).

WHAT IS SLEEP? *Sleep is very different from being unconscious. In sleep, you are still responsive to the environment. You can respond to the phone ring. Though we sleep right on the edge of your bed, we rarely roll off. During sleep, the body is more or less at rest (sleep walking and night terrors are exceptions), but our brain wave activity is as perky as when we're fully awake! We organize and store memories; enter drowsy wakefulness periodically to scan the room for danger (like smoke or someone opening a window); and, of course we experience the surreal thrill of dreaming.*

You can be awake and asleep... at the same time! When you're exhausted some brain cells fall asleep, even though you are still awake. Over the past fifty years, though we better understand the sleep experience, we are getting less of it. The average adult nighttime sleep has dropped from eight to about seven hours. For weary moms and dads, a good night's sleep shimmers in their minds like a desert mirage.

*A 2004 National Sleep Foundation poll found that **20% of parents of infants and 12% of parents of tots and preschoolers get less than six hours of sleep a night.** Like a rock thrown in a lake, exhaustion triggers waves after wave of quarreling, accidents, overeating, illness, worry and depression. Over just a few weeks, that level of sleep deprivation impairs the brain as much as being drunk, leading to car accidents and bed-sharing tragedies!*

Debunking myths offers help for parents of babies/young children. *"Be quiet! The baby is sleeping!" We used to think babies needed total silence and preferred sleeping in a flat still bed. However, we now know that the womb surrounds fetuses with a symphony of sensation. And, imitating these sensations, for example, using swaddling (for at least the first four months) can reduce night waking and reduce the temptation*

---

46 Harvey Karp, MD, FAAP, Author, The Happiest Baby Guide To Great Sleep: Birth – Five Years *www.happiestbaby.com/about-dr-karp*

HOW PARENTS CAN HELP THEIR CHILD

parents have to place babies in the riskier stomach position. In addition, white noise (similar to the deep, loud rumble babies hear 24/7 in the womb) may help enhance sleep.

Studies have shown that establishing better sleep patterns early in infancy leads to fewer nighttime struggles during the toddler years. And, longer sleep has also been associated with a reduced risk of a variety of health concerns (including overweight at one year of age and symptoms of attention deficit/hyperactivity).

***Establishing good routines promote improved sleep.** Those include daytime practices (outdoor play; sun exposure; avoidance of caffeinated beverages, dark chocolate, stimulant medications) and nighttime practices (**reduced brightness of artificial lights**; reduced screen time – **the bluish light of computer screens reduces release of the brain's natural sleep hormone, melatonin; avoiding stimulating play before bedtime**; ventilated rooms that are neither too hot or cold; establishing a caring, predictable bedtime routine – such as massage, reading, lullabies, rumbly, low-pitched white noise).*

Of course, even if you have established a successful sleep routine, it's highly likely that your child will have periodic struggles. Resistance going to bed; difficulty falling asleep; and night waking can be provoked by a variety of common life events (such as trips - especially those that require time zone changes; discomfort of teething or illness; new home/school/sibling; traumatic events – witnessed/experienced or seen in media).

***Notes for better sleep: White noise isn't just for your baby.** The brain has a hard time paying attention to two things at once, so a strong, rumbly white noise can cover over disturbing sounds from the next-door neighbors or passing trucks...or your own inner voice of worries and concerns. (Start it softly, an hour before sleep to give your brain a few days to get used to it.)*

***Light is the enemy of sleep.** For thousands of years, darkness was the brain's cue to get ready to sleep. (Electric lights have only been around for a hundred years.) Your house lights (and especially the bluish light from your computer screen, phone or TV) trick your brain into thinking it's still afternoon. The brain then shuts off your natural melatonin, which delays your drowsiness until much later at night.*

Implementing your sleep plan – improving sleep hygiene

Once you've asked and answered these questions in Table 12.2 and read Dr. Karp's "Pearls" above, you can start developing a strategy to help your child sleep better. This type of thinking also will help your child to cope better. The following nine points are good guides for better sleep.

PAIN IN CHILDREN AND YOUNG ADULTS

1 Set a schedule. Your child should go to bed at a set time each night and get up at the same time each morning. Many adolescents are sleep-deprived during the week with homework, late nights, and early mornings for school. Weekends are their "catch-up" time. However, for some children, weekend sleep patterns may make it more difficult to wake up early on Monday mornings. See what works best for your child.

2 Exercise. Your child should exercise 20 to 30 minutes a day. Daily exercise will help her sleep, but it is best to exercise about 5 to 6 hours before going to bed since exercising too close to bedtime can interfere with sleep.

3 Avoid caffeine products. Your child should avoid (soft) drinks as most sodas do contain caffeine; it is a stimulant and will keep her awake.

4 If your child is napping during the day, interrupt this pattern so that she will be more tired at night.

5 Don't lie in bed awake. If your child can't get to sleep, he shouldn't just lie in bed. Let him do something else, such as reading or listening to soft music, until he feels tired. The worry about "trying to fall asleep" will keep him awake.

6 Sleep until sunlight. If possible, wake up with the sun, or use very bright lights in the morning. Sunlight helps the body's internal biological clock reset itself each day. It is often helpful for a child to get at least an hour of morning sunlight if he has problems falling asleep at night.

7 Control the room temperature. Maintain a comfortable temperature in the bedroom. Room temperatures that are too hot or too cold can prevent your child from falling asleep or can wake her up during the night.

8 For younger children, setting up a bedtime routine with a parent is very helpful. For example, the last thing that your child might do before sleep is for you to read him a story while he is in his bed, or massage his head and back..

9 If the above steps do not help your child get restful sleep (or even if they do), teach her any of the relaxation techniques for use in bed: progressive relaxation, breathing exercises (see below).

RELAXATION TECHNIQUES

Relaxation techniques are ones that you and your child can use throughout your life, even when there is no pain. Susmita Kashikar-Zuck, Ph.D[47] offers this metaphor:

---

47 Susmita Kashikar-Zuck, Ph.D., Professor of Pediatrics and Clinical Anesthesiology Research Director, Behavioral Medicine and Clinical Psychology, Division of Pain Management. Cincinnati Children's Hospital Medical Center *www.cincinnatichildrens.org/bio/k/susmita-kashikar-zuck*

HOW PARENTS CAN HELP THEIR CHILD

"Practicing your relaxation and biofeedback skills is like a fire drill. Fires don't happen very often, but you don't want to wait until one happens to practice how to save yourself. Pain can come and go, but the time the pain is bothering you is not a good time to learn anything. You need to practice all the time, so when the pain comes, you will be ready. So have fun, learn well, and enjoy!"

Breathing Exercises, Especially for Panic

Depending upon how it is done, breathing may reduce pain or accentuate pain. Improper breathing techniques can greatly increase the pain. Some children hyperventilate when they become anxious or during a pain episode. This means that their breathing pattern changes to shallow, rapid breathing. When this happens, your child breathes out too much of the "exhale gas" called carbon dioxide (CO_2) too quickly. Getting carbon dioxide out of your body too quickly causes your body to lose acid. These chemical changes might cause your child to feel dizzy, feel like he can't catch his breath, or is choking and his fingers or lips may begin to tingle or even become numb.

The following breathing exercise should help your child feel more in control, allow him/ her to get rid of the "funny feelings," and feel more relaxed.

Have your child breathe into a paper bag for about thirty seconds with very slow, long exhalations.

If your child is anxious and has difficulty concentrating, suggest that he imagine a balloon that needs to be blown up.

Ask him to purse his lips to blow up the balloon and to slowly start blowing so that he can make the balloon bigger and bigger.

Suggest that as he blows up the balloon, he notice its size, color, and shape, and whether there is any writing or pictures on the balloon.

After a few moments, let your child rest until he feels more relaxed and his breathing pattern has returned to normal. The exercise above is a good one to use during an acute pain or panic attack when there isn't much time to get your child's breathing under control.

Relaxation Breathing Exercise for Parents

The breathing exercise below requires a little more planning and time, but is excellent for helping your child to develop patterns of self-soothing and feelings of control over the pain. This is an excellent pain preventive strategy to teach your

PAIN IN CHILDREN AND YOUNG ADULTS

child. But now, we want you to practice this first alone for yourself to experience what happens in your body as you develop these breathing skills. This is part of your learning to take care of yourself so that you can continue in your role as the major support for your child.

You can practice this technique with your child later, prompting him or her to take the next step, until she can do it on her own. Younger children may benefit from a time each day when you and your child do this technique together; older children and adolescents can learn this technique for themselves. A daily practice of 10 minutes a day will be a useful prevention strategy.

Preparation Directions:

Find a quiet room where you can get into a comfortable position to relax. The room should be fairly warm. When you become deeply relaxed, your body temperature drops and you can feel cold.

Close the door and tell other family members that you will need to be left alone for the next half hour (or as long as you would like). Put up a "do not disturb" sign, if you think that will help.

To use this technique to relax but not sleep, do this exercise sitting up, either sitting on the floor while leaning against a wall to support your back or sitting in a straight-backed chair. Your arms can drop comfortably in your lap.

If the intent is to use this technique to go to sleep, do this exercise lying in bed ready for sleep.

Eyes are closed. Arms and legs should not be crossed. This might cut off circulation and cause numbness and tingling.

After you first go through the exercise below, you can then guide your child with the following directions:

Breathe in deeply and exhale slowly as though you were whistling. Breathe deeply and exhale slowly three times.

Count in your mind as you breathe out and see if you can get to a higher number each time that you breathe out (allowing yourself to breathe just a bit more slowly each time you breathe out).

Notice your body beginning to feel more relaxed with each breath out.

After three nice long breaths, you should begin to notice that tension in your body is moving through your body and out through your breath as you exhale.

194

HOW PARENTS CAN HELP THEIR CHILD

Notice your body becoming heavy and limp, as if it were too much effort to even think about moving it. Conversely, you may notice your body feeling weightless, or comfortably warm, as if you were floating in warm water.

You might notice that your breathing is nice and slow. At the end of your breath in, pause for a moment. Then, let the breath out again, nice and slowly. Continue breathing in this way for a few minutes.

Notice your breath pushing down gently on your diaphragm. As this happens, you might notice your stomach begin to rise with each breath in. This is called "diaphragmatic breathing" and is the type of breathing that allows the most air into the lungs, with the least effort. (You can imagine your belly is an accordion, moving up and down as you breathe.) You can put one hand on your belly and feel it rise as you breathe in. The other hand can be placed on your chest and shouldn't move very much. When you breathe out, press the small of your back against the wall of floor depending upon whether you are sitting or lying down.

To end the breathing exercise, you should first go back to breathing normally and effortlessly. Then focus on taking three purposeful long breaths by extending the exhalation nice and slowly.

If you are in bed lying down and are using this technique to fall asleep, you may have fallen asleep somewhere in the middle of this exercise. If you have, this is fine. If you do this every night, your brain will learn to make the connections that indicate that it is time to fall asleep.

As you practice this breathing exercise, your brain will learn how to change to diaphragmatic breathing and your diaphragm muscles will get stronger and stronger. This will bring more air into the lungs and you will begin to feel more and more refreshed at the end of the day, rather than fatigued.

With this personal experience under your belt, you can then help your child to notice his breathing… that it can be as simple as asking him to pay attention to the beginning and end of his breathing out (exhaling) and breathing in (inhaling). He can be reminded to just notice his breathing but not try to change it. He can notice his belly moving up and down as he breathes.

For younger children, ask them to place a stuffed animal on their belly to help them notice the up and down movement of their belly as they breathe. You can ask them to breathe in and out slowly and notice how they feel, and then breathe in and out more quickly and see how that feels, and then go back to normal breathing where they just notice their breath but not try to change it, just notice it and their stuffed animal moving up and down on their belly as they breathe.

PAIN IN CHILDREN AND YOUNG ADULTS

Breathing is the easiest thing to do and pay attention to during times of stress. Next time you feel stressed, stop and take three long slow breaths and see what happens in your body when you do that.

MUSCLE RELAXATION TECHNIQUES

Chronic pain can cause children to tense their muscles and even hold their body in abnormal ways to protect themselves from stretching or injuring the painful body part.

However, pain in one body area can create pain in another area because of muscle tension. This set of muscle relaxation exercises is meant to encourage muscles that are already tense to relax, prevent the build-up of stress in the muscles, and prevent muscle-related pain from developing.

So now, begin this exercise yourself first. It will help you to personally experience the feelings in your body as you carry out this muscle relaxation program before you guide your child in this exercise.

Muscle Exercise #1: Progressive Relaxation

Allow yourself to be in a quiet place. If you are doing this exercise to help you sleep, it is best to do this in your bed just before you are ready to go to sleep. For relaxation but not sleep, it is best to do this in a comfortable chair upright or in a recliner chair.

Take three slow deep breaths and then just continue to breathe normally. Notice your breathing.

You will begin to feel tension in your body flowing through your body and out through your breath. Notice energy from the air coming into your body through your lungs when you breathe in and feel it flow to the parts of your body where you need the most energy.

As you continue to breathe normally, focus your attention on your big toe on your right foot. With each breath out, notice that toe relaxing and feel its warmth as the circulation increases and more warm blood begins to flow through it.

Notice the relaxation beginning to spread to the big toe on your left foot and notice that toe begin to feel relaxed and warm.

Notice the relaxation spreading in turn to each of the next toes on both feet... first the toe next to the big toes and the next toe and so on until all of the toes on both feet feel relaxed, warm, and comfortable.

196

HOW PARENTS CAN HELP THEIR CHILD

Notice the relaxation beginning to spread up to the top of your feet and under to the soles of your feet... spreading upward to your ankles, your calves, and shins, and up and around to your entire thighs... your feet might begin to feel so heavy that they can't even think about moving... they can just stay there and relax.

Now notice, with each breath out, this wave of relaxation continues to move up your body... to your buttocks... lower back and around to your pelvis... you might notice your body feel as if it is sinking deeper into your bed or chair. Allow the feeling to flow in that direction... but whatever you feel is fine... just notice it.

As the wave of relaxation continues to move up your back and around to your belly, notice how your abdomen and back muscles feel when they begin to relax... this is a different feeling... warm... relaxation spreading up your body to your upper back and chest... to your shoulders and the area between your shoulder blades... around to your neck... front... sides... back of your neck.

Feel the relaxation spreading up into your head... the back of your head... sides... top... forehead... eyebrows... eyes (if they haven't closed by now, they may just want to close because the lids might feel too relaxed to be able to work to keep your eyes open... but whatever happens is fine).

Notice the relaxation spreading down your face to your cheeks... your nose... the area above your lip... your lips.... your chin... around to your ears.

Now take a moment to enjoy the feeling of deep relaxation... feel yourself becoming deeper and deeper relaxed with each breath out... allow your body to become as deeply relaxed as you would like to be and spend a few moments noticing how good it feels to be relaxed.

As you notice this feeling of relaxation, your brain will record it. This will become a new memory that can be called upon when you need it. Each time you practice this relaxation exercise, that memory will become stronger and stronger. In time, you will just need to take three deep breaths and your brain will know exactly what to do…you will find yourself automatically going into a deep state of relaxation. You might find this happening even when you are busy doing other things. That is, you no longer will need to go through this exercise.

Muscle Exercise #2: Relaxation/Muscle Contraction

Some people have a difficult time knowing what it feels like to have a muscle "relax," especially people who have been in pain for a while. Chronically tense muscles use up energy when they are contracted. When you learn how to relax muscles, you free up energy so that you feel less tired and have the strength to get better. The exercise below will help you to feel the difference between muscle tension and muscle relaxation. It may be practiced on its own or in preparation for the progressive relaxation exercise that we described above.

To begin, lie in your bed or sit in a comfortable chair, as above, depending upon whether you are using this technique to help you (or your child) sleep or to relax and become energized.

Begin by taking three deep breaths as in the previous exercise, breathing out very slowly so that any tension in your body flows out through your breath and oxygen flows into your body with each breath in.

Contract your toes first by bending them down and squeezing as hard as you can and then just let them relax for a moment while you take two slow breaths.

Next, contract your ankles by bending your feet forward firmly for as long as you can and then bending them back upward firmly towards your shins for as long as you can. Then allow your feet to relax while you take two very slow deep breaths. Also take a moment to notice how relaxed your feet feel when they no longer have to do anything... just relax.

Contract the muscles of your entire legs. If you are sitting, stretch your legs out straight in front of you and hold them as long and straight as you can until it takes too much effort to keep them there; and then you can let them go and just allow them to feel heavy and relaxed.

If you are in bed, bend your knees and bring your knees to your chest if you can, or bend them as much as you can and hold that position for as long as you can until it takes too much effort to continue. And then allow them to drop and become straight again, heavy and relaxed. Again, when you are finished, take two very slow deep breaths and just notice how relaxed your whole body is beginning to feel.

Next, if you are sitting in a chair, bend your upper body down toward your lap or below your knees if you are able to and hold that position and keep pushing your upper body down... down... until it takes too much effort to keep it there... then come back up and allow your whole body to sink deeply into the chair and relax... again take two very slow deep breaths and allow your body to just "be" without having to do anything during this time.

If you are in bed doing this exercise, take three deep breaths and fill your lungs as your belly expands and just hold each breath for as long as you can before you slowly let out each breath. Notice your chest and belly muscles beginning to relax

HOW PARENTS CAN HELP THEIR CHILD

as you breathe out each time. Again, take two very slow deep breaths and allow your body to just "be" without having to do anything during this time.

> *Now expand your chest forward while you bring your shoulders back as close together as you can get them, making as deep a fold between your shoulder blades as you can... also bring shoulders downward... they should not be up by your ears... hold this position for as long as you can until it takes too much effort and then release the pose. Again, take two very slow deep breaths and allow your body to relax without having to do anything during this time.*

> *Bend your arms by bringing your hands up to your shoulders with your palms facing your shoulders and squeeze your arms in that position for as long as you can until it takes too much effort and then drop your arms at your sides and allow them to relax while you take two slow deep breaths.*

> *Now stretch your arms up as high as you can (if you are in bed you can stretch them upward toward the ceiling) and keep your hands fully open, palms facing each other, and your fingers outstretched wide apart. Keep your arms and hands that way until it takes too much effort and then drop them at your side and allow them to relax while you take two slow deep breaths.*

> *Finally, bend your head forward to touch your chin to your chest as far as you can go and hold it for as long as you can until it takes too much effort and then bring your head back up to a normal position. Do the same to the right and to the left, by turning your head to one side as long and deeply as you can and then to the other side as long and deeply as you can and then allow your head and neck to relax while you take two slow deep breaths.*

> *Take just a few moments to be still and notice your breath as it returns to normal breathing again and notice how deeply relaxed, warm, and comfortable your body feels without having to do anything and just relax for a few moments while you breathe.*

As you do this exercise with your child, you can turn it into a game. For a young child, you might want to suggest that she name her toes. Then your child can decide when each one has "had enough" and is ready to relax. Or you might want to create a challenge for each muscle that is being contracted. For example, when your child bends over, you might want to see how far downward he can bend... or how close he can get his chin to his chest, etc.

Spending the time with your child carrying out this exercise will be helpful in itself. Remember, these exercises work best for your child, if you first learn them for yourself, even if you don't have a pain problem. These are healthy exercises to enhance feelings of well-being.

12

FAVORITE PLACE

When your child is stressed or the pain has escalated, you can help him go, in his imagination, to a "favorite place." He can be encouraged to really let himself "be there" and look around, listen, and experience what it feels like being there. The point of having a favorite place is to develop somewhere a child can "go" to feel safe and comfortable. This is especially important for children with chronic pain because they often feel off balance and uncomfortable. Feeling good and having positive emotions can help in the healing process and deep relaxation also helps reduce the stress response in the body during pain.

One girl who had been in a wheelchair for two years because of total body pain was too anxious to picture herself dancing in her favorite place (she used to dance before her chronic pain problem), so she imagined herself at the dance studio "watching" herself dance and over time the watching gradually merged into the experiencing... when she was ready. In this way, the favorite place can also be used by a child to learn coping skills and to try a feared activity in small increments.

MINDFULNESS MEDITATION

Mindful awareness can be a useful tool to help children and adolescents with chronic pain. Often chronic pain invokes fear: fear of the unknown, fear that something is terribly wrong with one's body, fear of what school peers might think, and fear of losing control. Being able to cultivate mindful awareness of one's pain can help a child accept many of the feelings associated with the pain as well as give him insight into ways of actually controlling and regulating the pain.

Steven Weisman, M.D.,[48] talks about "mindful awareness" and offers a meditative exercise.

So how does one learn mindful awareness? I believe that this door is opened through learning the practice of mindfulness meditation. Long ago described by the Buddha as one of the means to overcome suffering, mindfulness meditation has been used extensively as a stress reduction technique as well as in pain treatment plans. Traditionally, mindfulness meditation uses simple awareness of the breath to help focus the mind as it runs and jumps from thought to thought or sensation to sensation. It literally takes only 1 to 2 minutes to learn the basic fundamentals of mindfulness meditation.

Simply find a comfortable, upright posture. If it is too uncomfortable to sit upright, lie down. The sitting posture tends to keep you from falling asleep. Some people find

---

48 Steven Weisman, M.D., Jane B. Pettit Chair in Pain Management, Children's Hospital of Wisconsin

HOW PARENTS CAN HELP THEIR CHILD

it helpful to sit on a cushion, but sitting in a chair or on a bench is perfectly fine. The arms can comfortably drop down from the shoulders and then the forearms can be placed on the thighs or in one's lap. You may keep your eyes open, gently gazing ahead, possibly at a spot on the floor or a wall. You might also choose to close your eyes. After a moment or two check in with yourself so that you feel comfortable, and direct your attention to your breath. Feel the air as it moves through your nostrils or mouth. Feel the breath as it fills your abdomen. Feel the abdomen rise up and then deflate down. Focus your slow comfortable breaths into the lower abdomen so that your breathing becomes regular and deep.

As you do this, it is natural for your attention to wander onto other thoughts or feelings. As you become aware of these thoughts and feelings rising up, acknowledge that your mind has wandered and then simply and gently, guide it back to your breath. Continue this for several minutes. If you notice some discomfort in your body due to your posture, with awareness of the body, shift to a more acceptable position. Try this when you awaken in the morning, or when you have a few spare moments. Surely you can find a few moments to practice in the evening or even before going to bed.

Below is a simple breath poem to help guide the breath during sitting meditation.

Breathing in, I know I am breathing in....

Breathing out, I know that I am breathing out.

Breathing in, I calm my body......Breathing out, I smile.

Breathing in, I am aware of the present moment.....

Breathing out, I offer love to my body.

Breathing in, I calm my mind....Breathing out, I am thankful to be alive.

Breathing in, I release my fears....Breathing out, I release my thoughts.

Breathing in, I know I am breathing in....

Breathing out, I know that I am breathing out.

Cultivating mindfulness can bring a profound relaxation to the body and mind. Over time, with the practice of mindful awareness, many children will notice a reduction in their pain and other symptoms. Often the "results" are not obvious. But it is precisely the moving away from the need to have "results" that often contributes to a lessening of the child's suffering.

PAIN IN CHILDREN AND YOUNG ADULTS

How does mindfulness work?

Mindfulness has been shown to alter brain connectivity pathways that lead to calmness and compassion; brain changes have been shown to be related to the length of mindfulness practice. As a busy parent, allowing yourself 20-30 minutes of mindfulness will provide tremendous benefits for you and your child. Mindfulness allows you to notice the present moment without being stuck in the past or worrying about the future. The practice involves just being wherever you are and noticing your breathing. In that process, you might notice thoughts, bodily sensation, emotions, sounds and smells, and you can notice them, let them go, and return to your breath. A mindfulness practice helps you to develop self-compassion and equanimity, among other positive states of mind.

To help your children learn mindfulness, we refer you to the book by Susan Kaiser-Greenland (*The Mindful Child*) published in paperback[13].

PAIN PREVENTION: STRESSES AND WARNING SIGNS

Stress increases the amount of pain, reduce pain tolerance, and can cause a pain relapse. The most common time for pain to relapse is the start of the school year.

- A viral infection in your child can set off a bout of irritable bowel syndrome symptoms or headaches.

- Lack of sufficient sleep, travel, or overdoing it with an activity on a weekend can also be causes.

- Other stresses can be related to family members: parental marital discord, death of a pet, illness in a parent.

Some of these have relatively easy solutions: more rest, sleep, or just offering your child an opportunity to talk about what is bothering her. Others may not be so easy to solve. Try these five steps:

1 Identify *sources* of stress and help your child learn how to deal with them.

2 Identify *warning signs*: new headaches, excessive fatigue, irritability, or "mopiness" can be warning signs of an impending relapse of chronic pain.

3 *Develop a game plan* that may include some of the following strategies:

  a Maintaining a normal schedule. Encourage your child to get out of the house and schedule plans with friends or go to school.

  b Helping your child seek distractions. Encourage him to read something he likes, watch a funny movie, call a friend, play videogames or work on the

HOW PARENTS CAN HELP THEIR CHILD

computer, go outside to play, be with friends, or do something physically active.

 c Encouraging your child to relax. Relaxation quiets the central nervous system and can reduce pain.

4 *Use medications wisely.* Drugs are not the only answer to pain and shouldn't be the first thing that you do when your child begins to complain of pain or becomes irritable. If the first thing that you do when your child has pain is to reach for medications or tell him to take a pill, this "medication first" plan will train your child to turn to medications rather than himself when he is not feeling well.

5 *Let your child know that you are confident he can get through this* and that it will pass. If you show that you have confidence in him, he will learn to have confidence in himself.

Now it's on to Section D and the actual, detailed, medicinal and behavioral treatments employed for children with chronic pain.

SECTION D

TREATMENTS—
WHAT ARE THEY?
WHAT DO THEY DO?

*"The greatest mistake in the treatment
of diseases is the thought that there are
physicians for the body and physicians for
the soul... the two cannot be separated."*

—PLATO

*My biggest frustration with chronic pain was not understanding
what was going on in my own body and not being in charge of
my own life. I still have my ups and downs but thanks to Dr.
Lonnie Zeltzer and her team, I have my life back.*

—GEORGIA *WWW.TEENPAINHELP.ORG*

CHAPTER 13

PHYSICAL THERAPY, MASSAGE, CRANIO-SACRAL THERAPIES, PERSONAL TRAINING:
HEALING THE BODY AND MIND

PHYSICAL THERAPY: WHAT IS IT? WHAT DOES IT DO?

- Traditional Physical Therapy (PT)
- Finding a Physical Therapist
- Transcutaneous Electrical Nerve Stimulation (TENS) Units.
- Mirror Therapy
- Aqua- and Dry Land Therapies

REHABILITATION PROGRAMS: WHAT DO THEY DO?

MASSAGE THERAPY: WHAT IS IT?

CRANIOSACRAL MASSAGE THERAPY

CHIROPRACTIC

A PERSONAL TRAINER FOR A CHILD/ ADOLESCENT WITH CHRONIC PAIN

PHYSICAL THERAPY: WHAT IS IT? WHAT DOES IT DO?

It almost seems counter-intuitive to tell a preteen soccer star who has had CRPS of her leg for six months, and hurts whenever she moves it— that the pathway to getting better is to exercise— under guidance from a physical therapist. But in fact the research evidence indicates that **exercise is exactly what is needed for CRPS, juvenile fibromyalgia and a number of other painful conditions.**

Examples of muscle tension contributing to chronic pain that we see almost weekly in our WholeChild LA clinic include headaches, back pain, and, even abdominal pain, where children grip their belly in a protective stance against the pain; the gripping tightens belly muscles thus adding to their abdominal distress.

The reason for physical therapy (PT) is that the pain *is* in our soccer player's head! In fact, it is in the areas of the brain that interpret pain suffering, such as the cingulate gyrus, and memory centers in the hippocampus. Active and strong connections in different areas of her brain emphasize feelings of pain in her leg and movement of the leg further activates those neural connections. It is not her imagination; and no, she isn't faking it.

Traditional Physical Therapy (PT)

So now let's explore what the different types of physical therapy are and what you need to know to help your child move back to 'normal'. We asked Kathleen Sluka PT, PhD, who is unique as she is both a registered Physical Therapist and PhD scientist[49]. Dr. Sluka's laboratory studies the peripheral and central mechanisms of chronic musculoskeletal pain and painful injury at the cellular level.

> *Injury Changes the Brain. Muscle and joint pain are very common and occur for many different reasons. Often there is a change within the muscle or joint itself, but there also can be changes throughout the nervous system in the pathways that transmit pain. This occurs in the nerves that transmit pain from the muscle up to the central nervous system, or in any area within the brain.*
>
> *The brain is changeable and is itself modified with input from injured muscle to produce enhanced sensitivity to painful stimuli. For example, nerve cells in the pain pathway become more excitable and respond in an exaggerated way after an injury. They produce chemicals called neurotransmitters that enhance the signal of painful stimuli, so that what used to not produce pain now does. These changes persist even after the injury has healed making the pain last much longer than expected. As you*

---

49 Kathleen A. Sluka, PT, PhD, FAPTA, Professor of Physical Therapy and Rehabilitation Science, University of Iowa Carver College of Medicine.

HEALING THE BODY AND MIND

will see below, regular exercise modifies these changes and makes the neurons less excitable.

Treatments: Myofascial and other types of muscle and joint pain are best treated with regular exercise. The exercises are often targeted to the area of pain, but they can also be more whole body. For localized myofascial pain conditions, exercises are designed to stretch the tightened muscle and strengthen the muscles surrounding the joint or area of pain. These exercise programs will increase the motion from a given joint like the neck or shoulder and will increase the strength around that joint putting less stress on the tissues.

Regular strengthening exercises are also useful to buffer against muscle fatigue. Muscle fatigue is a normal response to use of the muscle. However, if the muscle is weak, it is more easily fatigued. In fact, muscle fatigue releases chemicals into the muscle that activate pain fibers to produce more pain. Often people complain of pain during exercise, especially when initially starting a program. Increasing strength of the muscle allows the muscle to perform more activity at a lower intensity and thus it will reduce fatigue, release of these chemicals and then reduced pain with exercise.

How Exercise Changes You. Exercise activates our endogenous pain relieving systems by releasing the body's opioids to reduce the excitability of the pain neurons. Thus neurons in our brain are less sensitive to painful stimuli. Exercise also changes the immune system so that it releases cytokines that reduce pain. Both human and animal studies show that we can prevent the development of chronic muscle pain with regular physical activity or exercise. The changes with regular exercise can occur with strengthening and regular whole body exercises like walking, running or biking. It is important to realize that you don't have to exercise every day to see an effect – the American College of Sports Medicine recommends 150 minutes of moderate activity per week. That would equate to 30 minutes of exercise, 5 days a week. To monitor yourself and see if you are doing a moderate intensity physical activity, simply determine if you can talk but not sing during that activity.

Why Pain in Early Exercise Programs? While regular physical activity and exercise will reduce pain, initially there may be an increase in pain. The alterations in the muscle, nervous system, and immune systems produced by regular exercise may take 2-3 weeks to develop before you start to see a decrease in pain and a change in the systems themselves. Therefore, it is really important to consistently do the program for the first few weeks. It may also be helpful to add some treatments that will reduce the pain immediately after exercise such as hot pack, hot showers, or ice. Another treatment that can help in older children, adolescents, and adults is transcutaneous electrical nerve stimulation, TENS. This is a small unit that applies electrical current through the skin for pain relief. It activates the body's own pain relieving system and

PAIN IN CHILDREN AND YOUNG ADULTS

counteracts enhanced excitability in the nervous system. It is particularly useful for pain during activities and can also be used during exercise to reduce pain.

Summary *The most effective treatment for chronic pain is an active exercise program. It produces pain relief by 3 different mechanisms: 1) activating the body's pain-relieving systems to reduce neuron excitability, 2) creating alterations in the amount of muscle fatigue, and 3) altering the immune system.*

Diane Poladian[50] is one of our senior physical therapists who has helped pain patients recover for over 20 years; she shares her thoughts and experience with you.

What is Physical therapy? *It is a profession that specializes in evaluation and treatment of movement impairments /limitations due to pain, injury, or disease with the goal of returning the patient to normal activities.*

Physical therapists utilize specific exercises to enhance flexibility, strength, and function, along with interventions such as light therapy, ultrasound, and electrical stimulation to address pain and enhance healing. Manual therapy consists of soft tissue mobilization or massage, muscle energy techniques, or positional release techniques. Physical therapy interventions are research based and provided according to the patient's needs and expectations.

Evaluation: *Physical therapists evaluate function by assessing pain and sensory issues, joint motion, strength, muscle flexibility, endurance, and how a person moves. Compensation often occurs after an injury or when pain is present and must be addressed to restore normal function. Compensatory movement may be due to muscle imbalances due to loss of flexibility and/or strength or to pain inhibitory mechanisms that activate one group of muscles while inhibiting the opposite group. This is easily understood when looking at individuals with back pain. The core and hip stabilizers are inhibited while the muscles of the back are activated to guard the spine. This causes stiffness and pain in the low back that is perpetuated by the lack of spine stability due to the inhibitory response to the core muscles. This is addressed by retraining the core and hip muscles to activate.*

Treatments *Many children with chronic pain have stopped their normal physical activities and exhibit general deconditioning which further limits their ability to return to recreational activities and sports. Therapeutic exercises are specifically designed to improve endurance and to train for recreational and sports activity.*

General Approach: *In a typical physical therapy session, the child is instructed in therapeutic exercises based on the evaluation findings. They are coached to perform*

---

50 Diane Poladian PT DPT OCS, Director of Clinical Development, Progressive Physical Therapy, Inc.
   http://progressivept.net

210

HEALING THE BODY AND MIND

activities with normal motion and may require cues to activate or "turn on" specific muscles. The therapist may alter activities based on the child's response to allow a positive and enjoyable experience when moving their body.

Some children are afraid to move due to the pain they have experienced and may need encouragement along with distraction to perform the activities successfully. Activities and games are used to distract from the pain with focus on normal movement and normal sensations.

- *Using a drum beat while performing agility skills is fun and helps focus the child on the rhythm and movement of their body.*

- *Games such as playing "Simon Says" or throwing and catching a ball while on a wobble board are performed, depending on the age of the child, to help distract from the pain while enhancing physical activity.*

- *Music, dance, balance activities, coordination activities, and sports activities are utilized to help the child return to their previous activity levels.*

During physical therapy, the child is generally not questioned regarding their pain with activity as this may reinforce pain memory, although the child is allowed to report pain. Any activity that is painful is quickly modified to avoid focus on the pain.

Case Example: *Let's take a specific and common example: CRPS*

CRPS: *Children with Complex Regional Pain Syndrome (CRPS) sometimes present not with just pain but also with sensitivity issues and inability to tolerate touch to the affected region. This problem is addressed with desensitization training of the region using varied textures that are applied over the region and/ or mirror therapy.*

Mirror Therapy: *Sometimes, the patient is unable to move a limb due to pain, which limits their ability to walk. This may be addressed with mirror therapy, which retrains the brain to normalize the pain threshold of the affected region. The child places the affected limb in a box with the unaffected limb reflected in a mirror that is attached to the box. The child then moves their unaffected hand or foot; the brain is tricked by the reflection. The brain learns from the reflection that the 'affected limb' is moving and feeling normal. It is important that the child understands the goals of mirror therapy, including working on movement and retraining the nerve messaging to the brain. As the child transitions into more normal activity, the idea of learning what normal feels like in the unaffected limb can then be transferred into the affected side when performing more challenging activities, such as lunges, walking, or hopping.*

Physical Therapist Attributes: *It is important to find a physical therapist that is knowledgeable about central pain. Physical therapists do specialize in many different*

211

areas, including sports injuries, women's health, and pediatrics (for those children with developmental issues), geriatrics, and adults with neurological problems. It is therefore important when scheduling an appointment that the physical therapist has a background in working with chronic or central pain.

Upon the initial visit, the therapist should exhibit empathy for your child and establish trust prior to starting treatment. For example, when a child presents with CRPS of the foot, he may have fear of going through another painful exam. The therapist establishes trust by beginning the exam by having the child actively move their foot within their pain-free range of motion; this allows the child to be in charge. The therapist may encourage the child to be empowered in their healing process with participation in the treatment plan. This may include encouraging the child to be responsible for their home program, instead of the parent. The plan of care should include activities that are not painful. The concept of "no pain, no gain," is usually not appropriate with this population.

Home Program *This may consist of specific exercises, but may also include activities that the child enjoys, such as swimming or water play. It is important to allow the child to perform activities that they enjoy as they are then distracted from the pain while enhancing physical activity. Pain should not be encouraged as a limiting factor to physical activity. Any type of physical activity that the child wants to do, will most likely not aggravate symptoms and should be encouraged.*

Summary: *the primary role of the physical therapist is to help your child's physical structural body become normalized and in balance, including posture, tight or weak muscles, and muscle-nerve mechanics.*

Diane provides these references [14]

Transcutaneous Electrical Nerve Stimulation (TENS) Units

Many PTs also use TENS units for treating pain. This is an electrical gadget that your child can wear and place the electrodes on the part of the body that is in the most pain. The PT can teach your child how to increase the frequency or amount of stimulation so that she feels a comfortable "buzz" that doesn't hurt but feels good. This stimulation blocks pain signals and can be very effective. It also is typically covered by most health insurances.

Let's review an actual case study of a child we treated with Diane:

Case: *Joanne, a 6th grader with CRPS of her left knee, was in a wheelchair when we first saw her. She had seen other physical therapists before she came to our program and found physical therapy "too painful." She believed that it made her condition*

HEALING THE BODY AND MIND

worse, and she resisted it. Joanne's parents were suffering too with their daughter and were distraught; unsure whether making her go to physical therapy (PT) was the best thing to do for their daughter. When we suggested PT as a part of the treatment plan, Joanne and her parents became visibly anxious. We suggested that they just go for one visit and then they could decide if they wanted to continue. We had talked with Diane about Joanne and her previous experiences with PT. Diane knew that she had to form an alliance with Joanne before Joanne would do the physical work she needed to do.

Diane spent her initial session getting to know Joanne and finding out what her interests were. Diane used what she learned to develop games that interested Joanne so that Diane could get her to move her body in a therapeutic way. Diane also worked with Joanne's family to develop motivations and rewards for when Joanne reached certain milestones.

Once Joanne started working with Diane, her progress was immediate. She traded her wheel chair for crutches, and in two weeks she had no need for crutches either. Her pain significantly improved and she was playing ball and other running games with her friends within a few months.

Diane sensed that part of the original problem with PT was that Joanne did not trust her own abilities and feared the pain. As Diane showed *Joanne* that she could do certain things well without pain, physical therapy became fun, and Joanne was able to take increasingly greater risks with her body. She liked and trusted Diane, which helped her to trust herself. By seeing her own accomplishments, she felt more capable and could do more.

Finding a Physical Therapist

Diane suggests the following:

To find a PT resource in your area, use the website of the American Physical Therapy Association at www.apta.org. Once there, click on "Find a PT," put in your zip code and click on "orthopedics." There is also a section for aqua therapy. A list of therapists will come up in your area. Prior to setting up the appointment, inquire if the physical therapist has experience working with children with central pain. Physical therapists that you need should be familiar with mirror therapy and the research work of Butler and Moseley, who authored the book Explain Pain and numerous articles on pain research in physical therapy.

Unfortunately, there is currently only certification in pediatric PT, but not in pediatric pain physical therapy. As with all health care practitioners, the best physical therapist is one who instills trust, independence and confidence in a child and does

213

PAIN IN CHILDREN AND YOUNG ADULTS

not base treatment on a strict protocol that is applied to all patients. For example, Diane used a large ball and other props to engage a young boy with belly pain and chronic fatigue who was apprehensive about PT. She turned their sessions into a game and helped him begin an exercise program that was fun. Soon he asked his parents to buy him a ball and he began using it at home.

AQUATIC (WATER) THERAPY

We often recommend aqua-therapy for our patients who like water and are fearful of dry land PT or for whom weight-bearing physical activity is still too painful to undertake.

Celia deMayo[51] is our program Physical Therapist who specializes in Aquatic Therapy. She comments about what aquatic therapy is and for whom it is most helpful in the context of treating children who have chronic pain; she provides a case example.

Exercise in a swimming pool, instead of dry land, has been an effective treatment for patients experiencing functional limitations for many conditions, ranging from orthopedic and neurological conditions to chronic pain. Aquatic therapy is particularly helpful to children who have chronic pain, whether limited to a specific area or more generalized throughout the body. Aquatic therapy programs are designed specifically for each individual patient, depending upon his/ her particular needs.

What Is Unique About It? *Exercising in the water is beneficial because water's buoyancy limits the impact of gravity and physical activity on the joints. Therefore, the patient can exercise in ways that he/she might not tolerate on land, where gravity is present as a load throughout the activity. Water modulates the impact on joints and provides gentle resistance, thereby strengthening muscles as the person moves through the water. Resistance is easily controlled by the patient by altering his movement speed. That way, the exercise can be kept as gentle as necessary to allow the patient to work to his/her maximum potential, without overdoing it. As patients exercise consistently in the therapeutic pool, their endurance and overall activity tolerance improve, as does confidence in their ability to engage in and enjoy the activity.*

Psychological Benefits: *Although physical benefits of exercising in the water are well known, less familiar are the psychological benefits. Patients experience improved body image, decreases in depression, and improvements in their overall mood. Parents often report that their children sleep better on the days they exercise in the*

---

51 Celia Sabin deMayo MA, MS, PT, OCS, APTA. Board Certified Specialist in Orthopedics, Physical Therapist specializing in Aquatic Therapy. http://kernpt.com/celia/

HEALING THE BODY AND MIND

pool. Whereas children with chronic pain tend to avoid physical activity, exercise in the pool allows them to play and participate in physical activity at the same time. They are often distracted from their pain by the exciting and comforting medium of the water and benefit from age appropriate socialization.

The Evaluation: *Patients are evaluated thoroughly on their first clinic visit to determine the specific pain issues and its subsequent activity restrictions. From there, a comprehensive aquatic program is designed to meet the patient's specific needs. If the child can tolerate attending to the painful body part(s), the exercise/activity program will involve graded mobility, strengthening and functional exercises including and involving the painful body part(s). If, on the other hand, he/she is fearful of involving the painful body part(s), the exercise program will involve activity of non-painful areas, integrating painful ones only as tolerated, or by distraction during water play. Throughout the session, the patient's pace is monitored to allow maximum acceptable activity without overdoing. At the end of most sessions, patients are encouraged to float for relaxation, and to practice some meditation or breathing techniques they might be learning with other team members.*

The Ideal Aquatic Therapy Therapist: *Parents seeking pool therapy for their children should consider the experience and philosophy of the treating therapist(s) and the manner pool therapy sessions are conducted. The program needs to be tailored to the specific issues the child presents with. It is advantageous to work with a therapist who recognizes and communicates to you the interplay between physical and psychological issues existing with chronic pain, understands the mind-body connection, and ideally, one that works within a multidisciplinary team setting. The therapist should be patient, compassionate, and understanding of the causes of chronic pain and its effects on the child and the family. Aquatic therapy sessions are most helpful when the child is comfortable in the environment and when trust is established between the patient/ parents and the treating therapist.*

Case: *I remember fondly 9 year old Joseph who presented to me unable to walk or complete any activities of daily living, after having sprained his ankle while playing with his brother. He was the 'middle child' of 3 boys. Initially, he was hypersensitive to being touched, but immediately enjoyed the experience of being in the pool, even though the most he could tolerate was sitting on the pool bench. He hesitated initially, but within the first session was able to engage in gentle activity involving arm and leg movements while retrieving rings. Eventually, he became interested in swimming, and was able to push off the wall during swimming activities, whereas previously he had been intolerant of anything touching his feet. By the third or fourth visit we could practice standing and within a month he was walking in the pool and ambulating with crutches on dry land.*

PAIN IN CHILDREN AND YOUNG ADULTS

The pool allowed Joseph to explore activity in a non-threatening environment, and he realized that he could gradually increase his activity level without flaring his symptoms. A previously active child, he was able to exercise at a much more intense level in the pool than he could on land. With time, the gains Joe made in the pool certainly carried over to land, and he was willing and able to explore increasing his activity there as well, until he resumed all of his former activity without pain. The pool provided Joseph a safe place to try movements that were frightening on land. He was able to gain the confidence and reconnect with the joy of movement without the anxiety of his pain returning and limiting him.

If you cannot find a physical therapist in your area with experience working with children with chronic pain, tell the therapist that you want a gradual reconditioning program to help your child become more active. The therapist should assess your child for muscle strength and tone and for areas of muscle spasm; and work on these areas with a series of stretching exercises.

REHABILITATION PROGRAMS

Sometimes improvement does not happen for a while or things seem to be going downhill. We asked Dr. Deidre Logan[52] and Caitlin Conroy, Psy.D. at Boston Children's Hospital to give us their insights on how their program works and what are the expected results. See also the Program locator table in the Appendix.

Pediatric Pain Rehabilitation (PPR): PPR is the treatment approach for chronic pain that focuses on functional restoration of pain-related disability. It is collaboration among multidisciplinary providers in an inpatient or day-treatment model. It is helpful for children who have tried less intense treatment options and have not returned to functional activities or who need more frequent/ intensive therapy to achieve functional goals. Staff in PPR programs includes clinicians from physical therapy (PT), occupational therapy (OT), nursing, medicine, psychology, social work, or recreational therapy. Complementary therapies like acupuncture, Reiki, art therapy or movement therapy also may be included. There are benefits to receive combinations of therapies in a single program, including frequent communication among providers and the ability to work on interdisciplinary goals in a shared setting.

PPR programs can be housed within rehabilitative or acute hospital settings or outpatient settings; therapies typically occur throughout the day. Goals of treatment include

---

52 Deirdre Logan, PhD; Director Psychology Services, Pain Medicine Children's Hospital, Boston.Associate Professor, Harvard Medical School. Editor, Pediatric Pain Letter (*www.childpain.org/ppl*) & Caitlin Conroy, PsyD, Psychologist, Mayo Family PPRC Boston Children's Hospital. Instructor, Harvard Medical School

attending school regularly, regaining physical strength, mobility and independence, and learning coping strategies for pain and stress. Patients receive education about pain and a wide variety of management strategies. The focus is to treat pain from the Bio-Psycho-Social model, meaning that the physical and emotional aspects that impact family and friends are treated simultaneously.

Goals are achieved from using land-based and/or aquatic physical therapy to cognitive behavioral (CBT) pain management to community based activities, such as a school visit or practicing a social outing. Parents are involved in the model both in learning about their child's treatment as well as learning new parenting strategies. Programs typically have a group format that provides social support and exposure to peers who face similar struggles.

An Example Program: *The Mayo Family Pediatric Pain Rehabilitation Center (PPRC) at Boston Children's Hospital is one example. In PPRC children attend the program during the day (8a to 4p), Monday through Friday and either commute from their homes or find short term local housing. During the day, the patients (aged 8-young adult) participate in a combination of individual/ group based therapies of PT, OT, psychology and recreational therapy. They receive daily medical assessment and nursing care and have a block of time devoted to school work. The team works collaboratively to develop and achieve shared treatment goals. For example, if a child has not been attending school regularly, each discipline will work on complementary aspects of returning to school. PT will work on the child's ability to move within the school environment such as taking stairs or walking through halls. OT may work on proper sitting posture and backpack wear as well as desensitizing to noises, sights, and other stimulation within the school environment. Psychology will help improve coping strategies and address anxiety about attending school and recreational therapy may help the child reconnect with friends and develop a plan for returning to sports or other extra-curricular activities. The entire team works with school staff to provide education and recommendations so the child has a successful reentry to school.*

With group-based treatment the children with chronic pain conditions interact in a supported environment with other children with similar conditions. Group based treatments include group PT and OT, group psychology, music therapy group and recreational therapy groups. The PPRC also includes group-based support and education for parents in which parents observe their child's PT or OT or participate in family psychological counseling at designated "family" sessions. Average length of stay is 3-4 weeks.

Patients are discharged with a comprehensive plan to help them meet their goals: instructions on how to maintain physical progress, what to do if a flare-up of pain occurs, and recommendations for outpatient therapies upon their return home. The former patient, independently, should be able to manage pain with new and effective coping strategies and tools to reintegrate into their academic, social, and recreational lives.

PAIN IN CHILDREN AND YOUNG ADULTS

The PPRC schedules follow up visits with the first visit around one-month post-discharge and then subsequent visits as indicated. Follow-ups include re-evaluation by PT, OT, psychology and medicine. They are designed to provide a multidisciplinary view of the child's progress as well as any new recommendations.

Outcomes have been excellent to date, with patients achieving improvements in function and reductions in pain that are typically maintained/ improved at follow up. Outcome studies demonstrate these programs' successes[15].

MASSAGE THERAPY: WHAT IS IT?

Massage therapy is based on the belief that when muscles are overworked, waste products (like lactic acid) accumulate in the muscle, causing soreness and stiffness. The therapy improves circulation in the muscle, increasing flow of nutrients and eliminating waste products. There are different forms of massage such as Swedish massage, deep tissue massage, and craniosacral therapy. The type used will depend on the child's pain problem.

Dr. Kathi Kemper[53] offers her perspective on massage:

__Massage:__ Massage is commonly provided at home by parents and in clinical settings by professional massage therapists, physical therapists, and nurses. For example, infant massage is routinely provided in neonatal intensive care units to offer comfort and promote growth and development in preterm infants. Massage is beneficial for children suffering from colic, headache, insomnia, and juvenile rheumatoid arthritis. It helps athletes with sore muscles recover more quickly from an intense workout so they can continue training. Massage therapy is generally safe. Professional massage practice is regulated by state governments; over 44 states license massage therapists, while three offer state-wide independent certification. Combining aromatherapy with massage may offer additional benefits in terms of comfort, relaxation, and stress reduction. Massage can reduce heart rate, relax muscles, improve range of motion in joints, and increase production of the body's natural painkillers. It also can relieve headaches and lower blood pressure. Although massage is usually safe, it should not be done over an open wound, skin infection, phlebitis (inflammation of a vein), or in areas where bones are weak. If your child's joints are inflamed or if she has an injury, check with her doctor before she has a massage.

Nine-year-old Abe had chronic tension headaches. We referred Abe to Cara Amenta, our pain program massage therapist. His mother was taught by Cara how to massage

---

53 Kathi Kemper, M.D. Professor Pediatrics College of Medicine. Executive Director, Center for Integrative Health and Wellness, The Ohio State University http://fic.osu.edu/members/directory/k/kemper-kathi.html

218

HEALING THE BODY AND MIND

Abe's scalp, neck, shoulders and upper back, and they developed a 15-minute massage routine before he went to sleep. Abe describes this experience:

I used to get scared to go to sleep at night because I knew my head would keep hurting and I wouldn't want to be alone 'cause of the pain. Then Cara would come to our house and rub my head and back and that made my head stop hurting. My mom used to try to rub my head but she rubbed too hard and it hurt. Cara taught my mom how to do it just right and that felt sooo good that I went right to sleep.

We asked Cara Amenta[54], our pain program massage therapist, to talk about massage.

Massage therapy is an ancient form of bodywork that involves manually moving and shifting the tissues of the body to promote flexibility, relaxation, pain relief, and circulation. A massage therapist works directly with the muscles, tendons, and ligaments that attach to the bones. Massage helps children with chronic pain because it approaches pain management from both a mind and body perspective.

Nine-year-old Alyssa had tension headaches that were persistent for months. Massage therapy helped to relax and release the tight muscles and connective tissues that were causing the pain; it also helped to lower her stress level by reducing the stress hormone, cortisol, and by releasing endorphins, the feel-good chemicals in the body that block out pain signals and create feelings of euphoria.

When Should a Parent Consider Massage Therapy? *The easy answer is whenever their child has any kind of musculoskeletal pain that does not clear in 3-7 days. Children with chronic headaches, fibromyalgia, soft tissue injuries, and painful scar tissue sites, pain after surgeries, contractures, and nerve impingement caused by muscular tension are great candidates for massage.*

Massage can also be very supportive for children whose pain doesn't have a musculoskeletal source; for example: a child with irritable bowel syndrome (IBS). These children may be constipated and have abdominal pain. While massage may not solve the primary stomach or intestinal issues, the massage can gently shift the abdominal contents and encourage movement of the intestines that can facilitate the child having a bowel movement.

Criteria Parents Should Look for in a Massage Therapist *Consider both credentials and compassion in the practitioner. Parents should feel comfortable asking the potential therapists about their previous work and study with children, and what techniques they like to use when working with children versus adults. I have found*

---

54   Cara Amenta B.A., CMT, NCTM. Massage Therapist. Massage Therapy for Inner Peace, Relaxation and Therapy *www.amtamassage.org/famt/caraamenta*

PAIN IN CHILDREN AND YOUNG ADULTS

that my training in myofascial release and neuromuscular techniques have been crucial. These are gentle techniques that work with, and not against, the body. They are much less invasive than deep tissue massage and still create positive results. Parents should use their best judgment in gauging the compassion of their massage therapist, whose ability to empathize with a child and develop trust is crucial to success. Practitioners can develop trust by:

- *Allowing the child to be in control of the session,*

- *Letting the child know they can speak up at any time if they are uncomfortable or want to stop,*

- *Checking in frequently to see how the child is feeling in session.*

Case: Beverly was 16 years old and struggled her whole life with a 50-degree scoliosis that had caused a prominent "S" curve in her spine and a great deal of pain. When I started working with her, she already had successful surgery to correct the scoliosis, but she was still in pain, even though her back was now in alignment.

Beverly's enthusiasm and determination to feel better had an undeniable impact on our sessions. Her muscles would twitch and move involuntarily as they relaxed. By using neuromuscular exercises and techniques that encourage the natural movement of the body, she let go of her pain and was able to do the activities a high school girl should be able to do, like dancing at her senior prom without pain. The process itself took about one year of weekly sessions.

For Beverly, massage therapy, plus her determination to feel better and live a pain-free life, were what helped her heal. Massage therapy is a powerful form of bodywork that has been shown to have both positive physical and emotional effects. I encourage parents to explore massage therapy as an option if their child is in pain.

CRANIOSACRAL THERAPY: WHAT IS IT?

Craniosacral therapy is a type of body or manual therapy that is playing an increasing role in mind-body work that influences the nervous system and bringing it into better balance. We asked our program craniosacral therapist, Karen Axelrod[55], to comment on its uses and theories of action.

CranioSacral Therapy (CST) is a manual therapy that enhances function of your craniosacral system—i.e., the membranes and cerebrospinal fluid surrounding and protecting the brain and spinal cord. CST enhances proper central nervous system

---

55   Karen Axelrod MA, CST-D CMT. Diplomate-Certified CranioSacral Therapist, Redondo Beach, CA; certified CST instructor for Upledger Institute International; Craniosacral therapist.*www.karenaxelrod.com*

HEALING THE BODY AND MIND

function and can boost the body's ability to dissipate negative effects of stress. By softly touching the bones of the head and gently releasing restrictions elsewhere within the body's wide network of connective tissue known as fascia, CST can effect profound structural changes within the body.

How Does Craniosacral Therapy Help Children with Chronic Pain? Because of its light touch and inherently relaxing nature, CST can help reduce internal stress and negotiate the transition into a more parasympathetic state to eliminate improper pain signaling. It is ideal for children who have tender points in their muscles or whose pain is exacerbated by the slightest touch or movement. As the CST therapist gently releases restrictions within the musculoskeletal and nervous systems, he/she may also incorporate guided imagery or other relaxation techniques so children can learn to identify and self-regulate stress before it intensifies and triggers pain.

During the course of treatment, as the body softens and the child drops into deeper states of relaxation—and remains there for longer periods of time between CST sessions—the nervous system regains its ability to properly regulate pain signals. As underlying tension dissipates, bones, muscles, organs, and nerves that form part of the pain cycle eventually regain normal function. This process improves lymphatic flow to boost the immune system and blood flow within the cardiovascular system.

When Should Parents Consider Craniosacral Therapy? As with most complementary healing modalities, the sooner one seeks treatment the better. If the pain resulted from an accident or injury, seeking treatment within one week would be ideal. [The longer the child goes without treatment, the more her body starts to associate chronic pain as being the "new normal."] If your child has been suffering from pain for months or even years and other treatment modalities have failed to break the cycle, CST might be a next step.

A Typical CST Treatment Session The child may lay down on the treatment table; sit up (if capable) and draw, read, or play; or be held in a parent's lap. The therapist gently assesses for fascial, boney, and other inherent movements in the body, and then seeks to release restrictions and restore movement where it is lacking. The therapist often has older children feel the restriction; this gives the child a keener internal awareness of how that part of his/her body is held. As the child gains self-awareness and the therapist continues working through many layers of injured tissue, tight areas begin to soften. Pain sensations dissipate. The child re-experiences his/her body as a safe, pain-free container. The child regains trust that his/her body can heal.

Case Example: CST was effective in helping 15-year-old Kevin recover from chronic upper back and neck pain that resulted from a severe concussion following a skateboarding accident. In addition to upper body pain, Kevin experienced dizziness, loss of concentration, headaches, lethargy, and slight nystagmus. He withdrew from school for four weeks when he noticed that loud noises and crowds increased his pain.

PAIN IN CHILDREN AND YOUNG ADULTS

Kevin received five initial CST treatments in four weeks. The impact from his fall created a severe compression at the base of his skull, mostly on the right side. This may have led to agitation of the nerves in his neck and brain stem. The CranioSacral therapist helped to gently decompress the bones in his skull and to relax his neck and shoulder muscles.

Within one week, he no longer experienced dizziness or headaches. By week three, his ability to concentrate had returned, his eyes normalized, and the pain level was half that prior to treatment. He attended a birthday party after week 4 and reported no activation from the crowd or loud noises. Kevin's energy level was back to normal; he returned to school.

Kevin had two more follow-up CST treatments over the next two months. His mother reported, "Our son is doing really well, no symptoms of pain, and having a fun high school life. CranioSacral Therapy was an effective treatment for his concussion."

The State of the Science: *Numerous studies have shown CranioSacral Therapy to be effective in regulating the autonomic nervous system[16], decreasing anxiety and depression[17], and relieving chronic neck pain[18], headaches, migraines, and other pain syndromes[19,20]. While most studies have involved adults, empirical evidence has demonstrated similar results with children.*

To understand how CST can reduce chronic pain, it is important to understand how the central nervous system works. When we experience pain and stress, our nervous system moves into the "fight-or-flight"—or sympathetic—state. When we are stress-free, our body is in the balanced parasympathetic state. The parasympathetic state is what promotes relaxation and rejuvenation. This is the opposite of the sympathetic state, which prepares our body to fight, flee, or freeze in response to perceived danger.

Escape from "danger" is facilitated when the sympathetic nervous system activates the release of stress hormones that increase heart rate, flush muscles with blood, and prepare the body to fight or flee. When danger has passed, the normal response is a return to the balanced parasympathetic state at least until the next "threat" appears. In chronic pain, the threat is not knowing how serious that next wave of pain will be... or when it will go away. When we experience ongoing stress or chronic pain, our body spends more time in the sympathetic state.

Stress creates muscle tension. If muscles are always slightly contracted (i.e., ready to "fight or flee"), this eventually affects nerves, tissues, and organs that continue to feed the pain cycle. Until the body feels "safe" and is assured that the "danger" has passed, we will not move out of fight-or-flight and into a relaxed, balanced parasympathetic state that ultimately breaks the cycle of pain.

How Do Parents Choose a CST Practitioner? *CST is practiced by numerous types of healthcare practitioners: massage therapists, physical and occupational therapists,*

222

HEALING THE BODY AND MIND

> *naturopaths, homeopaths, acupuncturists, chiropractors, medical doctors, and osteopaths. Be sure your CranioSacral Therapist is certified by his or her educational institution. The Upledger Institute (www.upledger.com) and Biodynamic Craniosacral Therapy Association (www.craniosacraltherapy.org) are certifying bodies for paramedical professionals. Chiropractors and osteopaths often receive craniosacral training as part of their education. www.cranialacademy.org*

CHIROPRACTIC[56]

More than 50,000 chiropractors are licensed in the US, including licensure in all 50 states. Chiropractic care is covered by most major insurers. Up to 14% of all chiropractic visits are for pediatric patients, not including care provided by chiropractors working for athletic departments or professional teams. While chiropractic care may be useful for treating musculoskeletal injuries, **parents need to be cautioned not to rely on chiropractic as the primary treatment for serious conditions such as cancer or arthritis.** Severe complications are possible but are fortunately rare for chiropractic treatment of infants and children.

PERSONAL TRAINER FOR A CHILD/ADOLESCENT WITH CHRONIC PAIN

Many parents ask us, what happens after physical therapy (PT) has been completed or we have run out of insurance benefits? The problem is that some children are not athletic; and in some schools, physical education (PE) has become an elective or is not offered. What then? In almost every community in North America there are many private, franchised, or national 'work out' gyms, all with "personal trainers." The challenge is that most of the latter individuals lack specific education or know little about injury, pain or rehabilitation.

Choosing the Right Trainer

We posed questions to an experienced, certified trainer, Joe Garcia[57] of Arena Fitness, in Encino, CA, about his recommendations for the right time to start a training regimen for a child or adolescent with chronic pain: His philosophy is *"Move well first, and then you can move often."* Here are his views:

---

56 Kathi Kemper, M.D. Professor Pediatrics, Ohio State College of Medicine, contributed this section.

57 Joe Garcia NASM-CPT, SFG, FMS, Program Director, Arena Fitness Training Center, Encino, CA.
    www.arenafitness.com

PAIN IN CHILDREN AND YOUNG ADULTS

The answer to these questions is complicated and clouded by the child's pain and confirmed by the parent's protection of his or her child's pain. The "truth" is that it's never going to feel like the right time, but there is a way to determine the "safest" time to start Training. But first let's start with the "trainer."

Nine Key Points to Remember When Picking the Right Trainer and Training PROGRAM.

1 **Health Questionnaire.** *Health History or Athletic History should be the starting point for every Training Program. The #1 cause for injury in any person starting a Training regimen is "previous injury." The history can help the Trainer determine if he/ she is at risk for injury and where. It is a screen for any medications that may raise or lower heart rate. Oh yes, remember, adolescents should avoid energy drinks at all times.*

2 **Fitness Screening & Assessments.** *Is the Training Program individual or generalized? At the least, a 12-week Training Program designed in advance is the most effective and efficient for yielding the best results. Individualized Training starts with a screen and reassessment in about 6 weeks.*

3 *Get a **doctor's clearance** if there any doubts.*

4 *Train hard but **always train smart** first. How do we do that? We need to produce quick results for your child/ in order to show him/her that this is going to work. Sometimes we only have a small window of opportunity to convince him/ her that this is the right path for a better pain-free future.*

5 **Movement based Training Systems Vs Performance based Training Systems.** *What's the difference? Which one is right? Reassessment is the key. Performance based Training or Volume Training focuses on "capacity" of work- measured by integrity of postures and patterns against fatigue over time. Movement based Training Systems test "Competency" of the child's movement pattern prior to loading that pattern. This will start by identifying a dysfunctional movement pattern by using FMS or other form of Movement Screening tool.*

   *From there the Trainer designs an exercise protocol to establish Static and eventually Dynamic Motor Control resulting in competency of the specific movement pattern, before moving on to a Performance based training system. **Establishing which patterns of movement are being performed with competency Vs. which have a dysfunction is essential prior to starting your training regimen.** Dysfunctional Movement patterns in a Performance based Training System often result in injury. It is not a question of "if" it will happen; it is a question of...when.*

6 **Health & Medical Team Network.** *Who does he/she work with to keep you Healthy? Ask whom he or she is affiliated with. Call them. Often Trainers exaggerate their true relationship with people in the medical field, so make sure that it's a solid relationship.*

HEALING THE BODY AND MIND

7   **Program Description.** *Does he/she have a "System", a "Plan", a "Workout" that is easily explained to you. Are there handouts so you can review and understand the plan?*

8   **Credentials.** *Degrees and Training Certifications in the Health Industry can vary from Exercise Physiologists to Kinesiologists to Human Movement Specialists. Which Training degree/ certification do you want your Trainer to have for your specific needs? Are they current on all their educational requirements? Are they CPR Certified? This one is important and overlooked.*

9   **Experience.** *3 Years or more is useful, 5 years is needed for Special Populations. Professionalism. Punctuality and appearance will tell you much about the Trainer you have chosen. Results. What do his/her clients say about him/her?*

Reconditioning an Adolescent with IBS

We asked another trainer, Stacey Garcia[58] at Arena Fitness how she might counsel and set up a program for a 16-year-old adolescent with IBS who has become deconditioned:

Case #1: I met with Lois on a quiet Tuesday afternoon with very few clients in the gym. I wanted to be sure she felt comfortable as she seemed nervous as it had been some time since she felt well enough to exercise. I shared my own GI challenges and how I felt when exercising. Sometimes, it was that one hour a day where I had the most relief. I wanted Lois to know that I myself had experienced something very similar to what she deals with, that I understood and I was there to help. I asked her what her favorite activities were to ensure she was active every day for one hour, even when she was unable to come see me. She loved to dance so I made sure to incorporate some ballet bar work into our twice weekly sessions. I told her mom after her session that the secret to sustaining a long-term goal is by setting lots of specific, attainable short-term goals along the way with non-food related rewards: a new outfit after one month of consistently showing up to all workouts and doing her best.

We would start with the following exercises: self-myofascial release for 5 minutes then warm up with a minute each of squats, lunges, glute bridges and planks. Our circuit would include resistance band chest press, resistance band rows, dumbbell (8 lb.) squats, dumbbell (8 lb.) shoulder press, push-ups, plank, 1/4 mile on the treadmill, then abdominal cool-down of Pilates 100's, leg lifts and bicycle kicks.

---

58   Stacey Garcia, CPT, FNS, WLS; Shred Weight Loss Director. Arena Fitness Training Center, Encino, CA. *www.arenafitness.com*

225

PAIN IN CHILDREN AND YOUNG ADULTS

Lois committed to working out with me twice a week along with taking two dance classes and walking her dog on the weekends. I also customized a food plan to help her lose weight and keep her IBS symptoms at bay. IBS can sometimes be triggered by stress, and exercise is one of the best remedies. Lois left our first meeting feeling excited to start her new wellness journey.

Now we have covered the *physical* methods for the reconditioning and reprogramming of central pain... the reboot.

In the next chapter, let's move on to another critical component of the Bio-Psycho-Social model for eliminating the pain, *psychological* approaches. These methods address connections within the brain that, when repetitive loops form, continue the pain. Modern research has shown us that **how and what we think greatly influences pain circuits... and reprogramming the circuits will help to change the neural signaling responsible for pain.**

Table 13.1 Resources for Physical Rehabilitation Methods	
Find Physical Therapist	*www.apta.org*
Find Massage Therapist	*www.amtamassage.org/findamassage/index.html*
Find Craniosacral Therapist	*www.craniosacraltherapy.org/practitioner-referral*
Child Pain Letter	*www.childpain.org/ppl*

CHAPTER 14

PSYCHOLOGICAL AND BEHAVIORAL THERAPIES:
HELP FOR PARENTING THE CHILD WITH PAIN

"I'm not worried about my future.
I'm sad about everything I'm missing right now."

Two things happened when my daughter said that: my heart broke, and I realized... how right she was. It took some time for me to trust that she was feeling everything she said she was and she really couldn't go to school yet again. That I shouldn't push her to do things ... or that I should push her to do things when it seemed like she shouldn't...I wasn't giving her the space that trust requires. I wanted so much—for her to be well."

—JM, DAD.

THE INTEGRATIVE APPROACH-THE BIO-PSYCHO-SOCIAL MODEL

WHAT IS PSYCHOLOGICAL THERAPY?

- Cognitive Behavioral Therapy (CBT)
- Dialectical Behavioral Therapy (DBT), and
- Acceptance and Commitment Therapy (ACT)

ANXIETY, DEPRESSION / SUICIDAL RISK

PSYCHOLOGICAL TREATMENT FOR THE FAMILY:

- Family Therapy- What Is It?
- When Should You Consider Family Therapy?
- Family Therapy and Behavioral Plans
- How did my Child's Pain Become Family Pain?
- Kids and Parents Reflect on what they learned in Family Therapy
- Individual Parent Issues
- Marital Therapy
- Couples therapy, including Fathers
- Choosing a Therapist

227

So, when is psychotherapy helpful? This chapter answers this and other questions you may have regarding the roles of individual and family therapy for children with chronic pain.

THE INTEGRATIVE APPROACH – THE BIO-PSYCHO-SOCIAL MODEL FOR TREATMENT

Our experience is that for most children with disabling chronic pain, an integrative therapeutic approach has the best chance for success. That is, a treatment plan should include specific combinations of psychological intervention, physical therapy, complementary therapy, and, if needed, focused medication. Which ones are included depend on the *neurobiology*, that is, the temperament of the child with pain. It is the goal of the psychological intervention component to help children build the skills needed to cope, function, and feel empowered in this process.

Psychological parts of the treatment for chronic pain may include any combination of individual child intervention, individual parent psychological support, family work, or couples' intervention. All aspects of the psychological part of the treatment package for children are aimed at helping the child to increase function and quality of life, and to reduce pain. They are not aimed at "discovering some deep-seated psychological problem." Rather, **the combinations within the psychological treatment arm are intended to help the child climb out of chronic pain by learning self-help tools** as well as helping the family to most effectively and efficiently help the child in this process. If emotional, behavioral, or learning problems are uncovered, then the psychological intervention process helps with those issues that impact pain as well.

We have observed that **many children and teens with chronic pain hold in their feelings, especially negative feelings such as sadness and anger**. They are sensitive to the negative feelings of others but do not express their own anger. They are invested in "being good" and "well-behaved" and not causing distress for other members of the family.

Our team psychologist, Dr. Samantha Levy[59], provides advice to help teens who have chronic pain.

For every negative emotion that you feel but do not express, some "gunk" is put into a jar. What will happen if the jar gets too full? The lid likely will blow off. "That is your pain." What would happen if you poked a hole in the jar every day, just big

---

59 Samantha Levy, Ph.D. Clinical Psychologist, Member of UCLA and WCLA Pediatric pain team.
 www.wholechildla.org/clinical_team.php?pid email: *srlevy@aol.com*

PSYCHOLOGICAL AND BEHAVIORAL THERAPIES

enough to let some of the gunk ooze out? The lid won't blow because the pressure would be eased inside the jar.

Sometimes children have problems coping with day-to-day events. They may view certain situations as overwhelming or avoid those they feel incapable of handling. They "give up" readily with daily hassles so that when larger problems come up, they retreat and leave the problem to someone else, typically a parent, to solve. This passive coping style is especially problematic when these same children have to confront a pain problem. **Psychological therapies are there for children with coping difficulties to develop positive ways to appraise or view situations and to handle them with more effective tools.** In this way, the pressure cooker filled with negative feelings has an escape valve to allow the steam to release on a regular basis so the pot can be filled with more satisfying emotions.

WHAT IS PSYCHOLOGICAL THERAPY?

Even in the most cohesive, loving families, a child's pain can lead to family stress, frustration, helplessness, hopelessness, and discord. We asked one of our pain program psychotherapists, Azita Sachmachian, MFT,[60] to describe psychotherapy and how it can be helpful for the family that becomes stressed because of their child's pain.

In olden times when young people were sad or anxious, they might seek a compassionate person to disclose their most intimate feelings and thoughts. This wise, gentle and trustworthy individual (a grandma or a very good friend) could provide a shoulder to cry on and give good advice. Due to complexities of modernization, travel and industrialization, that role has now graduated from the informal table of grandma's kitchen to a more in-depth approach with "professionals" treating emotional pain in what we now refer to as "psychotherapy."

Psychotherapy is a science that sheds light into the interplay of our thoughts, feelings and actions. It helps us understand why we are anxious, depressed or fearful in our lives. It also makes us understand why we engage in behaviors that we know are not good for us and why we avoid doing things that we know will benefit us. Psychotherapy treats our emotional aches and pains. The core of psychotherapy is based on non-judgmental, compassionate understanding of human emotions.

There are many types of psychological interventions: this next section will discuss them. When a child has a pain problem that is not responding to medications, many

---

60 Azita Sachmachian, MFT, Licensed Marriage and Family Therapist; Board Certified Art Therapist LMFT, ATR-BC; Therapist in the WCLA and UCLA Pediatric Pain Programs *www.Azitasach.com*

PAIN IN CHILDREN AND YOUNG ADULTS

physicians will suggest a mental health specialist, with this referral suggesting to the child that the problem is not *physical* but *psychological*. However, as we have described throughout this book, **pain is *never* purely "physical" or "psychological."**

In Chapters 2, 11-13, we discussed the *mechanisms* of how emotional factors cause a pain problem to worsen if they are not addressed. In this chapter, we revisit some of those factors (such as anxiety, depression, coping problems, social skills deficits, and others) and see how to address them with psychological interventions aimed at the child, parents, and/or family.

Cognitive Behavioral Therapy (CBT)[21]

One of the common and most researched types of psychological intervention for children with chronic pain is CBT. CBT helps children to identify and resolve different situations that cause them stress and pain and helps them to adopt new ways to react. It teaches them how to be calm so that they can feel better, think more clearly, and make better decisions.

In the example below, Angela, a child with chronic pain, feels like a failure, is hard on herself, and tends to see the world through a glass half empty rather than half full. If she makes a mistake on a quiz, she often tells herself, *"I'm so stupid! I should have studied more and I'm going to fail the class now."* In CBT, Angela would learn to remind herself that everyone makes mistakes, that one quiz will not affect her grade significantly, and that she can stop all the "I should have's" on herself. CBT will help her learn how to do this effectively.

Often in CBT, children first practice being able to think about the things that make them anxious and then think or imagine themselves in the situation. They practice, first in their imagination and then in the real world, doing the easiest task and work their way up to the more complicated problems, as they can now remain calm at each level. This accomplishing a task in small increments is called *desensitization*.

Case: Angela is a 13-year-old with irritable bowel syndrome that was causing her such severe belly pain that she was unable to return to school after winter break. She had significant anxiety, with lots of worrying about missing school, getting behind, not getting 'A's, not being able to make the basketball team, her parents' health, her father's job, her sister's asthma to name a few of her worries. Angela began to focus on her belly pain in the morning before school and, according to her, she "tried to go to school" but was unable to and she worried that even if she forced herself, she would never be able to stay in school because of her pain. Soon she began worrying the night before school. All of these worries made her pain worse and worse, and she was missing more and more school, and getting further behind.

230

PSYCHOLOGICAL AND BEHAVIORAL THERAPIES

Since Angela had been a straight 'A' student and was a perfectionist, she worried constantly about getting behind and not being able to get 'A's. She then worried that her GPA in middle school and then in high school would be too low to get into a good college and she would never have the career that she would have wanted.

This type of catastrophic thinking (projecting worse and worse scenarios for the future) was causing Angela's body to be in chronic stress mode and we know that physiological stress will increase pain. So not surprisingly her pain worsened. This didn't mean that there was some "undiscovered disease" but rather that clearly her stress about missing school was exacerbating the pain and causing a vicious cycle that created more pain. We referred Angela to a psychologist for CBT to help her develop the tools to extract herself from the stress/pain cycle.

The Plan The psychologist first helped Angela figure out what kinds of situations made her feel tense and have more pain. It wasn't school in general that made her anxious, but some bullies at school who had made fun of her just before winter break. She had not been back to school since. She now had identified a significant and specific problem that was stressful for her.

Angela learned the technique known as "thought-stopping." When thoughts about school and seeing these students came into her mind, (e.g. they are going to laugh at me and get everyone in the school to laugh at me) now she would tell herself, "stop… this is not going to happen… I can handle seeing them."

Angela learned breathing exercises to calm herself when she felt her heart racing or her hands becoming sweaty. She now had a plan for what she would do at school when she saw the other students and figured out how she might react in a couple of different scenarios, depending on how the girls behaved toward her (e.g. if they looked at her, laughed, pushed her, etc.)

Angela practiced this plan in her mind first and then role-played it with her therapist. She was able to go to school and, even though the girls laughed at her, as she had feared, she was prepared for it. Now she was able to ignore them and feel OK. This made it easier for her to return to school the next day. As her stress about going to school lessened and she felt more competent, her belly pain also lessened and she could easily get caught up in the missed work and she continued to make all A's.

We asked Tanya Palermo, PhD, Seattle, WA[61], a leading pediatric pain psychologist, and expert in CBT for children with chronic pain, to talk further about CBT.

> ***How do you think about CBT?*** *Cognitive-behavioral therapy (CBT) is a type of psychological treatment that teaches skills to change the way we think and act. It is a type of "self-management therapy." This means that a person learns skills to use*

---

61 Tonya Palermo, PhD, Professor of Anesthesiology and Pain Medicine, University of Washington and Seattle Children's Research Institute, Seattle, WA. *www.seattlechildrens.org/medical-staff/tonya-m-palermo*

and manage his/ her own condition. For children and adolescents with chronic pain, the goals for learning CBT are two: A) To increase participation in important daily activities (such as going to school) and B) For the child and family to learn to cope and feel better.

CBT is usually brief and can be learned over several months. Major skills that children and their parents learn include relaxation strategies, sleep and healthy lifestyle habits, communication strategies, changing behavior through reward systems, and ways of thinking differently. An important component of CBT is the opportunity for regular practice to try out new skills. For example, when relaxation strategies are taught, children are asked to practice the strategies every day to encourage rapid learning.

How does CBT help? CBT has been used for over 30 years to help kids with chronic pain. There is scientific evidence that CBT is effective for reducing pain and improving children's physical functioning. As an example, CBT might help an adolescent with migraine headaches with its interference in her daily activities. Goals and interventions might include:

- using behavior plans to work on attending school regularly,

- learning sleep interventions to improve falling and staying asleep, and

- learning relaxation strategies to promote feelings of calm and decreasing stress.

When should a parent of a child with chronic pain consider seeking a CBT approach from a psychologist? Many children with chronic pain cope very well, but when chronic pain starts to interfere with important life activities like participation in school, social activities, extracurricular activities, consultation to learn CBT strategies can be enormously beneficial. For example, a parent might notice poorly adaptive behavioral changes in their child that last for weeks or months at a time; therapy can be helpful in this setting. Some children become very sad, hopeless, or withdrawn in response to having chronic pain. Other children experience increased worries. These behavioral changes are important to address because they make coping with chronic pain more challenging.

What is new on the CBT front for kids with chronic pain? Much of the current work on CBT for kids with chronic pain is focused on making treatment brief, and delivering it remotely to children and families in their homes. The goal is to improve access to pain treatment since many families cannot get appropriate treatment in their local communities. To overcome distance from Centers, several computer programs and Smartphone applications have been developed to monitor pain and teach CBT strategies to children and their parents. These programs use interactive components of the internet (such as videos and games) to teach CBT strategies. Several programs

PSYCHOLOGICAL AND BEHAVIORAL THERAPIES

are undergoing evaluation in research clinical trials and should become available to the public in the near future.

To learn more about CBT strategies that can be learned by parents to help their child or teen cope with chronic pain, see Managing your Child's Chronic Pain, by T.M. Palermo and EF Law, Oxford University Press: New York, NY. 2015

Dialectical Behavioral Therapy (DBT)[62]

Dialectic means accepting and balancing what seem like opposing views. For example, you can accept your child as he/she is in this moment *and* also expect him/her to change and make his/her life better. Similarly, adolescents with pain learn to do the same acceptance and balance with their parents. Both learn how to accept and tolerate painful feelings, their current life situations and themselves. DBT teaches that acceptance of "what is" will be needed first to create change later. DBT teaches other "balances" such as acceptance and hope, independence and assistance, choices and limits, giving in and choosing priorities, and for parents, firmness and gentleness.

The goal of DBT is to replace ineffective, maladaptive, or unskilled behavior with skillful responses. It was originally developed to help suicidal adults but has been adapted and studied for work with depressed and/or anxious adolescents and for those with chronic pain (who often have both depression and anxiety). It is a structured, didactic psychological intervention, often carried out in a group setting, with either adolescents alone or with adolescents and their parents. It has a heavy emphasis on modeling, instructions, behavioral rehearsal, feedback and coaching, and homework assignments. DBT provides training in mindfulness skills, interpersonal effectiveness, emotional regulation, and distress tolerance. Examples of DBT training include learning that two things that seem contradictory can both be true. That is, there may be a parent view and teen view of a situation that seem polar opposites. **In DBT, teens and parents learn to find ways to consider the other's thoughts and that both may have some merit.** The goal is to accept both views and yet develop a new path forward in interacting with each other. This new middle path is important between parents and children and also between each of the parents.

DBT teaches awareness and balance in language to avoid extreme words like always/never and no-one/everyone. DBT teaches the importance of validation... that is letting your parent (your teen) know you are listening, taking him/her seriously, understanding his/her feelings as well as the behavior within the context of those feelings. **This doesn't mean agreeing but rather learning how to communicate**

---

62 *www.amazon.com/Skills-Training-Manual-Second-Edition/dp/1462516998*

PAIN IN CHILDREN AND YOUNG ADULTS

with empathy and acceptance. DBT is thus a skills-based psychological intervention and is particularly helpful for the child with chronic pain who is depressed.

In the the story below, a teen who has participated in a teen DBT group at UCLA (evolved from Dr. Joan Asarnow's DBT research program), describes her experience:

Comments from a 15-year-old female with anxiety and depression:

It is easy to understand because it is specific instruction and skills that you can use. It is tailor made for anxiety and depression. It gives you tools and guidance for how to solve the problem the next time or how to take the pressure off. It helps in getting out of my head, like not letting my thoughts stop me from living life. Also it helps me recognize what are my rational thoughts and what are irrational thoughts. I recommend it mostly for teens with anxiety because it is tougher to use when really sad because you are not as motivated to follow through. It is helpful as a second step after you have figured out your deeper issues. You should deal with your inward issues first and then deal with the outside world through DBT skills. I recommend the teen group because everyone contributes and shy people can learn from questions that others have that they are too shy to ask themselves.

Dr. Joan Asarnow[63], a DBT researcher, comments:

DBT is a proven evidence-based treatment that combines the best of our science with the knowledge and compassion of Marsha Linehan—an exceptional researcher and clinician whose innovative work has advanced the field and shifted many individuals from lives of suffering to lives of hope.

*Chronic pain can lead to depression and depression reduces the child's ability to cope. While medications like anti-depressants can be helpful, **research has shown that a combination of medication and psychological therapies work most effectively**.*

Acceptance and Commitment Therapy (ACT)

ACT is a new cognitive-behavioral approach that extends classic CBT by placing more **emphasis on acceptance-based and experiential treatment methods, on committed action and patient values**. In ACT, reduction in pain is not a primary focus. Instead, ACT helps adolescents with pain to encounter their distress openly and without ineffective resistance ("acceptance"). **Its focus is on how to live a personally meaningful and valued life, despite the pain ("values-based living").**

---

63   Joan Rosenbaum Asarnow, PhD, Professor of Psychiatry, Department of Psychiatry and Biobehavioral Sciences,
      University of California, Los Angeles. *http://people.healthsciences.ucla.edu/institution/personnel?personnel_id=9712*

PSYCHOLOGICAL AND BEHAVIORAL THERAPIES

ACT differs from CBT by acknowledging the importance of thoughts and beliefs, but without any attempt to change them.

ACT treatment can be characterized as "exposure" to distressing emotions and physical sensations, and learning to accept and tolerate these while progressing toward one's goals. ACT tends to use more experiential tasks, metaphor, and behavioral experimentation rather than didactic explanation or instruction. The ACT model emphasizes a balance of mindful acceptance and committed action, including role-playing, even during physical therapy and other physical activities where pain might ensue. Training is also provided in mindfulness techniques to help the adolescent be present and notice distressing feelings and bodily sensations in an accepting, non-judgmental way without needing to put effort into changing them. Drs. Lance McCracken and Christopher Eccleston in the United Kingdom have provided the most research on ACT therapy for teens with chronic pain.[22, 23]

DEPRESSION AND SUICIDE

If your child attempts suicide or tells you about details of planning for a suicide, then you need to bring your child to an emergency department for psychiatric evaluation to see how imminent the danger is. The psychiatric evaluation will determine whether hospitalization is necessary for your child's protection or whether your child is safe to return home and begin psychological intervention. If your child is already seeing a psychologist, it would be important to notify the therapist immediately.

One teen with chronic muscle pain reported feeling so sad at night that she would cry secretly in her bedroom—too distraught and embarrassed to ask her parents for help, she was trying to handle it on her own. She also thought that if she told her parents how hopeless she felt her pain situation had become and how helpless she felt, they would think she was weak. She had always prided herself on being the strong one in the family.

It wasn't until she started to have thoughts about killing herself that she became frightened enough to tell her parents. They were understanding and brought her to a psychologist.

In our experience, **almost all children in pain at one time or another wish they weren't alive.** However, if you take time to listen to them, what they typically mean is that they wish that they didn't have to live with their pain. This is different from thinking about killing themselves; that is called suicidal ideation (SI) or thoughts. If your child appears depressed, it is important to talk with him/her and find out some details:

235

PAIN IN CHILDREN AND YOUNG ADULTS

- Has she thought about dying? About killing herself?
- About how she would kill herself?
- Has she made preparations for suicide (notes, giving possessions away, gathering pill bottles)?
- Has she had self-injurious behaviors before?
- What was the intent behind the past or current self-injurious behavior?

Commonly, depression stems from the pain, but often there are underlying issues of depression that have not been addressed and have caused or exacerbated the pain. When these are understood, the pain diminishes.

PSYCHOLOGICAL TREATMENT FOR THE FAMILY

Through therapy, families can work together to help themselves function better as a cohesive and supportive unit. In turn, this will help the child with pain to function and feel better. The five goals of family therapy are to:

1 Observe, identify, and alter family dynamics that may contribute to the child's pain perception and difficulty coping;

2 Participate in developing and implementing a behavioral plan;

3 Address family stress and other problems;

4 Improve family communication; and

5 Provide support and improve family coping.

How Does Family Therapy Help Parents?

Azita Sachmachian, MFT, offers these insights in how this therapy works on a practical level:

> *Parents of children with chronic pain may face the need for major alterations in their parenting style. Since chronic pain significantly alters their child's emotional state, parenting becomes a confusing task. It is not surprising to find many parents shift between becoming overly sympathetic or too harsh. They feel very sorry for their hurting child and start babying her—with major side effects. It takes away the child's power, the very thing that they need most throughout their life. Losing one's sense of power (agency) is dangerous, analogous to damaging a car's engine. With a compromised engine it will have a difficult time going uphill on a hot day. With a child having low or no sense of agency, she will not have sufficient horsepower to pull through life's*

PSYCHOLOGICAL AND BEHAVIORAL THERAPIES

challenges. Parents also can become critical and demanding and expect the child to get better... soon. In these situations, the child easily falls into the trap of shame, guilt and worthlessness. These feelings provide the foundation for anxiety and depression.

Family therapy will help parents in seven major ways:

1 *Identify poorly adaptive changes in their parenting style, guiding them to find more adaptive, productive ways of parenting with more positive outcomes.*

2 *Identify how their own fear and sadness may be shaping their behavior.*

3 *Learn how to set new expectations and new rules that are in accordance with their child's new state of being.*

4 *Minimize babying tendencies or inappropriate interactions with their child.*

5 *Build on their child's strength and rise above the difficulties.*

6 *Support parents to hold on tight without breaking down and provide the utmost support for the rest of the family.*

7 *Find new capabilities and resources they never believed that they had.*

Chronic pain alters behavior towards immediate family members and the medical establishment. *Each child responds differently towards parents in the context of chronic pain. Some might become hyper-vigilant about their parents' suffering. They might feel guilty that their pain has caused so many financial problems and stress for their parents. They may unconsciously decide to hide their true feelings, masking their fears, sadness and anger, simply because they do not want their parents to hurt even more.*

Chronic pain gives nonverbal permission to be angry and snappy. If the child has old unexpressed anger, the anger lashes out without control. Those children who did not get enough attention from their super busy, or emotionally unavailable parents develop other maladaptive behaviors. Chronic pain becomes the only reason for getting attention. Why should they get better, since that would mean losing their new loving and attending parents?

Parents have a very hard time adjusting to such complicated shifts in their children's emotional and behavioral responses. Family therapy or couples'/parents' therapy becomes a resource to alarm the parents of such internal transitions. Parents can learn new ways of interacting with their child such that the new maladaptive patterns do not become permanent.

In summary, once a child's pain has invaded the family, many factors are set into play that serve to maintain or increase a child's pain. As many parents have learned, the assumption that if you, as parents, just find the right diagnosis and cure for your child's pain, then things at home will go back to normal. Most know that it may not be that simple.

When should you consider Family Therapy?

There is often resistance to family therapy. It is easier to focus on the child with the pain problem rather than to examine other intra-family factors that may contribute to the problem. Parents often do not realize the inadvertent roles that they, or other siblings, play in aiding their child to cross the line from having a moderate pain problem to a pain-associated disability syndrome (PADS), a condition in which the child with chronic pain quickly spirals out of control and becomes low- or non-functional.

We recommend family therapy when individual psychological intervention for the child is not helping, or when there is clearly a family dynamic that is inhibiting the child from getting better. The general rule of thumb is that, if things don't improve with current treatment of your child's pain in a few months, you should consider what family factors might be inadvertently contributing to the pain.

For example, take a look at yourself and your spouse/partner (Table 14.1); see how many of the behaviors in the 10-point checklist below sound familiar? Notice how you react to your child when she is complaining about pain.

Table 14.1   Parent Self-Behavior checklist
1   Do you find that you get so anxious that you feel the need to "do something" immediately to make it stop?
2   Do you feel that you are suffering as much as your child? Is your suffering interfering with your life, causing you to lose sleep? Have you become irritable, depressed, or anxious?
3   Is it difficult to convince your child to do anything when he is in pain?
4   Do you have a hard time not asking your child how she is feeling?
5   Are you and your spouse/partner frequently in conflict over the best way to deal with your child?
6   Do you constantly monitor your child's face for signs of pain?
7   Are you sleeping with your child more than two nights a week?
8   Do you identify with your child because you have the same type of pain problem?
9   Do you feel that you are the one shouldering all the responsibility for your child's pain and that you are not getting the support you need from your spouse/partner?
10 Are other children showing signs of neglect? Are they "acting out"?

If your answer is "yes" to several of these questions, then you are probably a candidate for family therapy; ideally, that includes all of the family members who are living in the home. Treatment is focused on changing the family system within which the child with pain is trying to cope.

PSYCHOLOGICAL AND BEHAVIORAL THERAPIES

Typically, the therapist listens to and observes each member's perceptions of the child in pain, as well as the roles and behaviors of each member within the family. In this process, the therapist learns which factors contribute to the child's pain experience and behaviors. For example, in some families, the child in pain is inadvertently "forced" to maintain the role of the "non-functioning pain kid" so that the focus of parental attention is off more serious and pressing family problems.

Family Therapy and Behavioral Plans[64]

In the years that we have been working with children with chronic pain and their parents, we have come up with an informal list of "unhelpful behaviors" that parents engage in that seem to negatively influence improvement in their child (Table 14.2). We tell you this not to make you feel like a bad parent— you are not—but to illustrate how a parent can, unknowingly, add to a child's suffering. You also can do something about it by changing your behavior when necessary.

Table 14.2   Are you a participant in "unhelpful behaviors" ... sometimes?
1   Providing undue sympathy and attention for your child's pain complaints, creating secondary reinforcement for the behavior;
2   Being excessively emotional in response to the child's complaints/behaviors;
3   Continually looking for help outside the family to make the child's pain better (for example, bringing the child to more doctors for more tests);
4   Complaining a lot about your own pain or problems, and using your own pain to connect with your child;
5   Not functioning when you are in pain; or
6   Supporting your child's avoidance of every-day tasks and responsibilities "because of the pain" (e.g. chores and schoolwork).

Tom is a bright, witty 12-year-old with recurring abdominal pain. His pains reliably occurred every weekday morning when he had to get ready for school. Tom's morning pain symptoms often involved crying and screaming. His pains had caused him to miss significant amounts of school, but usually improved by the late afternoon, at which time he would go to play outside with his friends. Tom had developed anxieties about going to school, partly because of his mom's belief that the school staff was not sympathetic to his pain problems. Tom was convinced that he could not be at school and cope with his pain at the same time.

---

64   Samantha Levy PhD made significant contributions to this section and others in this chapter.

PAIN IN CHILDREN AND YOUNG ADULTS

Tom's dad would try to drop him off at school and they would argue, sometimes violently, when dad tried to push him out of the car. His dad thought that Tom "should be able to tough it out… and not be a wimp."

Goals The first goal of family therapy was to change Tom's mother's perceptions about school by developing an agreement (a signed contract) among the school principal, nurse, Tom, and his mother: Tom would be allowed certain privileges at school (e.g., lying down in the nurse's office when he was in pain). In return, Tom's mother was to get Tom to school every day. They agreed that for now Dad should not drive him to school for the next 6 weeks since the morning arguments were never productive.

The Plan In the beginning, Tom was to remain at school through first period. His time at school increased gradually each week, and he received incentives for his coping (extra screen time). [Part of the vicious cycle of pain and school absence is from feelings of isolation, so we always suggest not taking away social interactions as a consequence, or using them as a motivator.]

Soon Tom's mother was able to get him to school and was less anxious about what 'might happen' to him. Once Tom sensed his mother's changing attitude toward the school, he became confident in his own ability to remain for increasing amounts of time. He became interested in some of his classes, and his pain lessened.

David, a 3-year-old boy scheduled to have his second heart surgery after the first one a year ago, was becoming anxious in anticipation of the surgery, as were his parents. The first surgery was difficult because his postoperative pain was not well managed. His parents were worried that David would be in a lot of pain after this second surgery. However, this time Kaitlin, a Child Life specialist, helped David and his parents to develop a plan. She practiced the step-by-step pre-operative plan with David using play therapy, while parents watched and learned. Parents learned how they could be calmly supportive of David before and after his surgery. They learned how distracting David by engaging him in play or telling him stories was more helpful than reassuring him that "Everything will be OK." Their own anxieties influenced their child's anxiety.

Parental behaviors such as apologies, reassurance, and criticism, are typically associated with increased child distress. David recovered quickly from his surgery and displayed much less anxiety following the surgery than previously. He required minimal postoperative pain medication and had a much shorter hospital stay than the previous time.

David's story illustrates how behavioral plans can be implemented. In this case, the plan made the surgical experience for David better and reduced his parents' anxiety. For many children with chronic pain, a simple behavioral plan that addresses specific problems and sets a few goals for parents and child, such as helping the child return to school or increase his functioning in other ways may be all that is needed.

PSYCHOLOGICAL AND BEHAVIORAL THERAPIES

HOW DID MY CHILD'S PAIN BECOME THE FAMILY PAIN?

We would like to return to Carly, the 12-year-old girl, described in previous chapters, who had been in a wheelchair for several months with severe leg and back pain, as well as headaches and abdominal pain. Following physical therapy and some medication, Carly was beginning to improve. In fact, as we noted previously, her mom had called to tell us that Carly was no longer using a wheelchair. However, her mom was upset that Carly's belly pain had not gone away.

It was becoming clear that mom's lack of excitement about Carly's improvement in walking was not enough. Worries about her daughter's abdominal pain were related to the mom's own anxiety. She viewed Carly's refusal to eat when her belly hurt as a sign that something dangerous was not being discovered. **This worry about our missing the diagnosis of something serious caused mom to focus on the amount of food that Carly was eating and created mother/daughter conflict over food.** If we stand back and look at the situation more broadly, one of the ways that mothers nurture their children is through preparing and serving food. Carly's refusal to eat (she said that "food will make my stomach hurt more…") created feelings of helplessness in the mom and added to her worry.

The relationship between Carly and mom began to change. Carly became more irritable, snappy and wanted to be left alone; while mom was developing simultaneous feelings of worry, caring, and frustration with her daughter. Carly's dad saw his wife becoming more stressed, and his first response was to become stricter and demanding of Carly. He believed that Carly was exaggerating her pain complaints to get attention and he insisted that she attend school, even though she complained that her stomach hurt too much to attend. The more insistent Carly's dad became about school, the more protective of Carly mom became.

These disparate views on how to treat Carly created conflict between mom and dad. Carly's younger brother became angry at Carly because he saw her as the cause of the rising tension in the household. He became moodier, was causing problems at home and at school, and his grades began to suffer. Both parents were becoming increasingly stressed until the tension was palpable. Pain had entered the family through Carly and had invaded the entire household.

When we see a situation such as what evolved in Carly's family, we know that the child's pain has become the family's pain, creating feelings of stress, worry, anger, frustration, and helplessness. Family members see little hope for an end, and they worry that this is their "new life." Some families then focus on "finding a cure for the pain" so that everyone will get back to their prior state of functioning. They continue taking their daughter to doctor after doctor for more tests. They may look to the internet and talk with others to search for a cure that will "fix the pain."

PAIN IN CHILDREN AND YOUNG ADULTS

Not uncommonly, they travel to different healing centers in different parts of the country because they read or heard from a friend that the doctor or program there has "cures for this type of problem."

The family often returns months later after spending significant amounts of money no better off than when they began their wide journey looking for the "magic cure." At this point they feel discouraged and the child believes that she will spend her whole life in pain. No one can help her since "no one" has.

Parents of 10-year-old Melodie, in reading an early draft of this book, commented:

Having been on this journey for some time, we can absolutely relate to every word and concept you are imparting. When first confronted with Melodie's pain syndrome, our primary focus was alleviating her pain. Neither her pediatrician nor the other medical professionals we saw had the depth of understanding of what we were dealing with! The medical practitioners limited their efforts toward ruling out plumbing issues and prescribing traditional migraine medication. Candidly it is the incredibly myopic approach to the problem by our pediatrician and subspecialists that we take issue with. It was very late in the process that our pediatrician mentioned that he "knew" of a physician that ran some type of pain clinic and that he was going to contact Dr. Paul Zeltzer. Other than that, his last suggestion was, "we should consider taking her to a psychologist." This was incredibly offensive in light of the physical pain Mel was dealing with and emotional pain we were all suffering.

It wasn't until Melodie's second in-patient stay at UCLA when you (Lonnie) were rounding and spent time with Mel did we feel that there was light at the end of this tunnel. We feel strongly that we are where we are today solely based on Lonnie's kind and gentle manner in the hospital and your guiding us toward a Medical-Bio-Psycho-Social model toward treating her pain.

Lastly, dealing with this "monster" takes the entire family's understanding and commitment toward a comprehensive cure. Once we dropped our defenses and grasped the fact that we play a part in the recovery team the pieces started to fall into place.

What goes on in the family unit affects how a child responds to pain, how long it lasts, how the child copes, and, ultimately, how quickly he gets better. Changing the ways that family members communicate with each other and understanding the roles that individual family members play that maintain maladaptive family systems is a pivotal part of the treatment program. Families (this includes parents, siblings, even grandparents) who learn and understand the important roles of the family in helping the child with chronic pain to function will help children reduce their pain more quickly and effectively.

PSYCHOLOGICAL AND BEHAVIORAL THERAPIES

Neil Schechter, MD[65], comments:

> *"Many parents feel that we are saying that they are failures. Or they may say, 'I think we are doing pretty well... why do we need family therapy?'"*

A recommendation for family therapy does not mean that your marriage is bad or your family is dysfunctional. Typically, the recommendation simply means there are some behavioral patterns within the family that may be making it more difficult for your child with pain to function. Nobody is at fault; the system just needs "tweaking." We can promise you this: whenever a family makes a commitment to therapy, changes happen!

18-year-old Jennie reflects, below, on when she was 10 years old and had CRPS and was in a wheelchair because her legs hurt too much to walk:

> *I have an older brother and an older sister. It was very difficult. My brother was a freshman and my sister was going off to university. It was an important time in their lives and a lot of my parents' attention was focused on me, and I was completely dependent on them for my movement...I couldn't do anything on my own... I couldn't go to the bathroom on my own. I think there was some resentment, definitely, but they never showed it, and I am sure it was difficult for them to accept.*
>
> *We went to family therapy... it was difficult. But the sessions were helpful. It made my parents more aware that my brother and sister needed extra attention. It was an opportunity for me to tell them what I was going through, at a time when it wasn't an argument or a fight. It was Ok for them to say, "I am angry that this is happening."*
>
> *I think one of the reasons I have recovered is because my parents learned how to give me enough space and independence so that I could learn to trust myself. As much as it was a difficult time in my life, if I could, I wouldn't change a thing. I consider that I am the person I am today because of what I went through. I have an incredible relationship with my parents because we went through so much emotionally and physically together. It's kind of funny, because at the time I hated the psychologist, Shelley; she was the tough one. Getting me to talk... was torture. I was the kid who was the pleaser. I didn't want to cause any problems. I didn't want to talk about the things that were bothering me... my depression, or my anger. Those are the things I needed to do. I kept a diary as a release. I didn't keep track of improvements, because then I felt bad, like I wasn't trying hard enough if I regressed a bit. But having a place to release emotionally was helpful.*

It takes a lot of courage to allow a stranger to join your family circle and hear conversations that have only taken place behind closed doors. Most importantly,

---

65 Neil Schechter MD, Director of the Chronic Pain Clinic at Boston Children's Hospital. Associate Professor of Anesthesia, Harvard Medical School. Pediatric pain researcher and developmental specialist. *www.childrenshospital.org/doctors/neil-schechter*

PAIN IN CHILDREN AND YOUNG ADULTS

it is threatening to allow another adult to have an influence on your child's life. What if the therapist does not understand your point of view? What if the therapist contradicts you in front of your children or your spouse?

KIDS AND PARENTS REFLECT ON WHAT THEY LEARNED IN FAMILY THERAPY

In preparation for writing this book, Samantha Levy PhD[66] asked many of our patients and parents to tell how family therapy helped them. Below are some of their comments:

- I gained more self-confidence in my ability to tell my parents how I felt... I didn't have to keep my feelings inside.

- It was reassuring to know that if we had trouble handling something during the week, we could bring the problems up in the family session.

- When we try to talk about some issues at home, tempers get hot. It feels safer to try and tackle these with a therapist present.

- At least I know that there is one time a week when the family is together. With our different schedules... we keep missing each other.

- I get to hear from my daughter who doesn't have a pain problem in these meetings.

- The therapist helps our children speak up more easily.

- We learned to stop the Blame Game.

- I was finally able to tell my parents that I didn't want to play baseball anymore, and that relieved a lot of stress.

- I feel like now my parents know that I am scared about them expecting too much from me as I start to improve, so they are putting less pressure on me now and letting me get back to my activities slowly... as I am ready.

- We learned how to walk that fine line between empathizing with our child's pain and pushing her when she was ready.

- We learned how to praise our child for increases in functioning, while acknowledging that he was still in pain.

---

66   Samantha Levy, Ph.D. Clinical Psychologist , Member of UCLA and WCLA Pediatric pain team. *www.wholechildla.org/clinical_team.php?pid*

244

PSYCHOLOGICAL AND BEHAVIORAL THERAPIES

INDIVIDUAL PARENT ISSUES

Azita Sachmachian, MFT notes that sometimes individual psychological therapy for a parent may be helpful. She provides the following case to illustrate this direction that may be needed:

> *14-year-old Sandra had chronic migraines and was referred for psychotherapy because she was sleeping most of the day and was refusing to go outdoors. It became clear that her mother's non-verbal expectation to get better was playing an important factor in maintaining Sandra's depression. This unmet expectation made Sandra feel unworthy. Since Sandra was not getting better, she had made an unconscious decision that there must have been something inherently wrong with her. Feeling inherently flawed contributed significantly to her depression.*

While Sandra was referred to one of our team psychologists to help with both her depression and provide her with coping tools, the more than she progressed, the more depressed her mother became.

In this case, in discussion with Sandra's mother, it was felt by mom that she needed her own therapy to discuss feelings that would help her become more available and helpful to Sandra. With psychotherapy, Sandra's mother was able to realize the impact of her expectations on her daughter. This awareness helped her to identify sources of her expectations. She realized that it was her own fear that Sandra would never get better and suffer lifelong pain. **She did not know how to deal with her terrifying thoughts on a conscious level,** so she unconsciously wished and expected her daughter to simply get better. In other words, her daughter's improvement would have freed her from dealing with her own terrifying feelings.

Psychotherapy helped mom to deal with her own fears proactively. It gave her tools to fight her own fight with fear and take the pressure off her daughter. As mom's understanding of her own behaviors increased, her behavior and relationship with Sandra improved. Sandra then began to feel more at ease. In her own psychological intervention, Sandra's sense of being flawed was also challenged and slowly her depression lifted. With no intervention, this mother had a slim chance of gaining awareness over such complex intertwined dynamics contributing to her child's depression.

MARITAL (COUPLES) ISSUES

A family therapist may choose to work with the parents alone if she/he feels that marital issues are impacting the child. For example, marital/ **couples therapy may**

PAIN IN CHILDREN AND YOUNG ADULTS

be the most effective treatment if parental discord is creating tensions at home or aggravating the child's pain problem.

A couple's relationship is often strained by a child's chronic pain, and sometimes it is helpful for the parents to meet in sessions without the children. The focus of marital therapy in this context is to help both parents examine their goals and expectations of their child, and to learn how to work together. **Often parents have different ways of coping with their child's pain problem;** this leads to conflicts about how to treat the child.

The 14 major issues that parents frequently address with therapists are described by psychologist Dr. Samantha Levy in our pain program as the following:

1 Conflicting opinions/recommendations from various physicians.

2 Feeling resentful towards the "sick" child.

3 School reintegration—how to get my child back to school or to full days

4 Concern that my child feels guilty about the financial, emotional and overall impact her pain is having on the family.

5 Feeling helpless when my child is in pain.

6 Impact on other kids.

7 Balancing when to push and when to empathize or "coddle"

8 Feelings of isolation—other parents do not understand.

9 This major stressor has affected my marital relationship.

10 How to deal with my child regressing when she was making improvements or having a flare up after she was "cured."

11 How to deal with the reactions of others—having teachers, other parents, church/temple members, etc. not comment to my child about his illness.

12 Not knowing when my child is faking or exaggerating symptoms.

13 How to reconcile that my child seems fine when doing something he/she enjoys but says that school is too difficult to handle with pain.

14 How to decide whether to allow my child to engage in fun activities that I know will cause him to "crash" later.

When there is so much focus on children, some parents find that they neglect themselves and their partner, and their relationship suffers. They become distant. It is important to set aside specific times each week to nourish the marital relationship.

Divorced parents find themselves having increased contact with each other. They must come together to make important decisions about their child's treatment.

246

PSYCHOLOGICAL AND BEHAVIORAL THERAPIES

In Joint Legal Custody, both parents have the right and responsibility to make decisions relating to the health, education, and welfare of their child. If one parent has Sole Legal Custody, the other parent doesn't have that right to make decisions.

At UCLA, our legal department told me (LZ) that I could not give mother information about her child's diagnosis or treatment because the child's father had Sole Legal Custody and refused to give us permission to talk with her. This was very difficult for the child and was a factor in their child's pain problem.

Including Fathers

Sometimes dads take a back seat when medical problems arise. They may not feel the need to come to family therapy, especially if mom has been the primary caregiver. This may stem from the father's own reluctance, or because mothers automatically take over, leaving dad to question what more he can do.

Fathers, however, are crucial participants in family therapy. They provide a different point of view that balances the mother's perspective. Because fathers tend to be more objective and less protective (this is not always the case; of course, the roles can be reversed), dads are often more convincing in helping their child to become independent and cope with the pain. Often, however, the children complain that their fathers do not believe that they are in pain and push them too hard. The important thing is, if there are two parents (or caregivers) in the family, it is crucial to have them both take part in family therapy, especially if there are conflicts at home over what the parents expect from their child.

If parents have different expectations about how the child is handling pain or how quickly he is recovering, a child may feel he needs to take sides. One parent becomes the "good parent" and the other the "bad one". This kind of issue can be worked out if both parents participate. The ultimate goal of both couples and family therapy is to establish better communication within the family.

CHOOSING A THERAPIST

The first place to begin is by looking at the list of mental health providers covered by your health plan. Your child's physician may know child therapists to whom he has referred children and whom he thinks are especially good.

The therapist should be a licensed clinical child psychologist, child psychiatrist, licensed clinical social worker, or a licensed marriage and family therapist. You should ask about the therapist's training, credentials, and experience, especially in treating children with chronic pain. You and your child should like and feel connected to the psychotherapist, especially after several sessions. For guidance in finding a family therapist, see the websites: *www.apa.org* or *www.aamft.org/TherapistLocator*

247

*The greatest mistake in the treatment of diseases is
the thought that there are physicians for the body and
physicians for the soul... the two cannot be separated.*

— PLATO

*Very early on, I discovered that yoga makes you fix problems
yourself. It also worked much faster than any of the other treatments
and the results lasted much longer. I learned that my headaches
were a result of deeper problems and headaches were the way my
body let me know something was wrong. Yoga made me fix my
headaches myself and not rely on medication or a machine to solve
my problem. And if I ever get headaches again, I know what to do.*

— JL, A 14-YEAR-OLD YOGA STUDENT.

CHAPTER 15

COMPLEMENTARY MIND AND BODY THERAPIES

WHAT IS COMPLEMENTARY THERAPY (CT)? CAUTIONS ABOUT CT

COMPLEMENTARY THERAPIES INCLUDED IN WCLA & UCLA'S INTEGRATIVE PAIN PROGRAMS

- Acupuncture
- Therapeutic Yoga, including Iyengar Yoga
- Biofeedback
- Hypnotherapy
- Mindfulness Meditation
- Art Therapy
- Energy Therapy
- Music Therapy
- Massage Therapy
- Craniosacral Therapy

OVERVIEW OF "MIND-RELATED" INTERVENTIONS: Which is Best?

COMPLEMENTARY PRACTITIONERS—Checking Them Out

BOTANICALS AND NATURAL PRODUCTS

OTHER COMPLEMENTARY THERAPIES (CTS)

PAIN IN CHILDREN AND YOUNG ADULTS

Table 15.1 Major Areas of Complementary Therapies		
Domain	Therapies and Their Applications	
Alternative Medical Systems	1 Homeopathic medicine (HM) 2 Naturopathic medicine (NM) 3 Ayurvedic medicine (AM) 4 Traditional Chinese medicine-(TCM)	• Minute doses of plant extracts, minerals, nutrition (1) • Counseling (1); Pharmacology (2) • Hydro/ physical therapies (2) • Herbal medicine (2,3,4) • Massage (3,4); Acupuncture (4) • Movement (3,4)
Biologically-Based Therapies	Same as above plus 1 Herbs 2 Nutritional 3 Natural compounds 4 Special diets	• Herbal remedies, plant preparations (1) • Vitamins, dietary supplements • Macrobiotics (3)
Manipulative & Body-Based Methods	1 Chiropractic & Yoga 2 Osteopathic manipulations 3 Massage & Physical therapy; 5.	Touch, pressure (1,2,3,4) Movement (4,5)
Energy Therapies	1 Reiki 2 Therapeutic Touch 3 Electrical devices	Manipulate energy biofields within/ body w/o direct contact (1,2). Electro-magnet fields-pulsed, AC/DC current] (3).
Mind-Body Interventions	1 Art & Music therapies 2 Biofeedback 3 Hypnotherapy 4 Meditation; 5 Psychotherapy; 6 Spirituality.	Enhance the mind's capacity to affect bodily function and symptoms

In this chapter we will discuss the scientific evidence and experience for how these different therapies can help the child with chronic pain.

> *Jack is a five-year-old who has had chronic headaches for one year. Typically, he gets one every other day. When they occur, he cries continually and is usually inconsolable, demanding more and more attention from his mother. Jack was diagnosed with*

250

COMPLEMENTARY MIND AND BODY THERAPIES

childhood migraines. Medications provided by the neurologist gave intolerable side effects without relief. Recently, however, Jack's mother learned a series of relaxation and imagery techniques, which she and Jack practice together. When the pain first starts, Jack and his mom lie down together and begin by taking long, deep breaths. Jack's mom urges him to relax and think about something he likes to do such as playing on a swing in the park.

Jack's mom begins by describing the sights, sounds and feelings of the park and then asks Jack to describe them and also to notice how comfortable and relaxed he is feeling as he continues to breathe deeply. After several weeks of practice, Jack was able to relieve much of the pain. He has also discovered that he can sometimes stop the headaches on his own when his mom is not around.

As many non-traditional therapies have come into popular use, and as the public has become dissatisfied with the conventional medical approach to conditions like chronic pain, more research is being done to test the effectiveness of these therapies. Often we discount what is new to us or that we don't understand. **Many non-drug options have been found to be highly effective in the treatment of chronic pain in children.** Many non-traditional therapies have become so popular that the U.S. Department of Health's National Institutes of Health (NIH) established the National Center for Complementary and Alternative Medicine (NCCAM) to oversee funding and selection of research to be funded in this area. This name was recently changed to the National Center for Complementary and Integrative Health (NCCIH) at NIH because "Alternative" medicine indicated a totally different system of viewing and treating health and disease. Rather "Alternative" was replaced by "Integrative Health" to indicate the optimal therapies that combine traditional Western medicine with complementary therapies.

WHAT IS COMPLEMENTARY AND INTEGRATIVE HEALTH (CIH)?

Complementary Therapy is a general term for many types of therapy that are not part of the history and style of disease-based, Western medicine as practiced in North America and Europe for much of the last 100 years. NCCIH divides complementary therapy into three categories: mind-body therapies, botanicals, and other therapies used less often and less studied, such as energy therapies.

Complementary and Integrative Health (CIH) is the modern treatment approach to pain that uses these complementary therapies (CTs) in a patient-centric way, plus Western medicine, physical and medicinal approaches. This combination is referred

251

PAIN IN CHILDREN AND YOUNG ADULTS

to as *Integrative Medicine*. One of our nation's experts in pediatric Integrative Medicine, Dr. Kathi J. Kemper, offers her insights[67]:

*"**Introduction** Integrative medicine focuses on promoting physical, mental, emotional, spiritual, and social, well-being in the context of a healthy family and community. Integrative medicine emphasizes patient-centered care and the relationship between practitioner and patient. It is evidence-based, and uses appropriate therapeutic approaches, healthcare professionals and disciplines to empower patients to achieve optimal health and healing.*

*The foundations of an integrative approach to pain are **healthy habits in a healthy habitat**. This means attention to a healthy lifestyle, including optimal nutrition, physical activity, adequate sleep, skillful use of emotional self-regulatory strategies (mind-body skills and stress management), nurturing relationships and communication patterns, and a healthy environment. In addition, integrative approaches include bio-chemical therapies such as medications, vitamins, minerals, herbs, and other dietary supplements; biomechanical therapies such as surgery, osteopathic and chiropractic adjustments, massage and body work; and biofield therapies such as radiation, prayer, acupuncture, homeopathy, Therapeutic and Healing Touch, and Reiki.*

Overall, complementary therapies were used by 42%-71% of patients, according to current research. The most commonly used therapies were dietary supplements such as herbs, vitamins, and minerals; the most commonly used practices were massage, chiropractic, relaxation, and aromatherapy. Side effects were uncommon and most were minor. Use of complementary therapies is most common among youth with chronic, incurable, or recurrent conditions such as pain. This section will focus on dietary supplements, mind-body strategies, massage, and acupuncture for children suffering from painful conditions.[24]

__Toxicity and Mislabeling__ Dietary supplements are the most commonly used complementary therapies for children and adolescents. In the US, dietary supplements are regulated more like food than medications, so it is important to be informed about the quality and reliability of purchased products. Inaccurate labeling is a serious concern. Dietary supplement labels might not accurately reflect the contents or concentrations of ingredients. Variations of 10- to 1,000-fold have been reported for several popular herbs, even across lots produced by the same manufacturer using the same label. Herbs may be unintentionally contaminated with pesticides or microbes, and products from developing countries have been found to contain toxic levels of mercury, cadmium, arsenic, or lead, either from unintentional contamination during manufacturing or

---

67   Kathi J. Kemper MD MPH, Professor of Pediatrics, Nursing; Dietetics, Director, Center for Integrative Health and Wellness, The Ohio State University, Columbus, OH. *http://mind-bodyhealth.osu.edu*

COMPLEMENTARY MIND AND BODY THERAPIES

from intentional additions by producers who believe that these metals have therapeutic value. Approximately 30-40% of Asian patent medicines include potent pharmaceuticals, such as analgesics, antibiotics, hypoglycemic agents, or corticosteroids; typically, the labels for these products are not written in English and do not note the inclusion of pharmaceutical agents. Even mineral supplements, such as calcium, have been contaminated with lead or had significant problems with product variability.

Dietary Supplements for Pain *As with any medication, the toxicity of a dietary supplement depends on its dose, what it is taken with (other supplements or medications), and the age and other medical conditions of the child. Even when a product is safe when used correctly, it can cause mild or severe toxicity when used incorrectly. Many families use supplements concurrently with medications, posing hazards of interactions. For example, St. John's Wort induces liver enzymes that can speed elimination of digoxin, cyclosporine, chemotherapy, HIV medications, oral contraceptives, and numerous antibiotics, reducing their effectiveness.*

No single vitamin, mineral or supplement is right for everyone, but recommendations can be useful. Many pain patients have low vitamin D and iron levels, and returning them to optimal levels helps patients feel better. Approximately 65% of children and youth have sub-optimal vitamin D levels. Low vitamin D is associated with muscle aches and fatigue; it is also tied to increase rates of depression that increase sensitivity to pain. Restoring vitamin D levels can safely help many children and should be a first line strategy. Similarly, a number of children benefit from optimizing iron and magnesium levels; low levels cause fatigue, irritability, and reduced ability to cope with pain and stress. Specific nutrients that may be helpful in specific conditions are listed in Table 15.2 below."

Table 15.2 Nutrient Therapies for Specific Conditions	
Condition	Nutrient
Abdominal Pain (IBS)	Peppermint, enteric coated (Pepogest™), Herbal mixture (Iberogast™), Probiotics
Colic	Herbal mixtures (chamomile, fennel, vervain, licorice, balm mint), Probiotics
Headache	Vitamin B2 (200 mg twice daily), Magnesium, Butterbur, Feverfew, Coenzyme Q10
Inflammatory conditions	Vitamin D, Omega-3 fatty acid supplements
Insomnia	Melatonin, Lavender aromatherapy, Chamomile, hops, kava-kava, passionflower, valerian, Tryptophan and 5-HTP (melatonin precursors)
Nausea	Ginger

Complementary therapy in the United States and elsewhere is huge. According to the 2007 NHIS survey, 83 million U.S. adults spent $33.9 billion out-of-pocket on visits to CT practitioners and on purchases of CT products, classes and materials. In total, there were approximately 354 million visits to CT practitioners and approximately 835 million purchases. More visits were made to *unconventional* therapy providers than to primary care physicians (629 million vs. 386 million visits).[25]

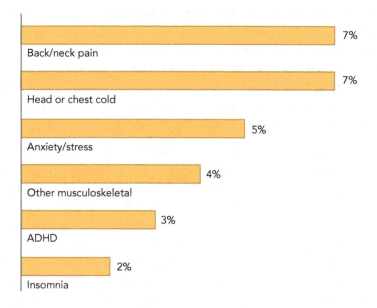

Figure 15.1. Diseases and conditions for which complementary and alternative medicine was most frequently used among children, 2007. (From the National Center for Complementary and Alternative Medicine, 2008; and Barnes PM, et al. CDC Natl Health Statistics Rep 2008[12]:1-24)

The conditions for which CT was sought are illustrated in the chart above. According to adult respondents who were asked about use by non-adults in their household, the use of CT was greater among children who:[14,15]

- had parents with higher education levels (15%) and who used CT (24%).
- were adolescents 12-17 years of age (16%).
- were Caucasian (13%) rather than Hispanic (8%) or African-American (6%).
- had six or more health conditions (24%).
- experienced delayed conventional care because of cost (17%).

COMPLEMENTARY MIND AND BODY THERAPIES

CAUTIONS ABOUT COMPLEMENTARY THERAPIES (CTS)

As mentioned in Chapter 16, in treating children's pain we rely on treatments (drugs) that have not been specifically studied in children, otherwise we would have very little to offer. This does not mean that many of the therapies are not safe and effective—they most certainly are.

There are, however, areas that fall under the umbrella of CTs that concern us; this includes the use of megavitamins, herbs, and other botanicals. Even though they are "natural," these are still potent substances and could have an impact on a child's developing organs. Herbal remedies also may interfere with the metabolism of prescribed medications or interact with these drugs to create a toxic effect. It is important to review with the prescribing clinician the other medications that your child is taking and to **insure that there are no toxic drug interactions or potentially harmful effects of the herb.**

We worry about invasive procedures such as "high colonics" and other "cleanse" remedies that claim to "remove toxins" in children, since such procedures could potentially sensitize already sensitive nervous systems in children with chronic pain, as well as remove needed nutrients and salts.

Beware of exaggerated claims about so-called "natural" drugs and therapies, especially on the internet. Also, personal stories of medicines or therapies that "worked wonders" for relatives or for the friend of the neighbor down the street may not be the right treatment for your child, even if he seems to "have the same pain problem." First, what *seems* like "the same thing" may not be. Second, even pain problems that bear the same name may represent different conditions in adults and in children. For example, **fibromyalgia in adults is different from *juvenile* fibromyalgia.** Use your best judgment and talk to your child's doctor about any concerns you might have (remember that talking with *your* doctor is different from talking with *your child's* doctor, unless you and your child have the same family medicine physician).

In this chapter, we would consider the term "complementary therapies" (CT) rather than "complementary and alternative medicine" (CAM) since we believe an integrative approach includes both biopsychosocial models and CT's where appropriate.

COMPLEMENTARY THERAPY (CT) PRACTITIONERS IN THE WCLA & UCLA PAIN PROGRAMS

We view chronic pain from a mind-body perspective, a continuum. This is why we use and recommend the integration of CT with more traditional psychological, physical, and pharmacological therapies for children with chronic pain. In our Pediatric

255

PAIN IN CHILDREN AND YOUNG ADULTS

Pain Program at UCLA and at WCLA, we incorporate CTs in an integrative way; we communicate with each other about patients.

Our team consists of an acupuncturist/Chinese herbalist, biofeedback therapists, physical therapists (including an aqua-therapist) with expertise in chronic pain, hypno-therapist, Iyengar yoga teacher, massage therapist, art therapist, music therapist, energy therapist, craniosacral therapist, a mindfulness teacher, and several child psychologists and psychiatrists.

Many CTs come from ancient healing arts that date back centuries. They all have the same goal: to restore balance and harmony within the body and mind (and spirit for some). In a somewhat different way, this is also the goal of Western medicine: to restore homeostasis or balance to bodily functions. In this chapter, we have asked our CT practitioners to describe their chosen therapy, how they work, how to decide which CT is right for your child, and some tips for finding the appropriate practitioner.

Many CT practitioners believe in an energy force that flows through the body. You can't see this energy, but if its flow is blocked or unbalanced you become sick. Different traditions call this energy by different names, such as "Qi" (pronounced "chi"), "prana" and "life force." Unblocking or re-balancing your energy force is the goal of these therapies, and each one accomplishes that goal differently.

Acupuncture

Acupuncture is intended to restore natural energy (Qi) through the insertion of needles into points along energy pathways (meridians) in the body. The needles help stimulate the energy flow. Acupuncture has been used effectively to treat headache pain, menstrual cramps, tennis elbow, fibromyalgia, myofascial pain, osteoarthritis, low back pain, carpal tunnel syndrome, and nausea and vomiting-related to chemotherapy.

Our UCLA /WCLA Pediatric Pain Programs acupuncturist, Michael Waterhouse[68], M.A., L.Ac., studied in China and helped us to establish this important part of our program. Mike not only understands acupuncture and Chinese herbs but also understands chronic pain and child development. Above all, he says, *"an acupuncturist must relate well to children and be able to communicate with parents how the treatment works and the goals of treatment."* Michael comments on his specialty:

> *What Is Acupuncture? Acupuncture involves the insertion of tiny needles in the body both near the site of pain and at a distance from the pain site on lines of acupuncture*

---

68   Michael Waterhouse M.A., L.Ac., UCLA /WCLA Pediatric Pain Programs acupuncturist,
     www.acupuncturehouse.com

COMPLEMENTARY MIND AND BODY THERAPIES

points called "meridians." What is important when considering acupuncture for children and adolescents is that these needles are extremely fine and unlike an injection or having blood drawn, they are not hollow and do not cut the skin or blood vessels. The insertion is practically painless neither leaving a mark nor causing bleeding.

Treated Conditions: Historically, acupuncture has been used to treat a variety of common conditions. The National Institutes of Health consensus conference on acupuncture concluded that it was effective in the treatment of the following conditions; headaches, menstrual cramps, elbow tendonitis, fibromyalgia, myofascial pain, osteoarthritis, lower back and neck pain, carpal tunnel syndrome and post-operative- or chemotherapy-caused nausea and vomiting. Additionally, acupuncture has been used to treat chronic abdominal pain, IBS, mild anxiety and depression, post-operative and post-procedural pain and PTSD. Chronic pain is best treated by a combined approach using a mix of modalities including western medication, relaxation therapies (biofeedback, guided imagery), PT, psychological counseling and acupuncture.

Mechanisms of Action: By needling acupuncture points, the brain releases enkephalins and endorphins; but even more importantly, needling enables the brain to increase its own opioid production. The increase in neurotransmitter production (serotonin and dopamine) enhances mood and allows those substances to calm down the pain receptor sites in the brain. By using modern imaging techniques (fMRI and PET scans), scientists have shown that needling acupuncture points caused observable increases in activity in the brain. This demonstrates the need for accurate needling!

Scientific Studies: The traditional idea for how acupuncture works is that it balances energy ("Qi") that flows through the meridians and unblocks stagnation that is the cause of pain. Particularly in cases of chronic pain, the purpose is to balance all the systems of the body (the cooling calming Yin energy and the hot metabolic Yang energy); such balance enables the body to heal itself. Traditional concepts such as Qi and Yin/Yang are unfamiliar and perhaps even off putting to the Westerner. Simply put acupuncture has a homeostatic or normalizing effect on the body.

Modern research provides a window to understand how acupuncture works. Acupuncture "points" are generally points of low electrical resistance on the surface of the skin. When a needle is inserted into an acupuncture point in a pain area, there is both an increase in blood flow to the area and an increase in the low amperage current that flows down the outside of the nerve sheaths; this causes cells to become more permeable allowing inflammatory material to leave and nutrients to enter. Additionally, by needling tight local muscles, it releases "trigger" points that causes the muscles to relax. It has been observed that needling the same acupuncture point has the effect of decreasing heart rate when it is rapid and increasing the rate when it is slow. One can see how acupuncture balances the sympathetic (fight or flight) and

257

PAIN IN CHILDREN AND YOUNG ADULTS

the parasympathetic nervous system which influences chronic pain syndromes where sympathetic arousal is a major contributing factor to maintaining pain.

Treatment of Children by Acupuncture: *Acupuncture has always been part of Traditional Chinese Medicine (TCM) and includes herbal medicine, therapeutic exercise (Tai Chi, Qi Gong), massage (Tui Na) and nutritional medicine. Today acupuncture is not only a stand-alone therapy, but demonstrates it's usefulness and versatility as an adjunct to Western Biomedicine.*

Side Effects: *The long history of the use of acupuncture is a testament to its efficacy and safety. Occasional there is a feeling of lightheadedness after treatment that is transitory and probably due to endorphin release. A recent review of acupuncture safety in children concluded that acupuncture is one of the safest modalities available. Minor bruising is rare. A 2001 study of 34,000 acupuncture treatments revealed no major incidents involving hospitalization; there was an occasional incidence of symptom aggravation, 86% of which resolved within 24 hours.*

When and How Often To Use Acupuncture? *Our experience at the UCLA and WCLA Pediatric Pain Clinics suggests that when approached delicately, the majority of children are very at ease being needled. It is important that the practitioner relates comfortably with the patient and takes time explain that these needles are "hair like" and do not cut the skin like getting a shot or getting blood drawn. It is also important to acknowledge that even grown-ups get a little apprehensive before a treatment and that it is normal to feel that way. I explain that if a needle feels uncomfortable, then they should say so and it will be adjusted or removed. While they lie with the needles in for 15 to 20 minutes, it should be a pain-free experience. Due to the release of endorphins, patients often feel very relaxed and consider the experience enjoyable rather than terrifying. From 6-15 needles can be inserted in one treatment; however, if a patient is showing hesitancy about being needled, it is advisable to agree to use one needle then see how the child feels, which is usually nothing or just a mild sensation, and then with their consent to proceed.*

The number of treatments required will vary, but as the treatments act cumulatively, one on the other, 2 treatments per week for a minimum of 4 to 6 treatments is advisable to determine if acupuncture is going to be helpful.

Recently acupuncture points have been stimulated by using a cold Laser that has the obvious benefit of not being invasive and therefore more acceptable to children.

Licensing: *Most states have their own acupuncture licensing exam to qualify practitioners, usually carrying the designate L.Ac (Licensed Acupuncturist) or D.O.M. (Doctor of Oriental Medicine). There is the National Certification Commission for Acupuncture and Oriental Medicine (www.nccaom.org) with a Dipl. Ac. There is a*

COMPLEMENTARY MIND AND BODY THERAPIES

Physician's organization, the American Association of Medical Acupuncture (www. medicalacupuncture.org) that can be contacted for a list of doctors trained in acupuncture in your area. The best referrals are by word of mouth from providers or acquaintances that have had beneficial experiences with local practitioners with experience in treating the child.

Case history #1: Three years prior to his first visit, Gary, a 15-year-old male, had been in a serious car accident. He sustained major injuries to his facial bones and a fracture of his right orbit. His chief complaint was chronic and debilitating right eye pain; this became so bad that one year previously his right eye was removed; this removal did not help the pain. He reported the eye pain to be "8/10," where 10 was the worst pain possible. The pain got worse with stress and fatigue. Sleep maintenance was poor and he was feeling unrefreshed upon waking. Since the accident he experienced generalized anxiety particularly when in a car and was hyper-vigilant about safety in general. He preferred to be with family members only; his affect was flat and depressed. His chronic pain was a significant family stressor.

Gary was treated with a combination of therapies including medication, relaxation techniques, psychotherapy, and a course of acupuncture treatment. This integrated approach addressed both the pain and the psychological stressors that increased his sympathetic arousal thus increasing his pain. This treatment combination caused a 50% decrease in his pain within 3 weeks and enabled him to integrate himself socially with greater ease.

Acupuncture is not usually thought of as a primary option for relieving pain in children and adolescents. One theory holds that because acupuncture treatment most often involves the use of needles, and because most children are afraid of needles, they would be unwilling to undergo (and their parents would not want to subject their children to) a form of care that involves needling. In our experience this is *not* the case. We have found that most children are accepting of acupuncture. This acceptance however depends heavily upon the acupuncturist's ability to relate to children.

Case history #2: Eight-year-old Sammy liked the "sleepy" feeling he would get after an acupuncture session. He said that in the beginning, he was a little afraid of the needles because it always hurt when he had needles at the doctor's office. But "Dr. Michael" let him hold one and even put it into his arm and that it felt "weird" ... but didn't hurt.

Sometimes he would get a little "buzz" when needles first went into his body but that went away and he felt calm and relaxed, "...kinda like I was sleeping or dreaming, but not quite." Sammy said "being in our acupuncture research study and having 'Dr. Samantha' talk with me and remind me to imagine being in my favorite place, together with the feel of the needles, was the "best feeling of all."

PAIN IN CHILDREN AND YOUNG ADULTS

Therapeutic Yoga

There are many different forms of yoga being taught today. In our program, we use a type called **Iyengar yoga** because it is highly therapeutic and safe for people with medical conditions, including chronic pain. In therapeutic yoga, the yoga series is matched to the healthcare needs of the child and changes as the child progresses. The **poses intend to correct health-related problems, both in body structure and internal organ function**. Iyengar Yoga teachers must have a minimum of five years training before they are certified.

It is important that a yoga exercise program is developed by someone who knows human physiology and can tailor the yoga program to the needs of the child with chronic pain. Beth Sternlieb[69] has been the certified therapeutic Iyengar Yoga teacher in our program. We asked Beth to talk about her practice with youth in pain:

Iyengar Yoga is a traditional form of yoga based on the teaching of the Indian Master B.K.S Iyengar. His method of teaching is orderly and progressive; the postures are adjusted to meet the physical conditions and needs of each student. B.K.S. Iyengar developed a method of teaching that enhances the therapeutic benefits and a way of doing yoga postures and breathing that could be adapted to students of all ages, levels of experience, and ability. His method brings awareness, circulation, strength, and flexibility to various parts of the body to maintain optimal health.

Iyengar Yoga stresses precision and correct alignment in all postures and makes use of props, such as wooden blocks, belts, and blankets. With the aid of props, students who are stiff, weak, or unable to hold a pose for the necessary amount of time can use physical support to get the desired result. A well-trained, experienced teacher can use props to address health problems. For example, lying in a backbend over a chair stimulates the adrenal glands, doing standing poses, like Trikonasana (Triangle Pose) against a wall, can teach correct alignment and relieve pressure on the lower back.

Case history #1 Adrienne, a 10-year-old girl with severe abdominal pain, came to me to learn yoga to help with debilitating pain, a result of many complications following abdominal surgery. She had developed the habit of gripping her abdomen in anticipation of pain. As she lay over blankets and pillows in passive backbends and named these poses (e.g., comfy pose, puppy pose), Adrienne learned to release, relax, and let go of abdominal tension. She began to understand how guarded she was and how vulnerable she felt when her belly was open and exposed. Over time she learned to tolerate more sensation there without instinctively gripping and guarding herself.

---

69 Beth Sternlieb, certified therapeutic Iyengar Yoga teacher. *http://inside.insightla.org/beth* and *www.wholechildla.org/clinical_team.php?pid=NA*

COMPLEMENTARY MIND AND BODY THERAPIES

I use Iyengar Yoga to help children, adolescents, and young adults with a variety of chronic pain problems. The combination of medical care, yoga practice and other therapies as needed, including psychological counseling, helps many children to overcome their obstacles to live full and productive lives. Kids with chronic pain problems have been betrayed by their bodies. At a time when they should be gaining more and more independence, their confidence and autonomy are undermined. One of the most important things that Iyengar Yoga offers these kids is a feeling of mastery. Through their own skill and actions, they can take charge of their healing and solve their chronic pain problem by virtue of their own effort.

Case history #2 Jenna, a young woman in her early twenties, came to study with me after being diagnosed with rheumatoid arthritis. Depressed and frightened by the prospect of living with a chronic, debilitating, and painful disease, she came to the UCLA Pediatric Pain Program looking for strategies that could improve her health. She decided, along with taking the medications recommended by her rheumatologist, to try yoga.

In the months leading up to her diagnosis, Jenna's quality of life had deteriorated rapidly. In September she was healthy and active, playing volleyball, hiking and rollerblading. By April, the smallest movements were painful. She walked slowly with a limp, it hurt to roll over in bed and she needed help to brush her hair. Jenna experienced pain, tenderness and/or swelling in almost every joint in her body—feet, knees, hips, shoulders, elbows, wrists, fingers, neck, and jaw. I wanted her to know that no matter how bad it got there was something we could do that would help. We might not make the problem go away completely but we could give her some relief.

We began with mostly passive inversions and passive backbends. She hung upside down on ropes, and lay over chairs and bolsters. The inversions would help her immune system and the backbends would lift her mood. Eventually I taught her poses, like handstand, to give her a feeling of confidence and optimism. Even for students without health problems, there is something exhilarating about kicking up into a handstand. When Jenna kicked into handstand, she used a slant board under her hand because of the problems she had in her wrists. She found that the pose actually made her wrists feel better and improved her range of motion. Soon she was doing standing poses with a quarter round [a wooden block that is a quarter of a circle and is used to ensure proper alignment in the leg] under her foot to help with the pain in her feet, ankles, and knees. If something in particular was causing her pain, I made sure to address it in class with specific poses that brought relief. I also encouraged her to practice on her own at home as she needed to.

Over the next several months, Jenna's health improved rapidly. By Fall, she was walking normally and, by the next Spring, she was pretty much back to normal— active and fully functioning. Most importantly, when she experiences pain related to

261

PAIN IN CHILDREN AND YOUNG ADULTS

RA, she knows what to do to bring relief. When she is feeling depressed she knows how to lift her mood. Iyengar Yoga gives Jenna a feeling of joy, accomplishment, and confidence.

Iyengar Yoga is a profound "meditation on the body" where kids, rather than avoid their problems and pain, can look at the underlying causes and habits that may contribute to these problems... and learn how to change them. For example, if a child has chronic headaches, it is quite possible that her neck and shoulders will be tight and contracted into a hard knot. She may have a rounded upper back and throw her head forward. She will probably be completely unaware of how much tension she is holding in her neck and how it has affected her posture.

Yoga is not just a series of exercises simply designed to build strength and flexibility. It is a vehicle to develop awareness. It is a process that develops strength of will, trust, confidence, and a willingness to look at one's self without judgment. Kids who practice Iyengar Yoga for their chronic pain problems begin to see that they can have some control over the underlying causes of their problems. Even kids who have conditions like rheumatoid arthritis, which yoga cannot cure, learn to see that yoga practice can greatly decrease or eliminate pain and reduce flare-ups. By doing yoga, those who feel betrayed by their bodies can learn some mastery over their problems and, by their own actions, develop a sense of competence and control.

Young people come to our pediatric pain program, and those who visit other similar pain programs, typically have sought medical help repeatedly, but without benefit. They are particularly vulnerable to feeling depressed and hopeless. We have observed the positive effect that Iyengar Yoga has on their mood.

Yoga Research

We developed an Iyengar-based yoga research program, initially for college students with depression. Our research demonstrated that yoga improved their *mood* and *function*. We also found a reduction in salivary cortisol, one of the body's major stress hormones. Subhadra Evans, PhD[70], the psychologist who developed with Beth our UCLA yoga research program, first studied young people with arthritis and found that the yoga program reduced fatigue and increased feelings of well-being. She then studied adolescents and young adults with irritable bowel syndrome (IBS) and found that there were major reductions in symptoms and enhanced energy and other positive outcomes. (See case #3 below). But... the only major change for the younger teens was improved physical function. The teens told *her "...I felt great*

---

70 Subhadra Evans, PhD; Assistant Professor, UCLA Pediatric Pain Program. David Geffen School of Medicine at UCLA. *http://ccim.med.ucla.edu/?page_id=155*

COMPLEMENTARY MIND AND BODY THERAPIES

at the end of class but the ride home with my parents 'undid' whatever benefits I got from the yoga class!" This led Subhadra to realize that including parents in the intervention for teens may allow for longer lasting and broader positive results[26].

Bottom line: Yoga needs to be tailored to the age and needs of students.

Iyengar Yoga for Irritable Bowel Syndrome

Case #3. Mary was a 14-y-old girl who had two surgeries for gastro-esophageal reflux disease (GERD), but had continued chest and abdominal pain, as well as vomiting, difficulty eating, weight loss, and anxiety. She was unable to attend school, sleep, socialize, or eat and had become wheelchair-bound. Despite evaluations and treatments by specialists over an extended period of time, her symptoms had not improved.

Mary was diagnosed as having irritable bowel syndrome (IBS), with esophageal hyperalgesia subsequent to sensitization following her GERD and two gastroenterological procedures, and conditioned food aversion. While the GERD had resolved, her fear of eating and conditioned vomiting food remained, as did the hypersensitive esophagus and stomach.

She was also diagnosed with a generalized anxiety disorder, which might have preceded or was subsequent to the IBS and vomiting. Mary was prescribed escitalopram, a serotonin selective re-uptake inhibitor and 4 months of individual treatment with Iyengar yoga. Her recovery was extraordinary. Midway through the intervention, Mary's abdominal pain eased, and she could eat in increasing amounts, gain weight, stand on her own, no longer needing a wheel chair for mobility. For Mary, taking charge of her own healing process though the practice of Iyengar yoga with props, helped her to feel optimistic and empowered. Her range of motion visibly increased, and she could extend and relax through supported postures.

By the end of the yoga treatment plan and sessions, Mary was no longer using a wheelchair, sleeping well at night, reported energy during the day and had gained back to her normal body weight. Her esophageal and abdominal pain had resolved completely; her eating patterns had returned to normal, with no vomiting or food aversion. Mary's mood had improved, feeling more content and less anxious. She also had developed a plan with gradual return to her school. By the following year, she was symptom-free and had an active social and school life. She was discharged from the PPP.

It is best to learn Iyengar Yoga with a qualified teacher. To find a teacher near you, consult the Iyengar Yoga National Association Web page at *www.iynaus.org* You can also call your local yoga studios and ask if they have a certified Iyengar Yoga teacher on staff. When you speak to the teacher, make sure you share with her your

263

PAIN IN CHILDREN AND YOUNG ADULTS

child's relevant medical history so that she can assess the most effective and safest way for your child to begin practice.

BIOFEEDBACK

Biofeedback uses a computer or other feedback device to assist your child in managing symptoms by becoming aware of and learning to voluntarily control physiological changes associated with the stress response. These monitored changes may include muscle tension, skin temperature, sweat gland response, brain wave activity, or breathing or heart rate.

During a biofeedback session, the trained therapist applies sensors to parts of your child's body. These electrodes connect with devices that monitor your child's responses and give him visual and/or auditory feedback. For example, he might hear tones and see colorful graphs on a monitor that display changes in his muscle tension or skin temperature. With this feedback, he will learn how to produce voluntary changes in body functions, like lowering muscle tension, sweat gland response or raising skin temperature. These are signs of relaxation. The biofeedback therapist also will teach different relaxation skills such as breathing, muscle relaxation techniques, or imagery.

Most parents have heard of "biofeedback" but often do not know what it is, how it works or why it might be useful in chronic pain disorders. We asked Bruce Levine, Ph.D.,[71], a psychologist in our team who is certified in Biofeedback, to discuss this modality for children with chronic pain:

How Does It Work? Let's consider that "biofeedback" includes "bio" (biological functions of the body), most of which are not in our conscious awareness (blood flow, heart rate, brain waves, or muscle contractions) while "feedback" is information within our awareness about the levels of these biological functions. So, biofeedback is a method to monitor and measure biological reactions in our bodies and then make those reactions known to us consciously in the form of "feedback."

An example: one device can monitor and record the temperature of a body part that is affected by the amount of blood flowing there (e.g. the more blood flow, the warmer the finger, toe or face). Normally, we exert no conscious control over blood flow or its effect on the warmth of any body part. However, with biofeedback devices, we do become aware of very small temperature changes and thus are aware of blood flow that causes the changes in temperature.

---

71 Bruce A. Levine, Ph.D., ABPP, BCIA, Board Certified in Clinical Psychology & Biofeedback Therapy. Beverly Hills, CA 90210. *www.drbrucelevine.com*

COMPLEMENTARY MIND AND BODY THERAPIES

Why Is This Important in Causing or Reducing Pain? *Biofeedback methods offer such a promise. By receiving sound or visual feedback that is directly correlated with slight changes in temperature (or muscle contraction levels, heart rate) the child acquires the ability to control these biological functions and their impact on the pain associated with these effects. Now, isn't that easy?*

Receiving feedback about changes going on inside our bodies allows us to gain conscious control over these functions! That's right, if you could become consciously aware of even slight changes in the temperature of a part of your body, then you could learn to control (voluntarily and consciously) the temperature of that body area by achieving the seemingly astounding ability to alter blood flow to it.

So, even if you could learn to alter your skin temperature, why would you want to and how might this be related to chronic pain? Let's say you suffer from chronic pain due to abnormal blood flow like in Reynaud's Disease (pain related to ice-cold hands or feet), CRPS (where decreased blood flow to some body parts often is associated with numbness and/or pain) or migraine headaches. Imagine for a moment how chronic pain disorders such as these might be impacted if you could actually learn to either direct or re-direct blood flow towards or away from the painful area, thus warming or cooling that area?

How Does the Fight or Flight Reaction Increase Chronic Pain? *Children with chronic pain disorders react to the pain in both emotional (fear, anxiety) and physical (heightened physiological responding) ways. Psychologists refer to this as a "stress reaction" known more commonly as the "Flight or Fight Response." It is the automatic, innate and protective response that we all have to signals that suggest danger; and it is mediated inside the brain. Of course, pain's major useful role in our lives is to signal us when something is wrong—when we are in danger, like when we mistakenly place our hand on a hot stove. But children with chronic pain often react to their pain with the same automatic responses triggered by the Flight or Fight Response... as if they were in danger. The brain does not distinguish the difference, even if there is no imminent danger.*

When part of the brain (called the "sympathetic nervous system") that responds to danger is activated by the perception of danger, many automatic and protective reactions are set into motion. Heart rate goes up (to move blood more quickly to areas that need oxygen and glucose), pupils dilate (to allow more light to enter the eye), perspiration increases (to help cool down the body during fight or flight), muscle contraction increases (to allow one to "spring" into action for defense or flight), blood flow moves away from the fingers and feet and towards the internal organs (thus the phrase "they got cold feet" when referring to people who make a decision to avoid something perceived as dangerous) and the intestines slow down their movement of food. This is all great and helpful if one is actually in danger. But when this cascade of reactions occurs in response to chronic pain, it paradoxically makes the child's symptoms even worse. For example, increased muscle contraction or decreased temperature is often associated with spasm and more pain.

One of the benefits of biofeedback therapy is to reduce activation of the sympathetic nervous system, thereby limiting or reversing arousal and the chain of physiological reactions linked to fear and danger.

How Can Biofeedback Change the Brain's Responses? *You are probably asking yourself, "How is this done exactly?" Biofeedback is a method of treatment that is painless and involves no pins, needles, shocks or any discomfort. Depending upon the physiological response that is being trained, a small sensor is placed on the body (e.g. a tiny thermo-meter may be attached to the finger or a small muscle sensor attached to the forehead) and the information is routed to a machine that measures slight changes in the response being monitored.*

The child is shown either a visual display or provided with head-phones through which some pleasant sound is relayed (e.g. music). When the child makes a slight alteration in the response (increases finger temperature or decreases muscle contraction level), the child gets immediate visual or auditory "feedback" telling the child of his or her success. So, if your child is being trained to raise his finger temperature, for instance, every time the temperature rises 1/100 of a degree, the child is reinforced by hearing music or seeing changes on a visual display! Through this repeated feedback, the child learns to control responses not normally under his control, in a direction opposite that occurring when autonomic sympathetic arousal arises. Magic...your child begins to produce physiological responses more similar to what happens when he is relaxed, rather than what happens when he experiences fight or flight-type reactions.

Case: *Recently, 10-year-old Reed was referred because he had recurrent head and abdominal pain for over a year. His pain was helped somewhat with medication, but he still missed many days of school and play-dates with friends. He had to refuse sleep-overs and day-trips with his friends because of fearing sudden, uncontrollable pain.*

Reed received a dozen biofeedback treatments over 10 weeks during which he learned to quiet his fearful arousal and establish a method to relax and gain control over the pain. He was taught breathing methods and cognitive strategies (ways to think differently and less catastrophically about his symptoms) that aided in his recovery.

Finding A Health-Care Professional Qualified to Provide This Type of Treatment. *The Biofeedback Certification International Alliance (BCIA) is the largest non-profit organization that credentials providers in this field and provides the public with a list of Board-Certified providers in their geographic area. To access their search site, place the following link into your browser: http://certify.bcia.org/4dcgi/resctr/search.html*

COMPLEMENTARY MIND AND BODY THERAPIES

The point of using biofeedback for chronic pain management is to help children learn self-empowerment: to be aware of how their body reacts to different experiences and to gain physiologic control of the branch of the nervous system that is activated by pain or stress. Everyone who has ever been in pain knows that the more pain you have, the more stress you feel. And the more stress you feel, the more pain you have. So, through biofeedback, we attempt to break the stress-pain cycle. Usually there are quick changes, but even if at first there is little change in the pain itself, as the child gains more control, the pain experience also becomes more manageable.

There are many practical methods of applying his new skills in everyday situations. A simple example is to use deep breathing before a test. A more complex example is having kids go into a stressful situation while they are being monitored with biofeedback instruments. We might suggest to a child who is anxious in crowds that he go to a mall and monitor himself in response to being around large numbers of people. Initially it might be hard for him to relax but eventually using biofeedback skills he can relax and be comfortable in that situation. It is a method of stress desensitization.

Habits of tension take some efforts to undo. Pain is a signal of wear and tear. Biofeedback is a fun and painless way for children to learn body awareness, relaxation, and pain and stress management skills that they will be able to use throughout their lives. As with any educational challenge, both timing and motivation matter. If the timing is right and motivation high, changes will occur during the first session and most definitely by the fourth. If no changes are noted after a month of treatment, it may be useful to stop and suggest alternative treatments.

Hypnotherapy

During my (LZ) fellowship in Adolescent Medicine at Children's Hospital Los Angeles in the 1970's, I became interested in the possible impact that hypnotherapy might have on pain.

> *Case: I worked with an adolescent, Gerald, who had sickle cell disease with many visits to the emergency department (ED) and hospitalizations for pain crises. I began to learn hypnotherapy and Gerald agreed to be my first "guinea pig" and undergo hypnosis while I learned. Typically, during our sessions, he would go in his imagination to a "favorite place" (usually that meant with his girlfriend, anywhere). He had always felt relaxed at the sessions but nothing dramatic had affected his pain episodes. After I had attended a workshop on Hypnosis and Pain at a national meeting, I suggested to Gerald that his mind would "know" when a sickle cell crisis was about to come, like an "aura" before a migraine, and that his mind would help him take slow deep breaths at those times to prevent the emergence of a pain crisis.*

PAIN IN CHILDREN AND YOUNG ADULTS

At the next session, rather than going to a "favorite place" of being with his girlfriend, Gerald began to have images of sewers overrun by rats, and a huge hose with high pressure water that would wash out the rats and garbage. He said that at home he would sometime notice a funny feeling in his body and his mind would take out the hose and wash out the rats. After four months, Gerald was going to the ED less often and was taking lower doses of pain medication. Several years later, Gerald received Emergency Medical Technician (EMT) training and became the first ambulance driver with sickle cell disease in Los Angeles.

We asked J. Kathryn de Planque, Ph.D[72], a hypnotherapist in our pain program, to discuss hypnotherapy in the context of treating children with chronic pain.

Children with chronic pain often feel powerless, as their lives have been greatly impacted by pain, and often they have not received the support and understanding from physicians, educators, family members and friends. They may experience a sense of isolation, confusion, anger, sadness and heightened anxiety and fear.

Goals of Hypnotherapy: *My specific goal as the therapist is to give my patients tools to help themselves so that they learn to utilize the techniques that are most effective for them on their own to provide the individual support they need. Often, children with chronic pain use hypnotherapy to break the chronic pain cycle and alter maladaptive neurological patterns.*

What Is Hypnotherapy? *Children and family members may have some misconceptions of what hypnotherapy really is. It is important to make the distinction between hypnosis, as simply an "altered state of consciousness" and hypnotherapy, a treatment that uses specific therapeutic techniques, often with the use of imagery, while the child is in an altered state of consciousness at least part of the time. The "altered state" is achieved with deep relaxation in combination with focused attention; this is the time when an individual is most available for suggestion.*

It is vital that all of my child patients understand how hypnotherapy works and why it is such a powerful mind-body tool. Once they establish understanding and trust for both the therapist and the techniques, they are then able to use the work more effectively.

How Does It Work? *Hypnotherapy is intended to help relieve the sense of power- lessness that children with chronic pain experience by learning methods to regulate physical and emotional pain, reduce side effects, and increase daily functioning in "normal" activities. Patients often suffer from a lack of sleep, so I usually begin therapy*

---

72   J. Kathryn de Planque, Ph.D., Simms-Mann Center for Integrative Oncology at UCLA; the hypnotherapist in our pain program. *www.simmsmanncenter.ucla.edu/index.php/profile/j-kathryn-de-planque-phd*

COMPLEMENTARY MIND AND BODY THERAPIES

by using guided imagery to help them experience deep relaxation and imagery. They are then given the option to take a CD that is similar to the imagery they just experienced for them to use at home to help induce sleep at bedtime, or just relaxation when it is needed. This often serves as a positive experience and introduction to how the "altered state" and door to the subconscious can be achieved.

It is important that rapport and trust be established in order for hypnotherapy to be utilized successfully. This is true in any psychotherapeutic interaction. But in order for children to "let go," they need to feel both safe and comfortable with the therapist and with the use of their own imagery.

When to Consider Hypnotherapy? *Parents may consider hypnotherapy when the child is open to it and receptive to using their imaginations. Some children may need to come to a session and have it explained to them by the therapist before making a decision. It is important that the children feel that the choice of hypnotherapy is theirs. When making a choice for a specific hypnotherapist, it is important for parents to seek a therapist trained and experienced in the health professions, certified in hypnotherapy, and specializes with children and teens.*

How I Use Hypnotherapy *An example with a child is in utilizing the classic imagery of "Special Place," in which the child establishes a therapeutic environment in their imagination, preferably outdoors, where he/she feels safe and comfortable. It is in that place that children can apply therapeutic techniques for healing and/or receive pre-determined suggestions in order to make the changes necessary to achieve their goals.*

*One specific example of a child's imagery was fly-fishing in a river where he could feel the movement of clear water and experience the tranquility and peace of the quiet surroundings. There he was able to reduce or eliminate his pain by the soothing nature of the experience; **the brain does not distinguish whether you are really in the river or you experience it in your mind and body as if you were there.** It is there that he was able to receive the suggestions about seeing himself returning to school and functioning in the classroom or going out with friends, depending on the goal he had established for that session. There have been many wonderful stories to tell of children with whom I have had the privilege to serve in hypnotherapy.*

Case Study. *Martha was a young lady who was fearful of going away to college the next summer, as she experienced severe nausea and abdominal pain impacting her ability to function. One technique that was exceptionally powerful for her was the use of an "inner healer," a lion named Mark. Whenever Mark came to her in her imagination and laid his body across her abdomen, the nausea and pain were decreased or eliminated.*

Once she was able to break that cycle of chronic pain, she was slowly able to heal and function. Her fear of going off on her own to college was eliminated, as she knew she had the safety and comfort of utilizing Mark if needed. She did successfully attend a college away from home.

OVERVIEW OF "MIND-RELATED" INTERVENTIONS: WHICH IS BEST?

Science has identified a number of "mind-related" interventions that alter neural signaling associated with pain. Biofeedback, described previously in this chapter, is one such therapy, and is particularly suited to children who need "physical proof" that their mind has some control to alter various aspects of bodily function. It is also helpful for children who especially enjoy computers and electronic gadgets.

Hypnotherapy, on the other hand, is most helpful for the child who has a good imagination and enjoys imaginative involvement. We describe both biofeedback and hypnotherapy as two different ways to "reprogram the pain circuitry" in the brain. We often say, "…if your brain were just a computer, we would turn it off and reboot it by turning it back on." However, the brain is more complex than a computer, so the brain needs to learn some mind-based strategies to reprogram those central neural circuits to reduce pain (see examples in chapter 12… things parents can do to help their child.)

Mindfulness Meditation

The goal of mindful awareness through mindfulness meditation is to help you learn how to "be present" and "in the moment." So many of us are worried about what we did, what happened, what we have to do, or what will happen. We spend much of our lives not enjoying or appreciating the present moment, being alive, and being with people we love. Learning mindfulness meditation helps us to focus. **Mindfulness is being present with what is happening, in a balanced and non-judgmental way.** When parents cultivate mindful-awareness, they develop more patience and acceptance when their child is in distress. This helps the whole family. (See Mindfulness meditation in Chapter 12)

Mindfulness helps parents find the right amount of distance with their child who has chronic pain. If parents get too close, too reactive, and become too involved, their child can feel that their parents do not believe that they (the child) have the ability to cope with the pain. This too-close distance can impair the child's recovery. Alternatively, if parents protect themselves because they feel helpless and hopeless, and pull too far back, their child can feel abandoned.

COMPLEMENTARY MIND AND BODY THERAPIES

The mindfulness practice helps parents to connect with their child and be with him in an adaptive and supportive way. When parents are worried about what will happen if their child can't sleep that night, or be able to attend school the next day, or that the pain will *never* go away (we've all been there...), mindful awareness helps parents return to the present moment, to the simple sensory awareness of what's going on in that moment. This **attention to the present moment allows parents to listen to their child, observe in a non-judgmental way, and have compassion without the need to "rescue."** By practicing mindfulness, **parents can learn to stay calm even in the middle of the storm of their child's pain**. Parents often are most helpful to their child by just being there, without the need to feel that they must take the pain away or make it better. Rather just be there, accepting, kind, and compassionate.

Susan Kaiser Greenland is a lawyer who cultivated mindful-awareness and gave up her law practice to develop what has become a nationally recognized program in mindful awareness for children, described in her book *The Mindful Child* (Atria publishers, 2013).[73] In the book, Susan describes a number of strategies to help children develop mindful-awareness. She talks about the little "heckler" that we carry on our shoulders and who criticizes us, or make us feel embarrassed, ashamed, or not worthy. The heckler makes us look outward to others to learn how we feel about ourselves. Susan describes how the heckler is the critical part of us and how a practice in mindful -self-compassion can override the heckler's messages, so that we learn to love and value ourselves. In this way, cultivating mindfulness in children can help them to become centered, calm, and confident, yet have compassion for others.

Case: Our daughter Carin was teaching 4th grade when Susan began her work teaching mindfulness to schoolchildren. Susan would come to Carin's class on Fridays for 30 minutes and create games that would help children learn how to be present, notice each other and themselves in the moment. Carin told us that the children looked forward to these visits and seemed truly calmer for the rest of the day after Susan left.

Carin wondered if she could take mindful-awareness a step further to foster connectedness and compassion for fellow students in her classroom. She set up a class website that she created on the school computer. The children could "earn points" by doing their homework, being helpful and kind to others in the class, and other positive behaviors. When they earned a designated number of points they could go to their class website on their classroom computer and write "something nice that they noticed about a fellow classmate." They lost points if they wrote something that

---

73 Susan Kaiser Greenland J.D. developed a nationally recognized program in mindful awareness for children, described in her book *"The Mindful Child"* (Atria publishers, 2013).

PAIN IN CHILDREN AND YOUNG ADULTS

was neutral or not nice and these writings were then erased. Writing something nice about someone else in the class became a sought after goal. They were writing about things that they noticed and appreciated about each other. They were becoming more aware and in the moment and more connected as a class.

Carin noticed that the classroom behavior began to change. The children seemed more considerate of each other and more willing to help each other. The cultivation of mindful-awareness had an impact on the whole class of nine year olds.

Art Therapy

We asked Esther Dreifuss-Kattan, PhD[74, 27], an art therapist and psychoanalyst in our Program, to discuss art therapy and how it is used for children with chronic pain.

One of the primary goals of art therapy is to understand the internal world of children. We strive to make it accessible for exploration and then search for the meanings that will ameliorate physical and psychic pain and foster growth. If we are to communicate effectively with our patients, it is essential to discover a common language. Long before the development of language, the infant has his own world with self-created images and sensory experiences. Sigmund Freud has suggested that children at play behave like creative writers or artists, developing a world that pleases them. He indicates art's curious ability to handle feelings and themes that in ordinary life are too painful to talk about directly.

The picture is a bridge between the inner and the outer world of the child. Both worlds contribute to the creation of the picture. Through their pictures, children express and project their inner images. Once the picture is finished, the art therapist, together with the child, will look at the finished product and invite the child artist to share his feelings, thoughts and associations about it. However, if the patient is too young or is not interested in talking about the picture, that is fine. Often the act of creation is therapeutic in itself. However, if a discussion is established, the child may share with the therapist a possible title or story or explain the individual parts of the picture. The better the therapist knows the child and his or her medical, psychological, and family history, the easier it is for her to interpret some of the content. This can relieve fears, allow for exploration of trauma, and elucidate family dynamics. Art therapy allows for externalizing on the paper the internal world and conflicts of the child.

Case #1: *Joe was referred to me through the pain clinic; he was a withdrawn, stressed, 16-year-old gifted high school student with severe chronic headaches. He completed*

---

74 Esther Dreifuss-Kattan, PhD ATR, Psychooncology, Psychotherapy, Art Therapy, Psychoanalysis, Beverly Hills, CA 90212. *www.dreifusskattan.com;*

COMPLEMENTARY MIND AND BODY THERAPIES

a scribble drawing in the first consultation. Filling in the colors, he recognized a bird with a huge head, with a red area, a small body and tiny wings. Joe's chronic, severe headaches, which had made him dependent on medication, were surfacing unconsciously in the big-sized head of this bird. Together, we realized how the oversized head made it impossible for the bird to take off, fly to his own place, away from his overprotective mother and the parents' marital conflicts. Joe's love of art and his ability to express his pain through artwork and also to "understand" his pictures brought him joy and relief.

Energy Therapy

Energy therapy, bioenergy, therapeutic touch, Reiki, and healing touch are all part of a system of non-touch (or light touch) healing treatments. Energy therapies assume the existence of a field of energy originating from within the body. Energy therapists perceive blocks or depletions within the patient's body. These blocks are assumed to be energetic reflections of pain.

The therapist manipulates energy fields with his or her hands to enhance the flow of energy, restoring and clearing these disturbances. Most energy practices have the underlying belief that illness occurs on the vibrational level before solidifying and manifesting in the body. It is believed that this *Life Force* is inherent to health and flows freely and fully when health is present. Energy therapists believe that as illness settles into the body, the flow of this life substance slows, stagnates, and becomes blocked. Energy therapy attempts to break up these blocks or unhealthy patterns both before and after illness is present and allow health to return to the body, mind, and emotions.

Many energy therapists offer training in their particular modality of working with energy. Some therapists work with the various body systems identified by Western medicine, such as the nervous, endocrine, and lymphatic systems as well as the major organs of the body. Others work with bodily systems identified by Eastern medicine including "Chakras" and "meridians" (see Acupuncture earlier in this chapter), which also correspond to the various organs and systems in allopathic medicine.

Music Therapy

We asked Vanya Green[75], MA, our pain program music therapist, to talk about music therapy.

> *What Is Music Therapy? It is a goal driven, evidence based practice in which the process of creating music in a therapeutic relationship promotes health and well-being. When parents and caregivers see "music" in the title, they assume that their child*

---

75   Vanya Green, MA, LPCC, MT-BC. *http://melodyworks.org/what-is-music-therapy*

is not a candidate, since he/she does not play an instrument; this is certainly not the case. The child does not need to have any musical experience or specific knowledge to participate and benefit since the therapy relies on the therapist's expertise and ability to make music accessible to anyone, regardless of age, training or experience.

Music therapists are trained in interventions and approaches to help patients tap into their potential, improve functioning, and take part in the healing process. Since music therapy does not depend on verbal communication, it provides a safe place within which to explore and express emotions and be particularly effective for working with children and adolescents. Sessions are a collaborative process—using music and arts to enhance therapy and help integrate the mind, body and brain.

I use the flexibility that music offers to help children and adolescents change the way they feel and think about their pain. Patients often take to vocal and breathing exercises as well as songwriting. Songwriting can be particularly effective for helping children experience some distance from their pain because they express how they feel about it within the confines of a song that has a defined beginning and ending. They can express a wide range of emotions, even within one song, in a way that reflects their process of dealing with the pain and hopes for recovery. In this way, creating and performing the song in a therapeutic environment is cathartic. When lyrics shift from negative, pain-ridden thoughts and feelings to positive, inspiring messages, this in turn helps patients shift their thoughts about their own pain.

Case #1: *Lisa, a young adolescent with cancer was initially very shy. However, in her work, Lisa decided to adapt the song "We Will Rock You" into an anthem against cancer. She ended up writing the lyrics out in poster form and posting it on her wall as inspiration. The work we did together was focused on Lisa's development as an artist as this helped her to feel less medicalized, more empowered, and less like a sick person needing therapy. We worked on singing skills, self-expression and songwriting. Whereas a teacher may have spent more time on ensuring that she could sing pitches perfectly, in therapy we worked more on breathing exercises for singing (and relaxation) and on 'perfecting' her songs until she was satisfied. She responded well to the ability to control the direction of the session.*

Through this, Lisa asked questions and created a listening audience with whom she could communicate, helping her to feel less isolated. She wrote, "Have you ever wondered why a baby bird is meant to fly up and out of its nest?" She also was able to express her feelings about family, writing, "When I'm sad and lonely, I think of mom. I know she's always there for me. She holds my hand..." While she used to be shy at recess and sit alone on the bench, music had transformed her life and as an artist, she could express herself and come out of her shell.

COMPLEMENTARY MIND AND BODY THERAPIES

Mechanisms of the Therapy: When we are injured, both the brain area corresponding to the part of the body that was hurt and emotional centers in the brain are activated. Consistent physical pain lowers our threshold for the amount of pain that can cause distress, leading to a destructive feedback loop. In order to decrease the amount of suffering that we experience as a result of injury, it is important to find ways to activate the brain's emotion centers in positive ways.

Music can be a particularly effective modality of treatment for working with people experiencing acute and chronic pain. Using non-musical and music therapy interventions, therapists tailor sessions to individual needs to decrease pain and facilitate coping.

Research: Singing in particular has been shown to significantly increase levels of oxytocin (a hormone important in bonding) and increase joy, self-expression, energy and relaxation (Grape, Sandgren, Hansson, Ericson, & Therorell, 2003). See [28] for more research articles on Music Therapy.

Complementary Practitioners—Checking Them Out

When you decide upon a CT, regardless of the type, interview the clinician first. (Conversely, if the practitioner doesn't ask you or your child any questions and "plunges into treatment," be wary!) We believe that it is important for a parent to ask the following nine questions:

1   What is your training in this therapy?

2   How long have you been practicing?

3   Have you worked with children before? If so, for what conditions?

4   What benefits can be expected from this therapy in general and given my child's particular pain problem?

5   How long before I can expect to see benefits and how often does my child need to come before benefits can be seen, on average?

6   What are the risks and side effects, if any?

7   Will the therapy interfere with conventional treatment?

8   Will the therapy be covered by insurance?

9   Are you willing to review your plans and the treatment with my child's physician?

PAIN IN CHILDREN AND YOUNG ADULTS

BOTANICALS AND NATURAL PRODUCTS[76]

Peppermint *(Mentha piperita)* *(www.mcp.edu/herbal/)*

The principal uses are for irritable bowel syndrome, other digestive disorders, and as a decongestant.

Overview: Peppermint is widely used in food, cosmetics and medicines. It is helpful in symptomatic relief of the common cold. **It may decrease symptoms of irritable bowel syndrome (IBS) and decrease digestive symptoms such as dyspepsia and nausea**; more research is needed.

It is used topically as an analgesic and to treat headaches. Peppermint is on the FDA's "generally recognized as safe" ("GRAS") list; whole herb peppermint has few side effects. However, peppermint oil can cause heartburn or perianal irritation and is contraindicated in patients with bile duct obstruction, gallbladder inflammation and severe liver damage, and caution should be used in patients with GI reflux.

Menthol products should not be used under the nose of small children and infants due to the risk of apnea.

Turmeric *(curcumin)*

In the U.S., turmeric is best known as a spice and one of the main components of curry powder; it gives Indian curry its flavor and yellow color. It is believed to have anti-inflammatory, antioxidant, and perhaps even anticancer properties.

Why do people take turmeric? Curcumin, a substance in turmeric, may help to reduce inflammation. Several studies suggest that it might ease symptoms of osteoarthritis and rheumatoid arthritis, like pain and inflammation. Other compounds in turmeric might also be medicinal. Turmeric (*Curcuma longa*) has been used for 4,000 years to treat a variety of conditions. Studies show that turmeric may help fight infections and some cancers, reduce inflammation, and treat digestive problems. But remember several facts when you hear news reports about turmeric. First, many studies have taken place in test tubes and animals, and turmeric may not work as well in humans. Second, some studies have used an injectable form of curcumin, the active substance in turmeric. Finally, some of the studies show conflicting evidence.

Curcumin is a powerful antioxidant that can scavenge molecules in the body known as free radicals that damage cell membranes, tamper with DNA, and even cause cell death. Anti-oxidants can fight free radicals and may reduce or even help prevent some of the damage they cause. In addition, curcumin lowers the levels of two enzymes in the body that cause inflammation. It stops platelets from clumping

---

76 *http://www.longwoodherbal.org/monographs.htm*

COMPLEMENTARY MIND AND BODY THERAPIES

together to form blood clots. Research suggests that turmeric may be helpful for the following conditions:

Indigestion or Dyspepsia: Curcumin stimulates the gallbladder to produce bile, which some people think may help improve digestion. One important placebo-controlled study found that turmeric reduced symptoms of bloating and gas in people suffering from indigestion.

Ulcerative colitis: Turmeric may help children with ulcerative colitis stay in remission, but the research has only been carried out in adults. In one double-blind, placebo-controlled study, adults whose ulcerative colitis was in remission took either curcumin or placebo, along with conventional medical treatment, for 6 months. Those who took curcumin had a relapse rate much lower than those who took placebo.

Osteoarthritis: Because of its ability to reduce inflammation, researchers have wondered if turmeric may help relieve osteoarthritis pain. One study found that people using an Ayurvedic formula of herbs and minerals with turmeric, winter cherry (*Withinia somnifera*), boswellia *(Boswellia serrata),* and zinc had less pain and disability. But it's impossible to know whether it was turmeric or one of the other supplements—or all of them together—that was responsible. Osteoarthritis is also uncommon in children.

Uveitis: A preliminary study suggests curcumin may help treat uveitis, an inflammation of the eye's iris. In one study of 32 adults with chronic anterior uveitis, curcumin was as effective as corticosteroids, the type of medication usually prescribed. Research in children is needed. Uveitis may be seen in children with juvenile idiopathic arthritis. Source: *Turmeric | University of Maryland Medical Center http://umm.edu/health/medical/altmed/herb/turmeric#ixzz32rFTkmPd*

St. John's Wort

This common meadowland plant has been used as a medicine for centuries. Early European and Slavic herbals mention it. The genus name *Hypericum* is from the Latin word hyper = "above," and icon = "spirit." The herb was hung over doorways to ward off evil spirits or burned to protect and sanctify an area. The species *perforatum* refers to the many puncture-like black marks on the underside of the plant's leaves. Some sources say the plant is called St. John's Wort because it blooms on St. John's Day (June 24); others say it was St. John's favorite herb; others note that the deep red pigment in the plant resembles the blood of the martyred saint.

St. John's Wort is reported to relieve anxiety and tension and to act as an antidepressant. It was once thought that hypericin interfered with the body's production of a depression-related chemical called monoamine oxidase (MAO), but recent research has shed doubt on this claim. Research now is focusing on other constituents, such

PAIN IN CHILDREN AND YOUNG ADULTS

as hyperforin and flavonoids. Wort extracts may exert their antidepressant actions by inhibiting the reuptake of the neurotransmitters serotonin, norepinephrine, and dopamine. The required dosage is three grams of powder per day, but it must be taken for weeks—and sometimes several months—before results are noted. Also the studies have been done in adults, and so the actual optimal and safe dose for children is unknown.

Coenzyme Q10

Coenzyme Q10 circulates in our blood and is a component of dietary phytoestrogens that display anti-oxidant activity. Soybeans are a primary source. Most clinical studies of coenzyme Q10 have focused on its prevention of oxidant-injury. See *www.mayoclinic.org/drugs-supplements/coenzyme-q10/evidence/hrb-20059019*

Antioxidant: CoQ10 has been studied for use as an antioxidant to protect cells from damage. CoQ10 has been used in combination with other antioxidants. Early study suggests that it may have antioxidant benefits in people with heart disease. More information is needed on the potential benefits of CoQ10 alone for pain.

Chronic fatigue syndrome: Early research shows CoQ10 may improve symptoms of chronic fatigue syndrome. More quality research is needed in this area.

Fibromyalgia: Fibromyalgia is a condition in which there is long-term pain and tenderness in the muscles and joints. Early study suggests that people with this disorder may benefit from CoQ10. More research is needed.

Nerve pain: Early research reports that CoQ10 may benefit people who have nerve pain. More research is needed to confirm these findings.

Melatonin

Melatonin is a hormone secreted by the pineal gland in the brain that responds to and regulates our day-night rhythms. It is used to initiate and enhance deeper sleep. Melatonin is generally a safe sleep aid for children, especially those whose ability to fall asleep has been disrupted by chronic pain. Chronic stress related to pain or not, can disrupt normal circadian rhythm cycles with the pineal gland not putting out nightly pulses of melatonin. Taking melatonin in 1-6 mg at 1-2 hours before bedtime can help your child with chronic pain fall asleep. There should be a "melatonin break" about once a month for a few days so that the circadian "clock" can reset itself.

Echinacea

Echinacea leads the list of herbs publicized for the treatment of colds. Many patients use Echinacea as an immune-stimulant with the hope of decreasing risk of infection.[29] No data exists on this use for children in general and especially those with pain. This herb

278

COMPLEMENTARY MIND AND BODY THERAPIES

is proposed to possess immune-stimulating properties that include increased phagocytosis, stimulation of interleukins IL-1, IL-6, and tumor necrosis factor (TNF). Research on Echinacea in the prevention and treatment of colds has yielded mixed results.[30, 31]

OTHER COMPLEMENTARY THERAPIES

There are other CTs used for children with chronic pain: Pet therapy, aromatherapy, hippotherapy (horse therapy), dance and movement therapies, creative writing, journaling, and others. There is little research to indicate how these work, for whom they may be most helpful, and what dose (how often and for how long) of these therapies is needed for effect. However, as with other CTs in which there is little or no research in children with pain, there may be little downside to any therapy that provides a means of expression and creative outlet to help empower children who suffer from chronic pain. In particular, pets are a source of comfort and support that might be considered as part of the treatment plan.

SUMMARY

Having good information is your first step to know if complementary therapies might be helpful for your child. Search out and evaluate the resources provided in this chapter. Are all these good sources? Unfortunately, there is no guarantee that questionable, false, or outdated information won't be found on the Internet. However, you can compare what these sources have to say and empower yourself with knowledge.

Table 15.3 Internet Resources for Complementary Therapies (CTs)	
Subject	Web Site or Contact Information
CT information	*https://nccih.nih.gov (government sponsored)*
CT in Children	*https://nccih.nih.gov/health/children* *https://nccih.nih.gov/health/pediatrics*
Botanicals in Children	*https://nccih.nih.gov/health/providers/digest/children* *https://nccih.nih.gov/health/tips/children* *https://nccih.nih.gov/health/tips/childsupplements*
Coenzyme Q10,	*http://www.mayoclinic.org/drugs-supplements* *https://nccih.nih.gov*
Melatonin	*https://nccih.nih.gov/health/melatonin*
Specific botanicals	*https://nccih.nih.gov/health/herbsataglance.htm*
Drug interactions- Side effects,	*http://www.quackwatch.com*
MedWatch safety alert	*www.fda.gov/medwatch*
Scams	*http://www.quackwatch.com*
American Academy of Pediatrics Section on Integrative Medicine:	*www2.aap.org/sections/chim/default.cfm*
Consortium of Academic Health Centers for Integrative Medicine	*www.imconsortium.org/*
Natural Medicines Comprehensive Database (requires subscription):	*www.naturaldatabase.com*
Natural Standard (requires subscription):	*www.naturalstandard.com*
US Department of Defense Total Force Fitness	*http://hprc-online.org/total-force-fitness*

COMPLEMENTARY MIND AND BODY THERAPIES

Locator for Complementary Practitioners & Services

Table 15.4 Locator for Complementary Practitioners & Services	
American Association of Medical Acupuncture	*www.medicalacupuncture.org*
National Certification Commission for Acupuncture and Oriental Medicine	*www.nccaom.org*
Bio-Feedback: Board-Certified providers	*http://certify.bcia.org/4dcgi/resctr/search.html*
Craniosacral Massage:	*www.upledger.com* *www.craniosacraltherapy.org* *www.cranialacademy.org*
American Massage Therapy Assoc.	*www.amtamassage.org/index.html*
American Physical Therapy Association	*www.apta.org*
Psychotherapist	*www.apa.org www.aamft.org/TherapistLocator*
Mindfulness meditation	*www.insightla.org*
Iyengar Yoga National Association	*www.iynaus.org*
Herbals/ Supplements	*www.longwoodherbal.org/monographs.htm*

On October 16, 1846, Gilbert Abbot, a Boston printer became the first human being to go under the knife without feeling any pain. After breathing in a new chemical called ether, the man was opened up by surgeon John Collins Warner, and a tumor was removed from his jaw while he slept, as doctors and medical students looked on. After the procedure, Warren addressed his Audience and declared, "We have conquered pain."

—ACCORDING TO PEOPLE'S JOURNAL OF LONDON, 1846.

Unfortunately, it was not to be as easy as that. ...
though surgery will never hurt the way it used to, pain remains.

CHAPTER 16

MEDICINES FOR TREATING CHRONIC PAIN

MEDICATION FOR CONTROLLING PAIN

PAROXYSMAL ORTHOSTATIC TACHYCARDIA SYNDROME (POTS)

OPIOID USE IN CHILDREN
- Addiction, Tolerance and Dependence

OFF-LABEL DRUGS AND FDA APPROVAL

ANTIDEPRESSANTS: WHY USE THEM FOR PAIN?

ANTI-ANXIETY MEDICATIONS

ANTICONVULSANTS

MUSCLE RELAXANTS

NEUROLEPTICS

TOPICAL AGENTS

NAUSEA AND VOMITING

OVER-THE-COUNTER (OTC)/ NON-PRESCRIPTION ANALGESICS

CONCLUSIONS

PAIN IN CHILDREN AND YOUNG ADULTS

There are four chapters in this Section D, each of which covers a specific aspect of an overall treatment plan for chronic pain. In the preceding three chapters, we discussed physical body-based therapies, psychological and behavioral mind-based therapies, and complementary therapies. Now, in this last section chapter we discuss the medications we use to treat chronic pain. In most cases, a treatment program will include more than one of these therapy types; often the program will include all four.

MEDICATIONS FOR CONTROLLING PAIN

Patients are referred to us by other doctors who seek our help in reducing patients' pain and enhancing their function. We find that often the primary approach used, after identified disease and disease-focused treatments have not resolved the problem, has been medicinal. In our experience, **only the most straightforward pain problems can be treated solely with medications or surgery**. A combined treatment approach is most often required.

> *Case #1: Thirteen-year-old Jane suffers from recurrent abdominal pain (unrelated to her menstrual cycle). Like clockwork every two weeks she ends up in the emergency department (ED) with debilitating stomach pains. Each time, the doctors treat her with intravenous morphine and the pain goes away (and she falls asleep), until the next bout. The doctors are stymied since their evaluations do not reveal a "cause" for the pain. They wonder if she is coming to the ED just to get morphine. However, Jane insists that the morphine makes her nauseated and that she would prefer that her stomachaches just go away so she doesn't have to come to the ED.*

Jane likely has functional abdominal pain (FAP), a brain/gut neural signaling disorder (see Chapter 5), and morphine was the wrong drug to give to Jane for this type of pain. Morphine stops the brain factory from making its own endorphins or "natural morphine," an important component of the pain control system. Jane was likely given morphine because her doctors didn't know how to diagnose or possibly how to treat FAP effectively. What she really needed was a better plan for pain control!

> *Case #2: Sixteen-year-old James has visited the ER multiple times in the past six months. He has sickle cell disease (see Chapter 6), which causes intense pain crises where his abnormally shaped blood cells clog small arteries, making it difficult for blood and oxygen to get to major body parts. The ER staff at his local hospital has become increasingly unsympathetic to his pain experience; they wait longer than they should to get him medication, and then give him a lower dose of morphine than is*

284

MEDICINES FOR TREATING CHRONIC PAIN

> *helpful for his pain. He is sent home with an insufficient supply and there is no plan for how to avoid ED visits and manage his pain better at home.*

In the case of James, the ED physicians wanted to do the right thing, but their biases about giving opioids to children, especially to a teenager, and maybe biases in relation to race, got in the way of proper treatment. They assumed that appropriate levels of pain relief would "*reinforce bad behavior.*" However, their approach did not bring about changes in James' behavior.

The best way to get an adolescent with chronic pain to keep asking for more pain medication or to keep coming to the ED is to under-treat his pain. If James had been prescribed the proper analgesic medication to take on a daily basis and had a plan in place to help him to cope with pain at home, he would have been able to reduce the pain before it got "*out of control.*" He would never have been in the ED getting opioids in the first place or at least far fewer times than without the home pain control plan.

The above case histories outline the problems. Now let's explore the range of medications that are important to control pain... when they are **used at the right time, for the correct condition**, and **at the appropriate dose.** First we want to discuss a common condition associated with chronic pain and the medication used to treat it, as long as the medication is used within an integrative biopsychosocial model of treatment.

POSTURAL ORTHOSTATIC TACHYCARDIA SYNDROME (POTS)

We find that about one-third to one-half of children whose bodies have undergone prolonged stress related to pain and other accompaniments (insomnia, mood changes) develop POTS. This means that, while blood pressure remains stable when sitting or standing, the heart rate increases by about 30 beats per minute from sitting to standing (or clinically tested on a tilt-table). POTS is more than anxiety. Deconditioning seems to play a role and a primary treatment is aerobic conditioning. POTS may cause the child or teen to feel dizzy upon standing.

Increased fluid intake, mind-body stress reduction strategies, and rarely a beta-blocker medication will reduce POTS over time in most cases. Beta-blockers are a group of medications typically used for people with heart problems, since they relieve stress on the heart by slowing the rate at which the heart beats. They reduce the action of certain sympathetic nervous system fibers. The most commonly used beta-blockers are propranolol, labetalol, metoprolol, and atenolol. If these POTS treatment strategies, as well as those addressing depression, anxiety, and/or sleep, are not effective and the child is symptomatic, then a pediatric cardiologist may evaluate

PAIN IN CHILDREN AND YOUNG ADULTS

and add other medications, such as a salt-saving steroid called Fludrocortisone (Florinef™) or midodrine (Proamatine™).

> *Case: Steven is a 15-year-old with systemic lupus erythematosus (SLE), an autoimmune disease that can affect different organs and be associated with pain. After a lengthy hospitalization because of severe headaches, Steven was discharged with no clear diagnosis for his headaches. It was thought that he might have had central nervous system SLE and had been placed on steroids, but they not only did not help his headaches, they gave him mood changes and hallucinations. So after a clinical trial for his SLE they were stopped.*
>
> *Steven was extremely anxious despite the high doses of an SSRI (fluoxetine) that his rheumatologist had prescribed 3 months earlier. He was quick to become anxious over even small changes in his breathing or heart rate and began focusing on his body. He told us that his face flushed readily and this scared him and that he was extremely sweaty all the time and thus always thought he had a fever. He also complained of dizziness, especially when getting up from a sitting position. On physical exam, his neurologic exam was normal. However, in checking his blood pressure and pulse in sitting and then standing positions, we found no change in his blood pressure but his pulse increased from 90 beats per minute (bpm) sitting to 120 bpm standing.*

We diagnosed tension headaches, anxiety and POTS. After conferring with his rheumatologist, we prescribed propranolol, because his sympathetic nervous system (SNS) had become hyperactive and his heart rate had increased 30 bpm when he stood up. He met criteria for a diagnosis of POTS and we assessed that his activated SNS was maintaining his tension headaches, his anxiety symptoms, and his dizziness. With high enough doses of propranolol, his heart palpitations, dizziness, and constant sweatiness improved, his headaches got better, and he stopped focusing on his body and was able to engage with friends and return to school.

It is worth re-emphasizing that POTS needs to be treated within a treatment strategy that addresses the underlying pain and stress that resulted in the POTS in the first place.

USING OPIOIDS IN CHILDREN

Paradoxically, many physicians use opioids for "pain management" in situations where this class of medications is not useful, yet they under-medicate when opioids are the right type of medication but higher doses are called for.

An opioid is a chemical substance that has pain control properties and sedative effects that dull the senses and induce relaxation. It may reduce the severity of

MEDICINES FOR TREATING CHRONIC PAIN

the pain and produce an *"I know it's there but I don't care"* attitude. Like many parents, doctors sometimes **fear giving opioids to children because of worries about harm to young children and addiction in adolescents.** When opioids are indicated as the correct medication, they should be given.

Addiction, Tolerance and Dependence

We emphasize that we use the term "opioids" here as the label for a class of analgesic medications, rather than "narcotics," which we view as a legal or police term. Opioid addiction, tolerance, and dependence are often confused with each other.

- *Tolerance* **is a physiological need for more opioids over time**. That is, the longer the child is on opioids (e.g. more than a week), the more likely that his body will acclimate to the medication and will need more to get the same effect over time.

- *Opioid dependence* **is the withdrawal that develops if the opioid is suddenly stopped after a week or more of use.** Withdrawal symptoms include sweating or rapid pulse, belly pain, increased hand tremor, insomnia, nausea or vomiting, physical agitation, anxiety, transient visual, tactile, or auditory hallucinations or illusions, and grand mal seizures. This is why opioids should always be weaned: removed gradually in lower and lower doses over time.

- *Addiction* **is the psychological craving for a drug**; that is, the individual wants it not for pain control, but for some other feeling that the opioid invokes, typically for euphoria or anxiety reduction.

- *"Pseudo-addiction"* occurs when the individual seeks opioids for actual pain control when past experience has shown that opioids have reduced the pain. Under-treatment of pain can create pseudo-addiction, as in the case of James who has sickle cell disease above. When pain is adequately controlled, the "addiction" behavior resolves.

Addiction is a rare problem in children, especially in children using medications to treat pain.

Opioids are *not* the medication of choice for most chronic pain problems because opioids do not directly re-balance nerve signaling. **Most chronic pain is caused by dysregulated nerve signals combined with a natural pain control system that is not working properly.** Opioids are aimed at what are called "opioid receptors" that normally respond to the body's natural opioids (e.g. endorphins, enkephalins), chemicals in the body's pain control system. If these receptors are filled with opioids from outside the body (such as hydrocodone alone or combined

287

PAIN IN CHILDREN AND YOUNG ADULTS

with acetaminophen), the body stops making natural opioids, resulting in a need for more and more opioids from outside. This delays the body's ability to get its own natural pain control system "up and running" effectively.

There are appropriate times for the short- and longer-term use of opioids to treat chronic pain. **We do not hesitate to use opioids for certain chronic pain conditions** where there is an ongoing nociceptive source of the pain, such as inflammation, pressure from a tumor, or ongoing severe active infection causing pain.

Case: Joey was in eighth grade when he developed chronic pancreatitis (chronic inflammation in his pancreas) of unknown cause. He had severe belly pain that he described as a "knife through my back from my stomach." He was not allowed to eat for months in order to give his pancreas a rest so it would heal. He received all nourishment intravenously.

In order to allow him to attend school and to not suffer, we gave him a patient-controlled analgesic (PCA) device with opioids in a little portable back-pack that he could wear to school. The PCA is a computer-driven device that allowed him to deliver a set dose of morphine into his veins when he pushed a little button at the end of a cord that was attached to the pump containing the morphine. We programmed the doses that he was allowed to give himself and the time intervals between doses. He did not give himself more than he needed to feel comfortable enough to function and reduce the pain

When his pancreatitis improved, we were easily able to wean Joey off of his opioid. Since this was a while ago, other delivery systems are now available for opioids. Now we might have provided Joey with a fentanyl skin patch on his back for transmission of the opioid fentanyl through the skin and into a reservoir under the skin to be gradually delivered to the rest of his body through his blood stream. The patch would need to be replaced every 3 days. This drug delivery method would have obviated the need for intravenous medication delivery. Also there are short-acting sublingual opioids that are absorbed through the oral mucosa for fast-acting pain relief.

For a chronic pain such as pancreatitis, ideally a longer-acting opioid, such as a fentanyl patch, would be ideal, with a fast-short-acting opioid for "break-through" pain, if there are some episodes of pain during the day that are not controlled by the baseline longer-acting opioid.

Below, we discuss different categories of drugs that are used effectively to treat chronic pain and describe when they should or shouldn't be used. One general caveat, from Dr. Elliot Krane[77]:

---

77   Dr. Elliot Krane Chief of the Pain Management Program at Packard Children's Hospital, Stanford Medical School, Palo Alto, CA.

MEDICINES FOR TREATING CHRONIC PAIN

"Drugs, per se, are seldom the answer or the solution. No drug works completely; most drugs carry with them a significant price in terms of side effects. Drugs are therefore used as an adjunct, but only inasmuch as they improve function. Except in hospitalized children and the terminally ill, the use of a drug that does not improve the level of function should... be stopped. For example, in a child at home with chronic pain related to most conditions, if an opioid leads to excessive sleepiness, depression, or decreases activity, it should be discontinued even if reports of pain diminish."

Off-Label Drugs and FDA Approval

*Most of the drugs that we discuss in this chapter have not been approved by the Federal Drug Administration (FDA) for the treatment of pain in children. In fact, **most drugs used to treat pain in children have not been approved by the FDA for children.** Prescribing drugs for something other than that for which they were originally intended is called "off-label" use. The FDA allows drugs to be sold and advertised for specific conditions for which they have been proven to be safe and effective. Once the drug is on the market, it can be used for any condition for which it seems effective. However, a drug cannot be advertised for any condition unless the manufacturer has proven to the FDA that it is safe and effective for that specific condition, and thus has acquired FDA approval. Many drugs used for chronic pain in children, such as low doses of antidepressants, have not been approved by the FDA for pain in children, even though such medications may be effective.*

The problem for those of us who treat chronic pediatric pain is that few pharmaceutical companies test drugs in children. From their standpoint, it doesn't make economic sense to do so, or unless the FDA will not approve their drug unless it is tested in children. This lack of FDA-approval may deter some doctors from using these drugs in children because they fear a lawsuit if anything happens that might in some way be tied to or attributed to the drug. However, physicians who treat children with chronic pain need to take these risks; otherwise we have few medications to offer.

More recently, the FDA has allowed pharmaceutical companies to extend their patent on a drug if the company will carry out the testing of that drug in children and gain an indication for use in children. Since pediatric analgesic clinical trials are expensive, pharmaceutical companies have to determine if their profits from the extended patent will be greater than the cost to carry out the pediatric clinical trials. However, with the addition of this inducement to extend clinical trials to children, there is an increasing array of analgesics and adjuvant medications now with indications in childhood pain conditions.

Many medications that are used to treat chronic pain were originally developed to treat something else, such as depression, anxiety, or seizures. These medications affect

PAIN IN CHILDREN AND YOUNG ADULTS

the neurochemical signaling in the central nervous system. Parents often become concerned or embarrassed when it is suggested that their child take SSRIs (anti-depressants). However, many of the chemicals underlying depression or anxiety are the same ones that are part of the body's pain signaling system.

If your child is prescribed one or more medications, you will want to find a method to keep track of the drugs, doses, and times you give the drugs. (Remember your notebook, Chapter 9.) As your child gets older, he may want to take his medication by himself and keep track of it all himself. This step toward independence can be anxiety provoking for many parents; but in fact, this form of responsibility is one of many important steps for your adolescent to regain a sense of control.

Kenneth R. Goldschneider, M.D.[78] emphasizes self-reliance and initiative in his patients. He tells children and adolescents:

"The pain is not your fault, but taking care of your body is your responsibility... This is one of those times when it is really 'all about you,' but that means you have to be the main one putting in the 'oomph' to get better."

If you choose to let your older child be in charge of taking his medicines, make plans to review how your son or daughter is doing about once a week, including how much remains in the medication bottles.

ANTIDEPRESSANTS: WHY USE THEM FOR PAIN?

Antidepressants raise the level of certain neurotransmitters—acetylcholine, norepinephrine, dopamine and serotonin (chemicals that the nerve cells use to communicate with or stimulate each other)—in the brain and in other neural pathways. By increasing levels of these chemicals at nerve endings, antidepressants seem to strengthen the system that *inhibits* pain transmission. Some antidepressants may be useful in treating chronic pain because they reduce depression and improve sleep (without being habit forming), and also because they reduce pain signals directly.

Tricyclic anti-depressants (TCAs) have been typically used in the past to treat depression. Examples include amitriptyline (Elavil™), nortriptyline (Pamelor™), imipramine (Tofranil™), desipramine (Norpramin™), and doxepin (Sinequan™). TCA's are used for pain control in low (not antidepressant) doses, typically given at bedtime. **Sometimes just helping a child to get good sleep is enough to help the pain problem resolve.** However, low-dose **TCAs have been shown to be effective for reducing abdominal pain in many cases of IBS or FAP,** as well as

---

78 Kenneth R. Goldschneider, M.D., Director, Pain Management Center at Cincinnati Children's Hospital,

290

MEDICINES FOR TREATING CHRONIC PAIN

in certain types of headaches. They are also typically used for pain that is directly "neuropathic" such as in Complex Regional Pain Syndrome (CRPS).

TCAs are non-addictive and do not lose their effectiveness once the body becomes tolerant of them, as is the case with opioids. Unlike most anti-inflammatory drugs (like ibuprofen), TCAs do not cause stomach inflammation and bleeding, and they do not interfere with the body's own natural pain control mechanisms. The most common side effects are drowsiness, constipation, dry mouth, blurred vision, and sometimes urinary retention (difficulty urinating). Rarely a person will have a condition where their heart rhythm or electrical conduction within the heart (called QTc interval) is different from normal when looked at on electrocardiogram (ECG). While this may not bother them, TCAs could worsen it. **An ECG is recommended, especially if there is a family history of heart rhythm problems or sudden, early death.**

Amitriptyline (Elavil™) is our first choice of the TCAs for abdominal pain, headaches, and CRPS. It is the most sedating of the TCAs (other than doxepin) and thus is useful for promoting sleep. We usually start with a lower dose of amitriptyline and gradually increase the dose if needed. Typically, we don't increase the dose to more than 50 mg at bedtime, since it is our experience that higher doses are more likely to bring about side effects.

Mirtazapine (Remeron™) is a tetracyclic antidepressant that increases the amount of noradrenaline and serotonin in the brain, both of which help with pain relief. While mirtazapine is often used as an antidepressant, it also is used to facilitate sleep. It is a potent histamine antagonist, which may account for its sedation properties. A major side effect is weight gain since it tends to stimulate the appetite. It would be a good medicine to prescribe for an adolescent who has lost significant weight related to a pain problem, is not sleeping, and is also depressed. **Trazadone (Desyrel™)** is another oral antidepressant that is used primarily to facilitate sleep.

Selective Serotonin-Reuptake Inhibitors (SSRIs) are both antidepressants and anti-anxiety medications and are used for treatment of chronic pain. Common SSRI's include sertraline (Zoloft™), *fluoxetine* (Prozac™), paroxetine (Paxil™), citalopram (Celexa™), escitalopram (Lexapro™), and fluvoxamine (Luvox™). Citalopram and escitalopram have the lowest gastrointestinal side effects among the SSRIs and have been studied as effective in IBS and FAP. Fluoxetine tends to be more activating than the other SSRIs and may be a good SSRI for children and adolescents with fatigue, pain, and depression and/or anxiety.

Unless your child's pain specialist has extensive training and experience with psychotropic medications that are used for chronic pain, it is ideal to work together with a child psychiatrist to prescribe this class of medications. The ideal plan would be for the pediatrician, child pain specialist, and child psychiatrist to communicate as the cohesive treatment team.

PAIN IN CHILDREN AND YOUNG ADULTS

Venlafaxine (Effexor™, Effexor-XR™), milnacipran (Savella™) and duloxetine (Cymbalta™) are medications called selective serotonin and norepinephrine reuptake inhibitors (SSNRIs) since they slow down the metabolism of both serotonin and norepinephrine, allowing increased levels of these two neurotransmitters. SSNRIs have indication for fibromyalgia in adults since they act in a broader way on central pain mechanisms. They may be useful for other widespread pain conditions since both neurotransmitters are involved in central pain inhibition. One study is currently underway on effects of duloxetine on juvenile fibromyalgia (in teens). The SSNRIs, like most anti-depressants, can cause nausea, headaches, anxiety, insomnia, drowsiness, and loss of appetite. The longer-acting form of Venlafaxine (Effexor-XR) is less likely to cause stomach upset, as is duloxetine

While most SSRIs have similar mechanisms of action, they all have slightly different profiles and may be prescribed for different reasons. Fluoxetine tends to be a more activating agent (increases energy) and thus is taken in the morning and is usually prescribed if fatigue is one of the primary symptoms. For children with abdominal pain, the newer SSRIs like citalopram and escitalopram tend to be used because they have a lower incidence of stomach upset than the other SSRIs and have been studied in children with IBS.

All of the SSRIs can have side-effects, such as nausea and fatigue early on. Starting with a low dose and gradually increasing it often prevents the development of side effects. These symptoms typically go away after about two weeks. Your child needs to be on the medication about four weeks before you will begin to see changes, and you will notice changes before your child does. **But it's best to not say anything until your child also notices the changes for his/her-self**. Some of the medications, like escitalopram, that are used to reduce depression or anxiety, can interfere with sleep in some children (in which case your child should take it in the morning with breakfast) or cause sedation (in which case your child should take it at night).

The way that antidepressants and SSRIs work to affect pain directly are not well understood. However, we like to think of them as giving boosts to the body's natural pain control system so that it will work more efficiently and effectively.

Some children with genetic contributors and neurobiology for anxiety disorders or who have a tendency to be worriers and perfectionists are at risk for the development of chronic pain. We know that when children are anxious, their nervous system gets "revved up," increasing the magnitude of their pain signals. SSRIs and related drugs can reduce anxiety and help lower the volume of pain signals to the brain. This category of medications also works directly on the emotional brain and can quiet fear centers and other reactive parts of the emotional brain. These medications act as a buffer to allow the child to learn other tools to reduce pain and anxiety, so that eventually he may not need to take the drug at all.

292

MEDICINES FOR TREATING CHRONIC PAIN

Case: Eleven-year-old Bonnie had fibromyalgia and problems sleeping. She was taking bedtime amitriptyline when we first met her, but the medication left her drowsy in the morning, even if she took it earlier in the evening. After months of sleep deprivation and chronic pain, Bonnie developed a depressed mood and appeared sad, even though she denied this. Her parents said that she had lost interest in her favorite activities and was often tearful. After taking a careful emotional history and evaluation from Bonnie alone, without her parents' presence, we determined that we would treat her with citalopram (in addition to a mind-based therapy), to determine if the sleep problem would improve if her depression lifted, and in turn if improved sleep and mood would be associated with reduced widespread pain. We knew that insufficient restorative sleep was also a product of and contributor to her fibromyalgia, as well as inactivity because of her pain and depression.

After six weeks when we saw her next, her mood seemed improved and her parents reported that they had their "old Bonnie" back. Bonnie was sleeping better, her function improved, and she was doing physical therapy and actively working with a psychologist in a cognitive-behavioral therapy skills-building intervention. If Bonnie were an older adolescent, we might have recommended the SSNRI duloxetine, as that has indications for fibromyalgia in adults, and would also be expected to have impact on daytime energy, mood, and pain.

ANTI-ANXIETY MEDICATIONS

The best way to treat anxiety is through behavioral, mind-body therapies, and, if needed, adding an SSRI. The SSRI's described under antidepressants also are used to treat anxiety. **We rarely use the group of anti-anxiety medications called benzodiazepines; we mention them here for completeness**. This group of anti-anxiety medications targets anxiety and may help pain indirectly by reducing anxiety. We might prescribe a benzodiazepine for a child who has panic attacks or to use early in treatment for a highly anxious child until the prescribed SSRI takes effect. Examples of benzodiazepines commonly used in children with chronic pain and concomitant anxiety disorders are lorazepam (Ativan™) or clonazepam (Klonopin™).

Benzodiazepines are *not* good medications to use for sleep because they block restorative sleep, the most helpful type of sleep to reduce pain. Common side effects include sedation and dizziness, among others. They are also habit-forming and should not be stopped abruptly, since withdrawal can take place. If anxiety does not respond to an adequate dose and trial of an SSRI combined with a psychological intervention, such as cognitive behavioral therapy, dialectic behavioral therapy, biofeedback, or hypnotherapy, among others, then a referral to a child psychiatrist should be made. For pediatricians without training in psychotropic medications, referral to a child

PAIN IN CHILDREN AND YOUNG ADULTS

psychiatrist to manage this part of the treatment plan should be made early on following diagnosis. Ongoing communication with a child psychiatrist is recommended.

ANTICONVULSANTS

Anticonvulsants are drugs that reduce central nervous system irritability. While most anticonvulsants typically are used to reduce or prevent seizures, they can be helpful for chronic pain, especially neuropathic/ central types of pain related to nerve hyper-excitability, like CRPS, and maladaptive brain neural connectivity patterns.

Gabapentin (Neurontin™) is the most common anticonvulsant with the least side effects that is used in treating *neuropathic* pain. It may cause drowsiness, but often it has minimal to no side effects when used appropriately. In children, doses start relatively low and increase until symptom relief is achieved.

- The liquid form of gabapentin comes as 250 mg/5 ml. However, the taste is awful and should be masked with syrups or food.

- Gabapentin can enhance entry into stage 4 (restorative) sleep and thus can be initiated just at night, or a higher dose is given at bedtime.

Pregabalin (Lyrica™) is an anticonvulsant that is used for neuropathic pain.

- Pregabalin does not come in a liquid form but capsule form with the lowest size being 25 mg.

- In adults, Pregabalin has indications for fibromyalgia. We often use it for central widespread pain in adolescents, if gabapentin is not effective.

Topiramate (Topamax) is another anticonvulsant, often used by child neurologists to treat headaches.

- Sedation can be a side effect and may be dose-dependent.

- Kidney stones have been reported with its use.

- Topiramate can have cognitive effects and impact memory.

MUSCLE RELAXANTS

There are a number of medications that relax skeletal muscle such as that in the back, neck, etc. These drugs are intended for myofascial (musculoskeletal) types of pain, such as low back pain, tension headaches, or other muscle spasm-related pain problems. The common drugs in this category include **cyclobenzaprine (Flexeril™), skelaxin (Robaxin™), zanaflex (Zanaflex™),** and **baclofen**. The common side

294

MEDICINES FOR TREATING CHRONIC PAIN

effect is sedation. Some doctors prescribe these for help with sleep or for children with ongoing severe muscle spasms, such as in cerebral palsy.

In our program, **physical therapy or Iyengar yoga has been more effective for myofascial pain than muscle relaxants,** and we use this group of medications infrequently. However, use of these medications differs by pain center and there are no studies comparing pain reduction with versus without the use of muscle relaxants.

NEUROLEPTICS

Neuroleptics are a group of medications that are used to treat severe anxiety, nausea and vomiting, or psychosis. They are not used to treat pain directly. We mention them here because some children have such extreme anxiety that they cannot sleep or function. Typically, this group of medications is prescribed by a child psychiatrist, when needed.

- The most common neuroleptics used for extreme anxiety in non-psychotic children are **quetiapine (Seroquel™)** and **olanzapine (Zyprexa™). Aripiprazole (Abilify™)** is an atypical neuroleptic used as an adjunct to treat depression as well as for elevated anxiety in a child on an SSRI.

- **Risperidone (Risperdal™),** another neuroleptic, acts by blocking subtypes of the neurotransmitters dopamine and serotonin. It is used often in children with tics, Tourette's syndrome, and as an antipsychotic drug. For children who have a neurobiology associated with tics, autism spectrum disorders (ASD), or other pervasive developmental disorders (PDD) and have chronic pain, Risperidone can be very helpful in altering behavior that can magnify pain. Used at bedtime, it can also facilitate sleep in this group of children. We tend to explain it to parents of children with ASD as a medication that "helps to unstick a sticky nervous system." That is, many of these children develop a neural circuit that keeps repeating itself, as if on automatic pilot. That is, the child notices the pain (headache, abdominal pain, etc.) and perseverates on it. He just can't get his focus of attention off the pain and continues to complain about it. Risperidone, as well as other neuroleptics, can cause weight gain and can stimulate the pituitary gland to produce prolactin, a hormone that can cause breast enlargement and galactorrhea (milk coming from the nipples). These side effects go away after stopping the neuroleptic.

Case: Francine is a 15-year-old with a five-year history of severe, super hypersensitivity to sound, touch, smells, and total head pain. She wore two pairs of very dark sunglasses even indoors, was in a wheelchair since changes in position and standing caused head pain, and wore a kerchief to protect her head. What also bothered Francine (and even

295

more so everyone around her) was a longstanding, chronic, loud, barking cough. She had been evaluated for her chronic cough by pulmonologists, allergists, and head and neck surgeons, and no one could find the cause. We learned that Francine had an early history of sensory sensitivities as a young child, had to have her food arranged a certain way on her plate, and had significant separation problems when attending preschool.

She was very bright and had special focused interest in various things, like "baby beanies," stamps, dolls from different countries, and other collections. School had been difficult for her socially and she had one friend who had moved away five years ago but still kept in yearly contact with Christmas cards. She and her mother were very close and she was on home-hospital with a teacher coming to her house since her pain and other symptoms prevented her from attending school.

She had seen a variety of child neurologists for her headaches, had been on a variety of "triptans" used for migraines, tricyclic antidepressants for her headaches, NSAIDS, and opioids, but not only did none of these medications help but she developed severe side effects to even tiny doses of each so that they had to be stopped soon after starting them.

After an extensive evaluation, we determined that Francine likely had the developmental neurobiology associated with autism spectrum disorders. That is, she was very high functioning, but had sensory sensitivity, difficulty with sensory integration (creating a buffer for being bombarded by internal and external sensory stimuli), had social difficulties since it was difficult for her to "read" non-verbal body language in peers and understand common social cues, and had a "sticky nervous system" in which she had difficulty with transitions and couldn't disengage from her headache by paying attention to other things. Her mother had learned what made her daughter anxious or upset and had developed a protective type of "mothering".

We thought that the headaches were myofascial since pressure on the muscles of her head, neck, and shoulders created pain, but her sensory sensitivities made her feel "overloaded" with trouble coping. We believe that the barking cough was a tic, a result of another repetitive neural loop that kept playing itself over and over. The more anxious she would become, the worse her cough (tic) would be.

The first thing we did was explain the neurological mechanisms underlying Francine's pain and her behaviors to both Francine and to her parents. We referred her to Dr. Samantha Levy, a psychologist on our team with significant experience working with children and families of children with chronic pain and developmental conditions, like autism spectrum disorders.

Samantha helped the parents work together to establish a daily routine for Francine and a behavioral incentive plan with the extra motivation encouraged by small rewards for the efforts.

MEDICINES FOR TREATING CHRONIC PAIN

> *We started Francine on a low dose of nightly Risperidone to help break her tic and perseverative (repetitive) behaviors. In time, we added low dose of the SSRI fluoxetine to reduce her anxiety.*
>
> *Francine liked being in the water so we engaged the help of Celia deMayo[79], one of our pain program physical therapists who was an expert in pool PT. Gradually, Francine's headaches resolved, her tic disappeared, she was able to slowly remove her sensory shields (sunglasses, wheelchair, head scarf, etc.), and was able to attend the independent study program and join the robotics club. In the latter, she found that she loved robotics and made some friends there who had similar interests.*

TOPICAL AGENTS

Topical anesthetics (for example, **Lidoderm™** patches) have a role in the treatment of chronic pain. The 5% lidocaine patch (Lidoderm™) is the only topical anesthetic agent to receive FDA approval for the treatment of neuropathic pain in diabetic neuropathy and post-herpetic neuralgia, both of which rarely occur in children. Off-label, we use these patches for CRPS-1 and applied over tender spots in myofascial pain or in fibromyalgia. They are applied for up to 12 hours (the patches must then be removed for 12 hours). Side effects are minimal and include skin irritation and swelling that usually disappear within 2 to 3 hours after the patch is removed. However, **many insurance companies will not cover the costs of these patches for conditions off label** and so other methods of topical pain treatment may need to be used, such as mentholated creams. We want to note that, unlike creams and other topical agents for chronic pain, there are many FDA-approved topical agents for numbing the skin for needle sticks in children.

NAUSEA AND VOMITING

Prochlorperazine (Compazine™) is probably the most commonly used of this class of drugs for nausea and vomiting, but also has the most side effects, including shakiness, the need for constant movement, and torticollis (where the head moves back in spasm).

There are other categories and types of medications that are more useful for preventing or reducing nausea and vomiting, such as **Diphenhydramine (Benadryl™), Ondansetron (Zofran™), granisetron (Kytril™),** and **Scopalomine.**

---

79 Celia Sabin deMayo, MA, MS, PT, OCS, APTA Board Certified PT Specialist in Orthopedics

PAIN IN CHILDREN AND YOUNG ADULTS

OVER-THE-COUNTER (OTC) OR NON-PRESCRIPTION ANALGESICS

These may be the most widely used and least understood of the medications available for people with chronic pain. This class of drugs includes: Aspirin, naproxen sodium (Aleve™), acetaminophen (Tylenol™ and others), ketoprofen (Actron™, Orudis KT™), and Ibuprofen (Advil™ and others).

Aspirin, ibuprofen, naproxen and ketoprofen belong to a subgroup known as nonsteroidal anti-inflammatory drugs (NSAIDs). They reduce inflammation caused by arthritis, connective tissue disease and injury by blocking prostaglandins, a chemical involved in pain signaling. **For their anti-prostaglandin effects, they are useful for menstrual cramps.** These drugs reduce adhesiveness or stickiness of platelets (a factor in the blood involved in blood clotting). Thus they should *not* be used for treating pain in children who also have a bleeding disorder such as hemophilia or in those who might have low levels of platelets, such as in children with leukemia or during the acute phase of mononucleosis or other viral illnesses. NSAIDs also can cause gastritis or stomach irritation and lead to abdominal pain and even to gastric bleeding.

Over-the-counter medications, such as the NSAIDs, are helpful in reducing relatively low levels of pain in a child who suffers from recurrent myofascial pain, migraines or daily muscle tension headaches, and menstrual cramps. As noted above, they can cause gastrointestinal upset or even bleeding and should be used with caution. They should also not be taken on an empty stomach.

Acetaminophen (Tylenol™ and others) does not have the same effects on platelets or on the gastrointestinal system as do the NSAIDs. While it is a mild analgesic, it also does *not* have the same effects on inflammation as do the NSAIDs. **Acetaminophen can be toxic to the liver and it is important to give only the dose recommended on the label.** Some medications, such as Percocet™ (oxycodone plus acetaminophen) or Norco™ (hydrocodone and acetaminophen), are combination drugs that include acetaminophen and can damage the liver if too many are taken in a day. These combination opioids with acetaminophen are prescription-only. You should check with your child's doctor about the total amount in a day that is safe for your child to take.

Some NSAIDs, such as naproxen sodium (Naprosyn), are available through prescription only. It is also worth noting that acetaminophen is often included in many "combination" drugs, both over the counter as well as prescribed, and so all ingredients in your child's medication should be checked for acetaminophen, since it is the total dose that can be harmful to the liver. **The American Academy of Pediatrics has expressed concerns about the amount of acetaminophen "hidden" in so many over the counter products.**

298

MEDICINES FOR TREATING CHRONIC PAIN

When using OTC drugs, be aware that **the brand name tells you about the manufacturer, not about the medicine.** For example, **Tylenol PM™ is in no way the same thing as Tylenol™.** It is important to read the medication ingredients to know what you are giving to your child, including the dose. Some newer types of NSAIDs, called cox-2 inhibitors, such as celecoxib (Celebrex™), are available by prescription and can be useful in children with an inflammatory component to their pain, since this group of NSAIDs does not have the gastric irritation effects that other NSAIDs do. Also, and most importantly, celecoxib has no anti-platelet effect so that it is useful before and after surgery and in children with bleeding issues (such as those with hemophilia, a low platelet count, liver disease, and others).

While we have said this earlier in the book, it is worth repeating here. **Medications alone will rarely solve a chronic pain problem.** For chronic pain, function returns gradually... before pain has resolved. It is crucial for parents—and the child if he is old enough—to understand that the goal of treatment is to help the child's body begin to function normally as it did before the pain occurred. To this end, various treatments, both drug and non-drug, are aimed at restoring balance and homeostasis in the body, and reversing the cycle of pain.

CONCLUSIONS

A key component in the healing process is the *expectation* that the pain will get better. **Quick solutions usually don't work for chronic pain problems.** Understandably, parents often anticipate that the medication will provide a significant reduction in pain, and hopefully right away. **Children who do the best over time make slow and steady progress in *function* first.** If a child has been in pain for a long time, it will likely take close to that amount of time for the pain to resolve.

We recommend that parents consider the basketball idiom, **"watch the feet... not the lips" for a hint in which direction to follow.** If your child's function is improving, even if he or she says that the pain is the same or even worse, be satisfied, silently. **Pain complaints are always the last to go.** Clearly as children begin to function more, they will be using muscles in ways that they hadn't before or not to that extent, and those muscles will be sore until they become used to the new activities.

299

SECTION E

GETTING BACK TO NORMAL... DAY-TO-DAY STUFF

The question is not how to get cured... but how to live.

—JOSEPH CONRAD (1857 – 1924)

CHAPTER 17

GETTING BACK AND STAYING IN SCHOOL

THE TRANSITION BACK TO SCHOOL

LEGAL RIGHTS OF EVERY CHILD WITH A CHRONIC PAIN CONDITION

- The Individual Educational Plan (IEP)
- The 504 Plan

SUBTLE LEARNING DISORDERS

WHY NEUROPSYCHOLOGICAL TESTING? WHAT IS IT?

WHICH ACTIONS AFFECT SUCCESSFUL SCHOOL RE-ENTRY?

- Parental Attitudes Affecting Successful School Reentry
- Preparation and support of the classroom teacher
- Potential problems in finding and using school resources
- Resources for parents and school

EFFECTS ON THE FAMILY

SIBLINGS AND EXTENDED FAMILY SUFFER TOO

THE TRANSITION BACK TO SCHOOL

Most children who have chronic pain actually tough it out and remain in school. There is, however, a significant group for whom multiple absences due to pain have interrupted their schooling. For some, there was a need to drop out or choose "home hospital" or on-line learning. It is for this group and those who might have a suspected learning disorder complicating their pain issues that this chapter will be most helpful.

For these kids, we know the pain is there, but there is no plaster cast or outward sign. To many peers, adults, and teachers it seems like the child could be "faking" it. For these children, whether due to a learning handicap, or a physical limitation(s), an individualized education plan (IEP) will be needed to maximize their school experience.

IEP-eligible students with chronic pain usually have serious *academic* and/ or *learning* problems that prevent them from meeting the standards of the class. They are not keeping up, often due to the multiple absences for doctor visits, therapy or pain that prevents them from leaving the house. Therefore, an **IEP will allow availability of instruction from resource teachers** in the Special Education Department and **program modification** and **accommodations**. The testing and steps in gathering this information are outlined in Table 17.1.

Table 17.1 Roadmap of Preparations for Return to School	
Evaluation/ Follow-up	Result
1 Medical (physical), Neurological, hearing, eyesight evaluation.	Treatment Plan for medical, physical, occupational, psychological therapies.
2 Neuropsychological assessment, if appropriate	Areas of strength, weakness → Individual Educational Plan (IEP) or 504→.
3 School/ Teacher receives IEP or 504	Implementation in class to benefit child.
4 Parents seek continuing retraining for short/long-term memory, organization, attention & processing skills	Periodic evaluations of progress, assessment of learning and improvement.

LEGAL RIGHTS OF EVERY CHILD WITH CHRONIC PAIN

"Other Health Impairment" (OHI) is one of the 14 *categories of disability* listed in our nation's special education law, the Individuals with Disabilities Education Act (IDEA). Under IDEA, a child who has an OHI is very likely to be eligible for special services to help address his or her educational, developmental, and functional needs resulting from the disability[80].

---

80 *http://www.parentcenterhub.org/repository/ohi*

GETTING BACK AND STAYING IN SCHOOL

Under Federal Law, P.L. 94-142 (1975), children with identified disabilities are entitled to a free and appropriate public education.[32] Children with chronic (pain) and handicapping conditions are guaranteed access to school by IDEA-2006. All children with special healthcare needs must be integrated into the regular school setting, and schools must modify and adapt their environment and programs to accommodate them. Discrimination based on disability in programs and activities is prohibited by Section 504 in public or private schools that receive federal financial assistance.

Children with chronic pain usually fall under the category of "orthopedically impaired" or "other health impaired". "Federal-ese" language reads that these children may have "limited strength, vitality, or alertness due to chronic or acute health problems which adversely affect educational performance." Remember Tom from Chapter 13, a bright and witty 12-year-old who had recurrent abdominal pain that had caused him to miss significant amounts of school:

> *Tom had developed anxieties about going to school, partly as a result of his mother's belief that the school staff was not sympathetic to his pain problems. Tom was convinced that he could not be at school and cope with his pain at the same time. He was out of school for over a semester.*

> *After participating in family therapy, Tom would remain at school through first period. His time at school was increased gradually each week and he received positive incentives for his ability to cope with being in school such as extra time outside to play with his friends.*

> *Soon Tom's mother was able to get him to school and was less anxious about what might happen to him while he was there. In turn, once Tom sensed his mother's changing attitude toward the school and he became confident in his own ability to stay at school for increasing amounts of time, he was able to go to school more easily, he became interested in some of his classes, and his pain lessened.*

This took place *without any need for an IEP or 504 plan* (below). **It did require detailed communication with Tom's school administration, however**. Once that was done the plan could be implemented.

The Individual Educational Plan (IEP)

So how does the formal technique work when the absences and informal adjustments aren't helping? In the public school system, the parent of a student with physical, emotional, or learning disabilities must submit a written "Request for Special Education Assessment." Within 15 days, he/ she should receive a written response. An evaluation determines if the student qualifies for *special accommodations* and/ or *modifications* under an IEP. **The Special Education Department of the school (District) is responsible for seeing that an IEP is followed and that the student's needs are met.** See below under Neuropsychological testing for more on this subject.

The 504 Plan

If a student does not need or meet the criteria for an IEP, he/ she might qualify for a *504 Plan that* **involves only modifications and accommodations in the student's program (no resource teachers).** An administrator or counselor and the classroom teacher, rather than the resource teachers in the Special Education Department, are responsible for carrying out the modifications and accommodations stated in the student's 504 Plan. The ultimate legal responsibility for implementation of either plan rests with the school principal. But the parent should be in continuous contact with the teacher to ensure it is carried out.

SUBTLE LEARNING DISORDERS

What sometimes is overlooked is that a subtle learning disorder can cause stress that aggravates any pain condition. Clues that this might be the cause are the following:

- A former good student makes poor academic progress as she gets older;
- Math becomes a big problem;
- All grades start to go downhill without other apparent causes;
- Problems on timed tests;
- Homework takes an inordinately long time (even if grades are A's).

If this is your situation, then in conjunction with your child's PCP, objective assessment of your child's strengths and weaknesses is necessary. This process usually starts with the following tests and evaluations and concludes with a plan of action— the Individual Educational Plan (IEP). The following studies will serve as the basis for developing the IEP that is specific to your child:

- Medical history and physical examination by a primary care provider;
- Neurological examination; and
- Neuropsychological assessment.

GETTING BACK AND STAYING IN SCHOOL

Why Neuropsychological testing? What is it?

If your child is suffering academically then additional testing may be warranted. Neuropsychological testing does *not* aim to mark you or your child as "crazy" or "retarded." It is a method to find out what portions of the brain and its circuits are working well and which ones are problematic. This will ultimately help you to understand and approve the resulting coordinated rehabilitation program and educational plan. See also Chapter 11.

Here are some concrete examples:

- If there is a subtle hearing-processing deficit, then schoolwork could be better presented in written form for visual processing.

- If concentration is affected, or there is attention deficit, then timed tests may need to be adjusted.

- If the child has IBS, then she may go to the bathroom without asking for permission.

Table 17.2   Seven Parental Steps to Promote Successful School Re-integration[33]
1   Request *in writing* a meeting to formulate & update your child's IEP. Insist that the IEP details the specific goals that meet his/her needs.
2   Provide the school with accurate and up-to-date medical information.
3   Communicate regularly with school personnel regarding the child's condition.
4   Encourage and facilitate continued interactions with classmates and peers.
5   Ensure that the child keeps up with his or her school assignments.
6   Encourage participation in ordinary tasks, responsibilities, school activities
7   Follow-up progress with the school.
8   Appreciate the teacher/ school efforts

Some school districts will perform neuropsychological testing, but the wait can be one to two years! If possible, have the testing performed privately to speed up the process.

Many parents tell us the importance of pursuing cognitive remediation or brain injury retraining in children who suffered concussions or other traumatic brain injuries. This retraining helps "beef up" mental skills such as short- and long-term memory, organization, attention, and processing skills. With this information, you will be able to get the help your child needs to attain his/her best chances of recovery and adjustment.

307

PAIN IN CHILDREN AND YOUNG ADULTS

Note: Even if your own insurance does not list neuropsychological testing, you can request or appeal for insurance coverage based on medical diagnosis. (See ombudsman Chapter 18.)

PARENTAL ATTITUDES AFFECTING SUCCESSFUL SCHOOL REENTRY

Returning to a normal routine is essential for the child, as "normality" has a significant effect on a child's general adjustment and self-esteem. School to a child is like work to an adult. **When a child is out of school for a long period of time, he or she is "unemployed"** and may experience depression, apathy, and poor self-concept.[34] **Parents can help socialization with invitation to after school 'play dates,' games, outings.**

The following *parental* concerns can affect the quality of the child's adjustment:

- Feelings/actions of uncertainty about the future.

- Expectations that emotional and physical efforts of returning to school will be "too much" for the child.

- Allowing him/ her to stay home. The pattern of absenteeism becomes a cycle and the child ultimately refuses to attend school.

- Separation anxiety by both parent and child manifests as school phobia.

- School may not be responsive to the child's needs.

- School is being unresponsive to concerns/requests for 504 plan or IEP.

Positive Actions for a Successful School Re-Entry

Both parent and child have been through a major illness trauma and their reactions of uneasiness are understandable. **Successful school re-entry depends on cooperation between the family and the school.** Seven factors become action items for the parent or child's advocate to resolve (see Table 17.2). Is it a smooth process? Not always. Read what one parent experienced:

> *The most important point for all of you is to not give up. This has been a harder fight than fighting the illness. After five years of fighting the school district, I am finally on the right track. At yesterday's IEP day 2, we finally got Speech, PT, Behavioral Planning and Vision Evaluation to get on board and recheck her status in three months. I have had as many as 25 people in my IEP meeting. I had reports contradicting just about everything that the District said. One therapist stated she had to*

308

GETTING BACK AND STAYING IN SCHOOL

ask permission to recommend service, since it would cost the district so much money to give it. This is against the law, and if I reported this she could lose her license to practice. Lucy, mom to Hayley. Morristown, NJ.

By following these guidelines (see Table 17.2), parents demonstrate to their child an optimistic expectation that their child will thrive in the school setting. Your worry about your child's ability to cope with school does not help in this adjustment.

Preparation for Child's Return to Classroom

There are several components here, including knowledge of all relevant information about the child and his or her illness. Sometimes, the privacy legislation (HIPAA) may, in fact, impede communication of key facts needed for teacher preparation. The teacher, school administrator, should be aware of the following:

1 Type of chronic pain that the child has, symptoms, and general course.

2 Treatments and their side effects.

3 Awareness of parents' wishes for what classmates and school personnel should know about their child's illness.

4 How effects of disease and treatments can affect skills needed for learning, such as attention, memory, language, nonverbal and motor skills (IEP review).

5 Psychological effects of chronic pain and issues such as anxiety, behavior problems, emotional difficulties, peer relationships and frustration related to school difficulties.

Teachers might receive a schedule of upcoming medical appointments to help the child prepare and anticipate absences. Sample letters by the child and parents to make the school more aware of the chronic pain issues are included at the end of this chapter.

Importance of Peer Support

Peer contact is important. Fear and lack of information can affect actual contact time of peers with the child. Research has shown the following for a variety of chronic conditions, while not just specific to pain:

1 Better social support from classmates is correlated with higher psychosocial adjustment for children with illness.

2 Peers who are knowledgeable and informed about the disease are more likely to accept and interact with children who have pain.

PAIN IN CHILDREN AND YOUNG ADULTS

3 **Peers influence treatment and medication compliance;** that is, the child is more likely to ignore treatment/medication rules, if they interfere with social situations.

4 Children often have misconceptions about disease. Preparatory conversations can dispel myths affecting the way peers treat the child.

5 Children's knowledge about disease varies with developmental level.

- Elementary school students ask questions such as "What is pain or IBS?" "Can I catch it?" "Can she still play?"

- Middle school and high school students ask harder, theoretical questions. "What will dating be like?" "Will he be able to work/ have a career?"

Preparing Class for the Child's Return

Absences of several weeks to months pose their own unique issues. The teacher should use the knowledge that he or she has gained in modifying goals, teaching methods and disciplinary practices. This is part of the specific IEP. The child may show academic and behavioral problems as a result of treatment for which the teacher may need preparation. **Appropriate expectations should still be maintained regarding the child's schoolwork.** If the child is unable to attend school, the teacher can facilitate classmate support by encouraging contact with the child, such as writing letters or cards or WEB-related technology, or suggesting home hospital or on line education.

In preparing the class for the child's re-entry after a long absence, especially in the younger grades, one designated individual (psychologist, school nurse, child life, social worker, and parent) might describe the patient's experiences, provide information about the child's specific illness in an age-sensitive manner and discuss support and teasing. Importantly, the patient can be the age-appropriate expert on his or her disease.[35] The school psychologist may offer support to school personnel or refer child and family to support groups, counseling, or social skills training.

Finding & Using School Resources—they may be rare

Many teachers express feelings of shock, worry, uncertainty and frustration by having a child with chronic illness in their classroom.[36] Some teachers seek support and information from the school nurse. However, teachers report that a lack of visibility, accessibility, and rapport prevent them from receiving support from the school nurse. Thus, the parent, school psychologist, child life, or social worker may be an alternative to establish a source of support and information for teachers.

310

GETTING BACK AND STAYING IN SCHOOL

Reintegration Resources for Parents and School

The needs for children with chronic pain are becoming better documented. But we know that their learning progress is aggravated by absenteeism that results from hospitalizations, treatments and treatment side effects. Children with chronic pain may be receiving services below, as part of their medical and IEP plan, to optimally benefit from their educational experience:

- Counseling, Cognitive behavioral therapy (CBT) or other psychological interventions, such as biofeedback or hypnotherapy

- Physical therapy; Massage therapy

- School health services (e.g. services provided by the school nurse).

- Medical pain management

The solutions discussed in this section require tremendous effort and cooperation with school personnel. Even if a student has an IEP or 504 Plan, the plan is only as good as the people who implement it. Caring school administrators, nurses, and teachers are often willing to accommodate students even without an IEP or 504 Plan. We need to continually acknowledge the individuals who are helping us every day. It is important to express appreciation periodically to those who are helping your child succeed in school.

GETTING BACK TO NORMAL

Getting back to school and reintegrating with the family is one way of getting back to normal. For most children with chronic pain, they will return to their pre-pain state. For some children, the term *normal* is relative. As they age, there sometimes is a new normal unlike the one before the illness. Perhaps this is the most difficult challenge for children and parents alike. Always remember your participation and championing will help your child attain the maximum benefit possible.

Brad, a survivor of childhood Hodgkin's disease and pain, who eventually received a PhD in sociology and is now a University Professor and researcher, talks about what he wanted from his physicians:

> *... to be understanding of the very deep needs... and to the authentic but often unspoken, expressions of... anxieties about physical and emotional pain, loss of control over personal destiny, and plain dread of dying and of the end of cherished relationships.*[37]

PAIN IN CHILDREN AND YOUNG ADULTS

SIBLINGS AT HOME CAN SUFFER TOO, NO MATTER HOW WELL PARENTS PREPARE

It is unavoidable. We found out about these effects in an unusual way. For over 15 years we have volunteered as summer camp physicians at the Barretstown Gang Camp[81] in Ireland for children with serious illnesses. This camp accepts children from all over Europe. Of eight sessions, we always had at least one 10-day camp session devoted only to siblings (no patients). Each year we recorded the number and types of visits to the camp medical facility. The "well" siblings had *more* doctor visits during the 10 days than any sessions of children with AIDS or cancer, 50 per cent of whom were actively receiving chemotherapy! We believe these siblings need as much attention as their sick sibling with chronic pain. *Normal* siblings may have medical and other needs that are not being met.[38]

SUMMARY

Is this an easy process? No. Our hope is that finding, learning and using the available information will make this journey a little smoother. **Most of our many patients do get back to their previous state and thrive, more mature with self-knowledge.** There is hope. As an example of surviving adversity, follow-up studies of more than 10,000 survivors of childhood cancer reported that only 11 per cent had an overall prevalence of significant psychological distress.[39]

---

81 *http://www.barretstown.org/*

CHAPTER 18

HMO'S, BENEFITS, INSURANCE & FAMILY MEDICAL LEAVE ACT:
GUIDELINES FOR PARENTS OF A CHILD WITH CHRONIC PAIN

Insurance maintains all rights to question claims from medical profession.
Insurance has no medical background or license.
Insurance maintains all rights to question therapist treatment schedule.
Insurance has no treatment training.
Insurance earnings depend on treatment limitation.
Negotiations proceed on legal grounds with insurance lawyers
reaching out to doctors.
Bargain for health.
Please pray

—EXPIRING EXTENSIONS: HEALTH INSURANCE POEM BY AURIN SQUIRE.

THE FAMILY MEDICAL LEAVE ACT (FMLA)

HIPAA

COVERAGE FOR PAIN MEDICATIONS AND MENTAL CONDITIONS

BASIC RULES OF INSURANCE BENEFITS

ECONOMIC BURDEN OF CHRONIC PAIN IN CHILDREN

SIX RULES TO OBTAIN YOUR BENEFITS

DENIALS OF COVERAGE THAT MUST BE CHALLENGED

FAQS ABOUT HEALTH INSURANCE

THE FAMILY & MEDICAL LEAVE ACT (FMLA) 1993

For the family of a child with chronic pain, especially in the beginning where it seems the days and weeks consist of waking up and driving to doctors or physical therapy sessions, the Family & Medical Leave Act (FMLA) might offer some relief, a breath of fresh air. It entitles the eligible employee parent to take up to 12 weeks of unpaid, job-protected leave in a 12-month period for specified family and medical reasons (Table 18.1). Let's explore the details so that its application can be an easier process.

Table 18.1 Family/ medical leave act guidelines
1   The employee must be eligible.
2   The employee (family member) must have a serious health condition.
3   The employee must work for a specific type of organization (employer).
4   The employee must have worked for a specified period of time and number of hours within an organization of a particular size and locale.
5   The employee must have specified reasons for taking leave.
6   The employee must take leave in acceptable ways.
7   The employee must work with a legitimate health care provider.

1   Terms of Eligibility

The employer defines "12-month period" as any of the following:

- Calendar year,

- Fiscal year,

- 12-months following commencement of leave,

- 12-months preceding the end of leave, or

- Fixed 12-week leave regardless of when it is taken.

Don't assume "they" will understand. You have to give exquisite details and information on your child's diagnoses from your child's physician, so that "they" understand you are dealing with a "serious health condition." The family member must have a "serious health condition," As detailed below.

2   **The chronic pain condition should qualify under federal guidelines of a "serious health condition,"** which means an illness, injury, impairment, or physical or mental condition that involves any of the following:

- Any period of incapacity or treatment connected with inpatient care (i.e., an overnight stay) in a hospital, hospice, or residential medical-care facility.

GUIDELINES FOR PARENTS OF A CHILD WITH CHRONIC PAIN

- Any period of incapacity or subsequent treatment in connection with such inpatient care.

Continuing treatment by a health care provider: any period of incapacity of the child (i.e., inability to work, attend school or perform other regular daily activities).

3 The employee must work for a specific type of organization (employer). Organizations that meet this condition include:

- Public agencies: federal, state, and local employers, such as local schools.

- Private-sector employers: employing 50 or more employees in 20 or more work weeks in the current or preceding calendar year and who are engaged in commerce.

Any industry or activity affecting commerce, including joint employers (two jobs) and successors of covered employers.

4 The employee must have worked for a specified period of time and/ or hours:

- For a total of 12 months. At least 1,250 hours over the previous 12 months at a location in the USA or its territories where at least 50 employees are employed by the employer within a 75-mile radius.

5 The employee must have specified reasons for taking leave. Acceptable reasons include:

- Caring for an immediate family member (spouse, child, or parent) with a serious health condition

- Two spouses employed by the same employer can take only a combined total of 12 work-weeks of family leave to care for the child.

6 The employee must take leave in acceptable ways.

- Intermittently—taking leave in blocks of time or reducing the normal weekly or daily workload.

- Choose to use accrued paid leave (such as sick or vacation leave) to cover some or all of the leave.

- This requires the approval of employers; the employer is responsible for determining whether an employee's use of paid leave counts as FMLA leave, based on information from the employee.

7 The employee must have a legitimate "health care provider." Approved health care providers include:

- Doctors of medicine or osteopathy

- Podiatrists, dentists, clinical psychologists, optometrists, and chiropractors.

315

PAIN IN CHILDREN AND YOUNG ADULTS

- Nurse practitioners and clinical social workers
- Any health care provider recognized by the employer or the employer's group health plan benefits manager.

From #1-7 above, any childhood chronic pain condition should qualify. But be prepared for a dark side. Family medical leave is not always honored in the way one would expect, as illustrated by the following report. This mom describes ambivalence that she sensed from her co-workers during her leave:

> Pardon my sarcasm. Although my fellow employees have been very supportive, there's a "we are doing you a favor" tone about the place. It's not a favor! It's the law and any time they want to trade places with me, even for a day, the offer is open! Darla, mom to Alexis, IBS and depression. Marietta, GA

PRIVACY: THE HEALTH INSURANCE PORTABILITY AND ACCOUNTABILITY ACT (HIPAA)

Ask any physician what they think of HIPAA and look how difficult it is for him/her to disguise his scorn. It makes our job so much more difficult. But it is here and we all have to deal with it. HIPAA is a privacy law that prevents doctors from giving out private medical information without permission from the patient. The Act is a set of standards to protect patients, given the widespread availability of electronic information on patients. It was purportedly designed to protect against researchers looking at data on patients for purposes other than health care. Scientists can use such data as long as it is *de-identified*, so that it cannot be traced to the original source.

This law presents serious challenges for patients with chronic pain and their doctors. It was not well thought out before implementation. You may not want your employer to know about your medical issues, but the law is so stringent that it prevents health care professionals from having *any* communication regarding your case, without your prior approval, even if it would be helpful to you.

HIPAA was first introduced in 1996 and mandates large fines up to $250,000 or imprisonment for violations. Most health care agencies are scared of the consequences. Hospitals are mandated to provide employee training in the implementation of HIPAA. All staff (which means everyone who works in a hospital, including the cleaning crew) must attend an hour of training. The training includes a video, with different situations about how a patient's confidentiality could be violated (talking in an elevator, reading a computer screen that you pass, telling a friend about a case, and so forth).

316

GUIDELINES FOR PARENTS OF A CHILD WITH CHRONIC PAIN

The original version of the Act was so restrictive that:

- Doctors' offices could not use waiting room sign-in sheets.

- Hospital charts could not be kept at bedside.

- Doctors could not talk to patients in semi-private rooms.

- Doctors could not confer at nurses' stations without fear of being overheard and reported.

HIPAA does not apply when your records are used for:

- Patient care/ government reporting (national statistics, cancer registries, etc.)

- Debt collection or internal hospital review of practice (quality assurance).

The Act has now been amended to modify a few of these restrictions, but the Act still affects how your doctor can communicate with you or your loved ones. The following example reflects the typical response since enactment of HIPAA:

> *I called my 18-year-old daughter's orthopedic surgeon to discuss her condition after surgery. He refused to talk to me because of HIPAA rules. Before he releases information or talks to anyone, my daughter Misty would have had to sign a paper authorizing him to talk with me. However, his office forgot to ask Misty to sign that form before her surgery. Faxes are not allowed, because I could fake them. Sharon, mom of Misty, St. Louis, Mo.*

If your child is 18 years or older, discuss with him/her about medical information sharing so that your child can provide written permission for her doctor(s) to talk with you about her condition.

Christy poses the following solution that worked for her:

> *We filled out a power of attorney written form stating, I as John's (23 years old) caretaker (mother), can have access to all medical information, labs, MRIs, X-rays, etc. related to John's medical condition. John signed it and we notarized it, and we have 10 copies of each. Carry it with you always. Even some of the nurses gave me a hard time when I asked for John's lab results during his last hospitalization. They shove these HIPAA forms in front of you and say "sign." We also added to the HIPAA forms my name but it doesn't matter because those forms go to medical records and no one can access them when you call and say "Can I get a copy of so and so's MRI? A down side to HIPAA. Christy, Santa Monica, CA*

BASIC RULES TO OBTAIN INSURANCE BENEFITS

This economic burden makes it imperative that insurance and other health coverage pay their appropriate portion to alleviate this hardship. In this section, you will find out how to negotiate to receive your benefits. It should not be this difficult, but *difficult* is the reality. The companies intend to keep the premiums that you have sent to them.

There are six principles for action you must understand to get your needs and services (see Table 18.2). Actual techniques and the appeal process are outlined in Table 18.3 (and examples below).

Table 18.2   Six Rules to Obtain Insurance Benefits
1   Arm yourself with knowledge.
2   Identify an advocate-representative to help you negotiate with the system.
3   Understand your policy, its entitlements & what is (and what is not) covered.
4   Know what can be negotiated, even if it is not covered.
5   Know the important federal rules that can protect and help you.
6   Do not assume they will understand your plight. You must make a strong case and be prepared to fight for your cause.

Health plan groups manage common diseases, like diabetes and heart disease, much better than they do for chronic pain in children. Pediatric pain medicine is a narrow specialty area that costs money and resources. Frankly, HMOs and prepaid health plans lack the motivation to provide this expertise. Nonetheless, **there are often dedicated and skilled medical professionals within these groups, who get little or no attention for their expertise.** Accept the challenge to seek them out. Much of the responsibility for getting the care your child needs is in your hands; it is you against *the system*.

Frustrations with insurance company

"It was the best of times it was the worst of times" when dealing with my employer provided medical insurance. For years we had very few issues as all her medical bills were being paid for and out of network visits were being authorized. However, I noticed periods of difficulty trying to get authorizations approved through the medical group for certain types of therapy. This required frequent interventions by pain clinic staff, the insurance company and even complaints filed with the Department of Managed Care. I found the medical group lacked familiarity with the providers in its own network. When she needed aquatic therapy, they would approve it then send her

GUIDELINES FOR PARENTS OF A CHILD WITH CHRONIC PAIN

> *to an office that only did physical therapy. It took four months to get an authorization approved for her wheelchair, a major embarrassment for them as an internal review had to be conducted. Debra, mother of Brianna*

Managed care policies are less expensive than other forms of health insurance. Why? **Managed care regulates how much health care you use, so that costs for your care can be controlled**. For example, one type requires that you obtain *written approval* from your insurance company *before* you are admitted to a hospital. This is to make sure that the hospitalization is necessary. If you go to the hospital without this approval, you may not be covered for the hospital bill.

Coverage for Pain Medications and Mental Conditions

Insurance companies typically divide payments for health insurance into "physical" (medical) and "behavioral" (mental health) benefits. (They do not see the symptoms affecting your child as a "continuum".) Thus, parents often have difficulty in obtaining insurance coverage for aspects of treatment for pain that the company deems a "behavioral health" benefit. **Most medical insurance programs do not ascribe to the biopsychosocial approach to chronic pain. Their view is to see health conditions and treatments using a pre-1960 model as *either* "medical" *or* "psychological."** They have different "carve out" benefits for each. Since many children with chronic pain also have anxiety and/or depression or elevated symptoms of each or both, parents find themselves in "denials" of benefits from their insurance company and spend endless hours in appeals to obtain needed services covered.

We asked Amy, a *Juris Doctorate* candidate, the mother of one of our patients, to share with us a summary of what she learned about insurance and health costs. She was researching the financial crossover from mental to physical illness in her Mental Health Law course. The following is an excerpt from her thesis:

> *Although pain has both physical and psychological components and both impact the child in pain, getting the needed "insurance approved diagnoses" and thus insurance coverage for the proper treatments, has been challenging for parents, medical care providers and insurance claims handlers. Psychological problems are not categorized in the same way as physical illness. Because insurance carriers are notorious for disparity in covering psychological conditions and physical illness, litigious confrontation between parents and insurance carrier often results. **Frequent denial of health care benefits for what is deemed "behavioral health" often results in children in pain not getting the full complement of therapy,** thus prolonging the pain problem and disability associated with the pain, such as school absenteeism.*

*Some states are more giving when it comes to treating mental conditions. In California, for example, the **Mental Health Parity Law**[82] protects members with certain conditions. For example, a health plan must cover the same or equal benefits for certain mental health conditions that it covers for other medical conditions. Specifically, if an insured's **plan offers prescription drug benefits, whether drugs are prescribed for a mental health or medical condition, they must be covered at the same rates.** The co-payments, deductibles, and maximum lifetime benefits charged for mental health conditions also must be the same as those for medical conditions.[52] This is an important issue for treatment of chronic pain since many medications used for mental health conditions are also the same ones used to treat pain.*

*The Mental Health Parity Law ensures the same medical care coverage for the following nine (9) mental health conditions: major depression; bipolar (manic-depressive) disorder; panic disorder; anorexia; bulimia; obsessive-compulsive disorder; autism or pervasive developmental disorder; schizophrenia; schizoaffective disorder; and, children's severe emotional disturbances. Psychological conditions that are not "severe" and do not carry any of the above diagnostic labels are not included in the Parity Act. **Chronic pain is often accompanied by elevated anxiety and/or depression, but neither may qualify for a categorical diagnosis** (e.g. major depressive disorder). Even "generalized anxiety disorder" doesn't make it into the 9 covered "mental illness" categories covered under the law.*

ECONOMIC BURDEN OF CHRONIC PAIN IN CHILDREN

As Amy noted, "diagnoses" count in what does... and doesn't get covered. We physicians do the best we can in trying to find the right labels and diagnoses for our child patients to get costs of their pain care covered by their parents' health insurance. However, treatment of chronic pain crosses the divide between "medical" and "behavioral health" coverage, so that costs of physical therapy might be easier to get approved than costs of biofeedback, hypnotherapy, or other psychological mind-based therapies. For example, it is often easier to get an interventional procedure, such as an epidural block, approved for a child with CRPS[83], than any psychological

---

82 *www.dmhc.ca.gov/LawsRegulations/MentalHealthParityandAddictionEquityActof2008%28MHPAEA%29. aspx#.VSmjT5NjfbU*

83 1: Simons LE, Basch MC. State of the art in biobehavioral approaches to the management of chronic pain in childhood. Pain Manag. 2015 Dec 17
2: Becerra L, Sava S, Simons LE, et al. Intrinsic brain networks normalize with treatment in pediatric complex regional pain syndrome. Neuroimage Clin. 2014 Aug 10;6:347-69.
3: Simons LE, Pielech M, Erpelding N, et al. The responsive amygdala: treatment-induced alterations in functional connectivity in pediatric complex regional pain syndrome. Pain. 2014 Sep;155(9):1727-42.

GUIDELINES FOR PARENTS OF A CHILD WITH CHRONIC PAIN

therapies. This is despite the fact that there is no published research to support the effectiveness of epidurals in childhood CRPS. There are many studies documenting the effectiveness of a variety of psychological interventions for treatment of chronic pain in children, including CRPS[36]. Thus, parents and their child's doctors alike are forced to spend needless time writing appeal letters and making phone calls to the insurer to try to obtain coverage for the needed services.

SIX RULES TO OBTAIN INSURANCE BENEFITS

1   Arm yourself with knowledge

The first denied insurance claim can be shocking and intimidating. Feelings of being overwhelmed and helpless can come flooding in. To convince insurance companies to honor your claim (and not deny it), you must understand who they are, their view of you as the consumer, how they process claims, and the terms they use.

Insurance is a business. As a business, the company has a mandate to manage your care effectively (We would say… to limit care) in order to provide a profit to its shareholders. A child pain client is an outlier (i.e. a money drain). Insurance companies know that in the marketplace your child's total therapy package could run upwards from $100,000. Your child is now viewed as a high cost item to be surveyed and flagged for more scrutiny. Your minimal past expenses for your child's routine care went under the radar screen. The company will not pay its full share or provide care… unless you provide the information and are prepared to fight for your case (see Tables 18.2 and Table 18.3).

Contact your local support groups and ask about others' experience with your HMO or insurance company. Go online and bring up the subject on all the chronic pain listservs or chat groups you may participate with (see Chapter 8: Searching the Web/ Internet and other resources).

2   Identify an advocate-representative to help you negotiate the system.

Identifying an advocate to help you carry this burden is a must. This is a difficult battle. You may be getting less sleep than usual, your son requires one to one attention both day and night, you are the monitor for his meds; major changes have affected your life. It is difficult to provide the care he needs and battle HMOs or insurance companies. The financial service person, social worker, or case manager at your hospital or clinic may be very helpful. Your spouse who was previously unfamiliar with personal finances and insurance can become a formidable champion for details of claim refusals and clarifications. Finally, your pediatrician or PCP can be a powerful ally.

PAIN IN CHILDREN AND YOUNG ADULTS

3 Understand your policy, your entitlements, and what is (not) covered.

Health care in America has changed in the last 15 years. Most people in the United States used to have *indemnity insurance* coverage. With indemnity insurance, you could go to any doctor, hospital, or other provider (who would bill for each service given); the company and the patient would each pay part of the bill.

Today, more than half of all Americans with health insurance are enrolled in some form of managed care plan or health maintenance organization (HMO), an organized way of providing (limiting) services and delaying payment for them. The organizational structures of such plans constitute a "word salad": preferred provider organizations (PPOs), health maintenance organizations (HMOs), and point-of-service (POS) plans. You've probably heard these terms before, but what do they mean, and what are the differences among them?

For people with Indemnity and other Plans, there are some ways to make the insurance dollars go even further.[40] This point relates to co-payments and deductibles. Any plan only pays up to its lifetime benefit. **Chronic illness patients frequently exceed lifetime coverage limits.** You can help yourself tremendously by comparing rates from different hospitals. All other things being equal (top-notch center, great expertise of your specialists, etc.), the lower the rates, the longer it takes to hit the maximum benefit limit and your dollar limit.

4 Know what can be negotiated, even if it is not covered.

How do you convince the insurance company to honor a claim? Our suggestion: **learn how to appeal *all* denials**. Generally, this requires a simple phone call or letter, yet only 30 per cent of claimants will appeal a denial. Remember, the insurance company is not expecting you to appeal. Times are changing, slowly. Aetna Insurance recently settled a $170,000 lawsuit and promised to interfere less with medical decisions and pay physicians more promptly.

When we physicians order an MRI scan or a medication, it often has to be "approved", and the person making this decision is not a physician. **The approval decision is not based on your medical need, or even if your doctor thinks is necessary.** Rather, **the decision is made by a clerk who uses a checklist**. If there is no code on his list or he does not understand, then it is denied. (And for children there are few drugs that are FDA approved.) The guidelines may be out of date; and if so, a strong case can be made for coverage to avoid not just your litigation but a range of challenges.

> *(Recently, I (PZ) had to spend 1 hour on the phone to Anthem-Blue Cross to get approval for Lyrica™ for a patient with chronic fatigue and juvenile fibromyalgia. The clerks had no idea that juvenile and adult "fibro" were different. How can doctors be expected to spend one hour for each prescription challenge?)*

322

GUIDELINES FOR PARENTS OF A CHILD WITH CHRONIC PAIN

Guidelines may be commercial—in which case the company will probably tell you which ones they follow. However, in *all* cases you want the plan to explain the *basis for the denial* in detail and to point to the section of your policy (in the booklet) that is used to support the denial. This makes it easier to challenge later. (As a pediatric neuro-oncologist (PZ) with more than 30 years of experience in treating children who have brain tumors, being informed by an insurance clerk reading from a list when I can and cannot order a brain scan incensed me!)

If you get a denial or restriction by message or phone, ask for it in writing. If they will not do this, then write an e-mail or letter memorializing what was said—make sure you always have the name and position of the person contacting you. It is very important to record the health plan's grounds for denial. Then if you can prove they erred on the original grounds, they can't switch it to another. ***Keep this in your insurance file!*** (Chapter 9)

A majority of states have mandated appeals for health coverage denials; you should take advantage of this. This gives you access to external independent review for reasonable and necessary care that can force coverage.

5 Dealing with plans that restrict physician access to those listed in their plan booklets.

If the care you need cannot be provided by those experts in the plan, the HMO has an obligation to let you have access to the level of care and expertise needed. For example, you should look at the resources available and check with your provider on what other resources have been accessible before; you then need to look up the physicians to whom you have uncontested recourse to see if they fill your need or not. **In most cases, once you get a medical director involved, you have a good chance to get the resources you need**—not always, but usually.

6 Do not assume they will understand your plight.

The insurance company has a mandate to limit care to the minimum that they must deliver in order to provide a profit to their shareholders or sponsors. With *chronic pain* you are now a high cost "customer" to be contained; they have little sympathy for your plight. The company will not pay its share or provide care *unless* you provide the justification and are prepared to fight for your cause.

The following is an example of what actions a patient took to prevail over her insurance company.

> *I very recently had a battle with a large insurance company. They raised our monthly rates to over $1000. I took this to Bill Nelson's office in Washington, D.C. He was a Florida senator who was the insurance Commissioner for years. I asked ABC to do*

323

PAIN IN CHILDREN AND YOUNG ADULTS

a story, and I contacted the largest paper in South Florida, the Sun-Sentinel; they ran a story. I won. Name withheld.

DENIALS OF COVERAGE THAT MUST BE CHALLENGED

When confronted with a denial of service, follow the examples below and Table 18.3. Also use the websites listed in Table 18.4 to better understand your rights and information to get maximum benefit from your insurance.

Example #1: Denial of Coverage for a diagnostic or follow-up test.

Ask your doctor to write a "letter of necessity." The letter should state that it is within the guidelines of standard care that a diagnostic or follow-up MRI scan be performed because it limits the radiation a child receives (as opposed to the cheaper, more radiation CT scan).

The following is real advice from George who tackled this problem:

The way an HMO works is that your primary care physician has to request the MRI. If the doctor doesn't believe that you need it, he won't ask for approval. The insurance company should not deny a diagnostic test in a case such as yours! Talk to the doctor who placed the request to find out what went wrong. You may also have to talk to the local "IPA," or the umbrella organization that administers the HMO funds in your doctor's group. If that fails, file a written appeal with the insurance company and send copies to your doctor and IPA. You will get your MRI, if you push all of them. Threaten to hold them liable if progression of your child's pain goes unmitigated because they failed to authorize proper follow-up. George, Paradise Valley, AZ

You might want to draft a letter similar to the one below and give it to your doctor to put on his/ her office stationery:

At UCLA, Boston and other Child pain treatment centers, the recommended MRI schedule is being followed. If your guidelines differ, can you provide me with the data to substantiate that decision? Otherwise we ask that you approve this reasonable request for routine diagnosis/ monitoring for my child's CRPS or Fibromyalgia or chronic daily headaches etc.

Example #2: Your "plan" does not have a Pediatric Neuropsychologist to perform this or other techniques.

Your second opinion neuropsychologist states you will need complete Neuropsychological testing because of probable learning disability and co-morbid conditions. Ask

GUIDELINES FOR PARENTS OF A CHILD WITH CHRONIC PAIN

your consultant Neuropsychologist to write a "letter of necessity" about Standard of Care to the Medical Director at the administrative address of your plan institution. Request to have your treatment covered by your out-of-network provider.

If this does not work, hire a lawyer or involve the local media (newspapers or television stations) in airing your plight. This can be a cure preventing situation, and you must act boldly in order to obtain the care you need and for which you have paid.

Example #3: Denial of a second opinion.

You can usually get them to pay if there isn't a qualified expert inside your plan, whether they say they will pay or not. If they are "steering" you to just local care, that is discriminatory. (See Table 18.3)

Example #4: A newer SSRI or anti-emetic is not covered under your plan.

Medications in common use are covered by most health insurance plans; however, newer drugs, especially those given as an outpatient, in pill or liquid form, are not always covered under these plans. Many insurance companies put expensive drugs in the same category as allergy medicine like antihistamines! Thus, when you consume the maximum, insurance pays no more. One course of Ability™ or Provigil™ will usually deplete the year's maximum for outpatient medications. Effective anti-nausea drugs used (like Zofran™ or Kytril™) are not usually covered and cost $5-20 per pill. The cheaper drugs that they do allow ($0.35-0.80) often do not work.

Example #5: Denial for coverage in a Clinical Trial

This is a big one and you will have to bring out all your "big guns." It was made easier in 2001, when California joined seven other states in supporting clinical trials for cancer; Governor Gray Davis signed a law that required health insurance companies to cover "routine services" of participating in Phase 1, 2, or 3 clinical trials. The covered costs include drugs, doctor visits, lab tests or hospitalizations as necessary. In 2004, at least 12 other states had the same law. There are also many clinical trials for different pain conditions and you should find out which ones apply to your child's pain and which require insurance coverage and which are free or which parts, such as the medication, are free.

In a highly publicized case seven years ago, the parents of a child refused care for an approved clinical trial lobbied the Department of Defense. The child's father was a military employee and the clinical trial was federally-sponsored. The parents won after seven months, using the Medical Care Ombudsman Program (MCOP), an independent referee. You can use this service to mount an argument against denials.

PAIN IN CHILDREN AND YOUNG ADULTS

If you are consistently denied service or coverage, you should appeal and threaten with newspaper or citizen advocates from radio or TV. Fortunately, there is a website that shows which drug companies and insurance companies have assistance plans (*www.needymeds.org*).

Table 18.3   Important Components of a Successful Reversal of Denial for Clinical Trial Treatment
1   Obtain copies of your insurance company agreements and guidelines for clinical trial participation. (Some companies do not even have them!).
2   Contact persons—Medical Care Ombudsman Program—Look up your state. *http://www.insurance.ca.gov/0500-about-us/02-department/10-cppib/omb.cfm*
3   Ask for form letters and guidance on appeals to your company.
4   Clearly state your purpose is to obtain coverage.
5   The label "clinical trial" may invoke initial denial because it is investigational. Call their bluff. If the trial is Phase 3, the drug is not investigational.
6   For military type insurance like Champus-Tricare, know your rights.
7   The Department of Defense and NIH programs include follow up care. This is important to lessen your health care costs later on.
8   Regardless what happens, remember that the insurance company may be ignorant. Their responses are not "personal."

FREQUENTLY ASKED QUESTIONS ABOUT INSURANCE & DISABILITY

1   In which ways can my health insurance provider (HMO, PPO) help me?
The system is not all bad news. Part of the organization's structure and economical orientation can actually help you. Your insurer might assign a *case manager* to coordinate your care; this is often a nurse or social worker who is experienced with chronic pain, pediatrics, or child neurology. **This *case manager* can be your liaison to facilitate your care.**

> *Case #1: My daughter Elise has headaches and a seizure disorder. The company I worked for changed insurance companies; they assigned a case manager to me; she takes care of lots of problems. This is a good thing… it is nice to know you have someone on the inside. This person knows your details, can go to bat for you, and can get the insurance company to take care of things that you need. Adrien, Wichita, KS.*

GUIDELINES FOR PARENTS OF A CHILD WITH CHRONIC PAIN

2 What are the important considerations in using a case manager?

If your insurance company offers you case management service, ask the following questions before getting involved:

- Can you leave the program if it does not work out for you?

- Can you switch to another case manager, if there is a personality conflict?

- Can you get a copy of policy explaining (in writing) how this will change your situation? In other words, what benefit is there to you to choose this program?

The Case Manager may negotiate with your health insurance carrier for a reduced price on drugs you need that are not considered as part of its pharmacy offerings. Also, check with your plan to see if it provides neuropsychological evaluations, rehabilitation services and equipment, and other things that you may need. If not, then use the tactic for denial of claims earlier in this chapter. Know what can be negotiated, even if it is not covered.

3 How do I fight a denial for home rehabilitation equipment?

Your primary physician or specialist could help you write a letter, or you could prepare it first and then send it to your child's physician to send it out on his/her letterhead. You would describe the special needs of your child, CRPS, depression, predisposition to blood clots from decreased leg movements, weakness, need for rehabilitation exercises, time spent in bed, and how this special rehabilitation equipment could prevent expensive complications like bed sores.

Look into aid organizations that will provide the needed equipment free or arrange for it at a deep discount; depending on whether equipment is owned or rented. You might find families who would be happy to recycle materials at a prorated cost or free after it has served its purpose; ask on chat rooms or local support groups.

4 Hidden costs to getting a second opinion

Our insurance will not cover out-of-state opinions. We have had major problems dealing with the financial department at our Medical Center. We live in Arizona and wanted a second opinion from X in Texas. As stated on their website, we paid $550 the day of the visit for the consultation. We met with a doctor for an hour for my child's evaluation and discussion of treatment options. Nothing extravagant was done other than a traditional appointment.

A month or two later, X sends my mom a bill for a balance of $350 remaining on our bill for the visit. They claim that the $550 fee that they charged us the day of the visit only covered the doctor, not the facility charge. Mary, Scottsdale, AZ.

PAIN IN CHILDREN AND YOUNG ADULTS

This surprise might have been avoided if the initial inquiry had included the question "What are *all* the costs of getting a consultation?" or the confirmatory correspondence had been read carefully. If this information was not included, then you may have an argument for getting the institution to void or eliminate its charge.

5 Medical expenses and tax deductions

You may deduct the portion of your medical expenses that *exceed* 7.5 per cent of your adjusted gross income. For example, if you earned $20,000, you could deduct any medical expenses that go over $1500. Therefore, if your medical expenses were $1,800, only the portion beyond $1500 would be deductible, that is $300.

Accordingly, if you earned $100,000, you could deduct the part of medical expenses that exceeds $7,500. If your medical expenses were $10,000, only the portion beyond $7,500 could be deducted; that is $2,500. The exception is if you are subject to alternative minimum tax.

Our healthcare systems are complex and have many components to master. This chapter has outlined the basic organization.

Table 18.4 Web Resources- Insurance & Health Care	
Type of Information	Contact Information/ Website
50 States mandated coverage Consumer Insurance Guide-HIPPA	*www.insure.com*
Understanding HIPAA	*www.insure.com/health-insurance/HIPAA-tools.html*
Obamacare- affordable care act	*http://obamacarefacts.com/affordablecareact-summary.php*
Denial of coverage- Legal rights	*www.healthcare.gov/ how-does-the-health-care-law-protect-me/*
Family medical leave act FMLA	Tel: 1-866-4-USWAGE *https://en.wikipedia.org/wiki/ Family_and_Medical_Leave_Act_of_1993 http://employment.findlaw.com/family-medical-leave/ family-and-medical-leave-act.html*
Medications help	*www.scbn.org www.needymeds.org/index.htm*

CHAPTER 19

THE ABC'S OF RECEIVING GOOD CARE FOR YOUR CHILD

We thought long and hard about how to end and summarize this book; it was a difficult task. Both you, as the parent and the child or young adult with pain, did not ask to embark on this journey and likely it has not been easy. What we can tell you is that **most children with a chronic pain condition do recover and go on to lead productive lives, better equipped to handle the stresses of adulthood.**

We leave you with our choice of 18 tips, "pearls", for you to receive optimal care in our current healthcare environment.

1 Find a doctor who listens.

2 Find a doctor who believes that your child is in pain.

3 Ask your child's physician and other clinicians to whom your child may be referred for treatment (e.g. physical therapist, etc.) if they have experience dealing with pain problems in children and adolescents.

4 Make sure that there is a treatment plan.

5 Choose a doctor with whom you can have open communication (talk, e-mail, phone calls etc.), and set up a plan for how to best communicate.

6 Try to establish a method for contacting your child's doctor with non-urgent questions or write down the questions to be addressed during a visit.

7 Don't make the doctor "king" (or "queen"). Doctors do not know everything.

8 Your child's doctor should have humility to admit when he/she doesn't know something and be willing to learn more, and then get back to you to discuss it; or to refer you to a doctor who is more familiar with your child's pain problem.

329

PAIN IN CHILDREN AND YOUNG ADULTS

9 Ask your physician to explain her diagnosis of the problem so that it makes sense to you. If you don't understand, tell the doctor and ask to explain it again.

10 You should not have to hear one diagnosis of your child's problem from the physician, another from the acupuncturist and another from the chiropractor.

11 Always ask about the side effects of a new medication, when you should stop giving that medication, and what to do if you observe side effects.

12 Ask your child's doctor to talk with the other clinicians who are caring for your child, so that they are all familiar with and up to date on your child's case.

13 Seek out all resources. Get as much information as you can through books and the internet. Use this information to raise questions with your child's physician.

14 Be an informed parent. This is the best way to advocate for your child's care.

15 Always consider complementary therapies, physical therapy, psychotherapy, or family therapy, not just medications. With rare exceptions, medications alone do not work for most children with chronic pain.

16 If you are dissatisfied with what your doctor has explained to you about your child's pain, and/or the treatment plan doesn't make sense to you, then it is allright to get a second opinion.

17 Doctors need to take children seriously. Your child's physician should not belittle or make fun of your child (this is different from having fun with your child and you during an evaluation)

18 You should never continue with a doctor who talks down to you. Your job is not to massage his/her ego.

APPENDIX A
PAIN CENTER LOCATOR

Pain Center Locator For the latest updated list of Centers go to *http://americanpainsociety.org/uploads/get-involved/PediatricPainClinicList_Update_2.10.15.pdf*

+ =AVAILABLE EXPERTISE 0 =Not available

		No. New Patients/ Year	Patient Age range	Multidisciplinary.	Bio-Psycho-Social Model..	Physical Therapy	Psychology-Psychiatry	Complementary Therapy	Neuropsychology	Additional expertise	Intervention Procedures	In-Patient Rehab	Day Treatment Rehab	Clinical Trials	Comments
		1	2	3	4	5	6	7	8	9	10	11	12	13	
AR	Sarah Tariq MD, Michael Schmitz MD, Mandy Horn RN 1 Children's Way, Slot #203, Little Rock AR 72202; T: 501.364.3100 hornak@archildrens.org www.archildrens.org/Services/Pain-Medicine-Clinic-Pediatric-.aspx	110	0-18	+	+	+	+	+	0	0	+	+	+	0	restoration of function. Inpatient rehab available
AZ	Dir.: Jonathan Jerman MD Pain Medicine Prog., Phoenix Children's Hospital 1919 E. Thomas Rd Phoenix, AZ85016 T: 602-933-1537;http://valleypediatricpain.org	250	0-18	+	+	+	+	+	+	0	+	+	0	+	Coordinated inpatient/ outpatient programs
CA	UCSF Benioff Children's Hospital, San Francisco, IP3 – Integrated Pediatric Pain/ Palliative Care Clinic: 1825 Fourth St., 5A, San Francisco, CA 94143, T: 415-353-1328, F: 415-353-3729, ip3.ucsfbenioff@ucsf.edu www.ucsfchildrenshospital.org	400+	0-21	+	+	+	+	+	+	+	+	+	0	+	Coordinated in-out patient/ programs
CA	David K. Becker MD, MA, MFT UCSF Osher Center for Integrative Medicine 1545 Divisadero St., San Francisco, CA 94115 T: 415.353.7720 www.osher.ucsf.edu/ patient-care/treatments-services/pediatrics-2	60	0-18	+	+	0	+	+	0	+	0	0	0	0	abd. pain, headaches, amp pain, chronic fatigue

Pain Center Locator For the latest updated list of Centers go to http://americanpainsociety.org/uploads/get-involved/PediatricPainClinicList_Update_2.10.15.pdf

+ =AVAILABLE EXPERTISE 0 =Not available

		#/yr.	Age Elig.	Multidisci.	BioPsySoc.	PT	Psy	Comp. Rx	NPsy	Exprt	Interv. Proc.	Rehab-in	Rehab-out	Trials	Comments
CA	Dir.: Dr Padma Gulur: Pain Mgmt Services pgulur@uci.edu UCI: Gottschalk Medical, Plaza, 1 .Medical Plaza Dr, Irvine, CA 92697 T: 949.824.7246 www.anesthesiology.uci.edu/pain														
CA	Prog. Dir.: Lonnie Zeltzer MD UCLA Ped. Pain Program, Dept. Pediatrics, 22-464 MDCC, 10833 Le Conte Ave. Los Angeles, CA 90095-1752; lzeltzer@mednet.ucla.edu www.uclahealth.org/pedspain T: 310-825-0731	200	0-21	+	+	+	+	+	+	+	0	0	0	+	Complex chronic pain of any type
CA	Co-Dir.: Paul Zeltzer MD, WholeChild LA Inc. Encino, CA 91436;www.wholechildla.org ; T: 310 489 3119 DrZeltzer@wholechildla.org	80	0-26	+	+	+	+	+	+	+	0	0	0	+	Same team as UCLA Program
CA	Dir.: Jeffrey I. Gold, PhD Childr. Hospital Los Angeles, Depar, Anesthesiology CriticalCare Medicine, 4650 Sunset Blvd., Los Angeles, CA 90027 T: 323.361.7686 jigold@chla.usc.edu; painclinic@chla.usc.edu	300	0-21	+	+	+	+	+	+	+	+	0	0	+	biofeedback CBT, peer group counsel occup Th.
CA	Prog. Dir.: Elliot Krane MD; Stanford Children's Health, 300 Pasteur Drive, Stanford, CA 94305; ekrane@stanford.edu T: 650-498-7000	700	0-20	+	+	+	+	+	+	+	+	0	+	+	Neuropathic pain

Pain Center Locator For the latest updated list of Centers go to http://americanpainsociety.org/uploads/get-involved/PediatricPainClinicList_Update 2.10.15.pdf

+ =AVAILABLE EXPERTISE 0 =Not available

	Pain Center Locator	#/yr.	Age Elig.	Multidisci.	BioPsySoc.	PT	Psy	Comp. Rx	NPsy	Exprt	Interv. Proc.	Rehab-in	Rehab-out	Trials	Comments
CO	Medical Dir.: Robin Slover MD Clinical Dir.: Sheryl Kent, PhD Children's Hospital, 13213 East 16th Ave, B615 Aurora, CO 80045 T: 720-777-6700 painservices@childrenscolorado.org	210	3-20	+	+	+	+	+	0	+	+	+	0	+	-CRPS -Functional Pain Disorders
CT	Prog.Dir: William T. Zempsky MD MPH Laura Miele, RN. Connecticut Children Medical Ctr.282 Washington Street,Hartford, CT 06106 www.Connecticutchildrens.org T: 860-837-5207 F: 860-837-5209	200	0-18	+	+	+	+	+	0	0	+	+	0	+	Sickle cell disease Complex Post Op Pain Widespread pain
DE	Prog. Dir.: Katherine S. Salamon, PhD Nemours A.I.duPont Hospital for Children, 1600 Rockland Road, Wilmington, DE 19803 Appointments: T: 302-651-5642 katherine.salamon@nemours.org	150	0-18	+	+	+	+	+	0	+	0	0	+	0	: AMPS, CRPS, POTS, chronic fatigue,
GA	Dir.: Claudia Venable MD. Children's Healthcare Atlanta, 1001 Johnson Ferry Rd. NE Atlanta, GA 30342 T: 404-785-6220; F 404-785-6223www.choa.org/ Childrens-Hospital-Services/Pain-Relief	150	5-21	+	+	0	+	0	0	+	+	0	0	0	Out-in patient CRPS
IL	Prog.Dir.: Patrick K. Birmingham MD. Lurie Children's Hospital of Chicago, Dept. Ped Anesthesia, Chronic Pain Management Prog. 225 E. Chicago Avenue, Chicago, IL 60611. T: 312-227-5157 www.luriechildrens.org PBirmingham@luriechildrens.org	91	5-21	+	+	+	+	+	0	+	+	+	0	+	

Pain Center Locator For the latest updated list of Centers go to *http://americanpainsociety.org/uploads/get-involved/PediatricPainClinicList_Update_2.10.15.pdf*

+ = AVAILABLE EXPERTISE 0 = Not available

	#/yr.	Age Elig.	Multidisci.	BioPsySoc.	PT	Psy	Comp. Rx	NPsy	Exprt	Interv. Proc.	Rehab-in	Rehab-out	Trials	Comments
IL — Gadi Revivo, DO, grevivo@ric.org Rehabilitation Institute of Chicago Center for Pain Management, 980 N Michigan Ave, # 800, Chicago, IL 60611 T: 312.238.7885; Diane Amstutz, PhD, damstutz@ric.org T:312.238.7827 www.ric.org/paincenter	100	8-21	+	+	+	+	0	0	0	+	+	+	0	
IN — Prog Dir.: Eric Scott, Ph.D. Riley Hospital for Children; Riley Pain Center, 705 Barnhill Dr. Indianapolis, IN 46202 erlscott@iupui.edu http://iuhealth.org/riley/pain-management/ T: 317-948-7040; F: 317-948-7041	200	0-20	+	+	+	+	+	+	0	+	0	0	0	
KY — Children's Health/Inness Recovery Program Directr: Bryan Carter, Ph.D.Kosair Children's Hospital/Bingham Clinic, Univ. Louisville School of Medicine, Dept. Pediatrics, Div. Child Psych. 200 E. Chestmut St., Louisville, KY 40202 T: 502 588-0811 F: 502 588-0801 bryan.carter@louisville.edu http://louisville.edu/chirp	75	8-19	+	+	+	+	+	0	0	+	0	0	0	manualized CBT/ 12 session out-pt prog, medical mmmgt PT, academic advocacy
NJ — Dir.: Katherine Bentley MD, Pediatric Chronic Pain Center Children's Specialized Hospital 200 Somerset Street, New Brunswick, NJ 08901 T: 888- CHILDREN www.childrens-specialized.org KBentley@c-childrens-specialized.org	130	7-21	+	+	+	+	+	+	+	0	+	0	0	In/ outpt. prog. EDS CRPS fibromyalgia abd pain, headache amplified pain

Pain Center Locator   For the latest updated list of Centers go to *http://americanpainsociety.org/uploads/get-involved/PediatricPainClinicList_Update_2.10.15.pdf*

+ =AVAILABLE EXPERTISE 0 =Not available

		#/yr.	Age Elig.	Multidisci.	BioPsySoc.	PT	Psy	Comp. Rx	NPsy	Exprt	Interv. Proc.	Rehab-in	Rehab-out	Trials	Comments
MA	Boston Children's Hospital Pain Treatment Service Dir.: Charles Berde MD 300 Longwood Avenue, Boston, MA 02115; Chronic Pain Clinic: Dir.: Neil Schechter MD. T: 617-355-7040 ; Pediatric Pain Rehab Center, Dir., Navil Sethna T: 718-216-1650	494	0-18	+	+	+	+	+	0	0	+	+	0	+	CRPS; Abdominal Pain, Headaches Day Hospital admission
MA	Pascal Scemama MD, MA General Hospital for Children 55 Fruit Street,Boston MA 02114 T: 617-6434086 *http://www.massgeneral.org/children/ services/treatmentprograms.aspx?id=1619 pscemamadegialluly@partners.org,*	100	0-18	+	+	+	+	+	+	+	+	0	+	+	
MD	Prog. Dir.: Sabine Kost-Byerly MD. Kennedy Krieger Institute, 707 North Broadway, Baltimore MD 21205 T: (888) 554-2080 *www.kennedykrieger.org/patient-care/ patient-care-programs/outpatient-programs/ pediatric-pain-rehabilitation-clinic-outpatient*	84	6-18	+	+	+	+	+	+	+	0	+	+	0	CRPS,-Fxnl Hyper-mobility, -EDS,-Abd pain,Chronic fatigue POTS, -Intens inpt/ day rehab
MI	Prog. Dir.: Suresh Thomas MD. Children's Hospital of Michigan, Pediatric Pain Management Clinic, Children's Hospital of Michigan, 3901 Beaubien, Box 181, Detroit, MI 48201; T: 313-745-4049, F: 313-745-5448, Contact: pediatricpainmgnt@dmc.org *www.childrensdmc.org/?id=1814&sid=1*	175	0-18	+	+	+	+	+	+	+	+	+	0	0	

Pain Center Locator For the latest updated list of Centers go to http://americanpainsociety.org/uploads/get-involved/PediatricPainClinicList_Update_2.10.15.pdf

+ =AVAILABLE EXPERTISE 0 =Not available

		#/yr.	Age Elig.	Multidisci.	BioPsySoc.	PT	Psy	Comp. Rx	NPsy	Exprt	Interv. Proc.	Rehab-in	Rehab-out	Trials	Comments
MN	Progr Dir: Stefan J. Friedrichsdorf, MD, FAAP. Childrens Hospitals/ Clinics of Minnesota. 2525 ChicagoAve S, Minneapolis, MN 55404 https://www.childrensmn.org/ painpalliativeintegrativemed; Contact: CIPPC@childrensMN.org T: 612-813-7888; F: 612-813-7199	150	0-17		+	+	+	+	+	+	+	0	+	+	https://vimeo. com/12265481
MN	Mayo Clinic Pediatric Pain Rehab Center (PRC) Clinical Dir., Karen E. Weiss PhD Mayo Clinic Chronic Pain Clinic, 200 First Street SW; Rochester, MN 55905; T: (507) 255-2412 Weiss.Karen1@mayo.edu	400	0-18	+	+	+	+	+	+	+	+	+	+	+	all pain and problematic symptoms, (POTS); 3 wk intense pain rehab
MO	Dan Millspaugh MD; Dir.,Comprehensive Pain Management Prog., Children's Mercy Hospitals, 2401 Gillham Road, Kansas City, Missouri 64108 cmhpain@cmh.edu	400	0-18	+	+	+	+	+	+	+	+	0	+	+	
MO	Lynne Sterni MD Charles Schrock MD St Louis, Childr. Hospital Pain Management Clinic #1 Children's Place # 5S 31 St. Louis, MO 63110 www.stlouischildrens.org/ourservices/ painmanagement-clinic	150	0-18		+	+	+	+	+	+	+	0	0	0	emphasis on less pain, improved quality of life/ fxn

Pain Center Locator   For the latest updated list of Centers go to *http://americanpainsociety.org/uploads/get-involved/PediatricPainClinicList_Update_2.10.15.pdf*

+ =AVAILABLE EXPERTISE   0 =Not available

	Pain Center Locator	#/yr.	Age Elig.	Multidisci.	BioPsySoc.	PT	Psy	Comp. Rx	NPsy	Exprt	Interv. Proc.	Rehab-in	Rehab-out	Trials	Comments
NJ	Dir.: Katherine Bentley MD, Ped.Chronic Pain Center Children's Specialized Hospital 200 Somerset Street, New Brunswick NJ 08901 www.childrens-specialized.org T: 888-CHILDREN KBentley@childrens-specialized.org	130	7-21	+	+	+	+	+	+	+	0	+	0	0	CRPS fibromyalg EDS, abd pain,head- ache ,amplified pain
OH	Prog. Dir.: Michael Joseph MD Center For Pediatric and Adolescent Pain Care 5080 C Bradenton Ave, Dublin, OH 43017 T: 614-889-6422; F: 614-453-8863 www.pediatricpaincare.com	120	0-26	+	+	0	+	+	0	+	+	0	0	+	Personal chronic pain & symptom mngment
OH	Dir.: Sarah Friebert MD, Haslinger Division f Pediatric Palliative Care Akron Children's Hospital, 1 Perkins Square, Akron, Ohio 44308, T :330-543-3343 F: 330-543-3539														
OH	Dir.: Timothy P. Smith MD, Comprehen. Pain Services Nationwide Children's Hospital, 700 Children's Drive, Columbus, OH 43205 T: 614.722.4205, F:614.355.2878 www.nationwidechildrens.org Anjana.kundu@nationwidechildrens.org														
OH	Prog. Dir.: Gerard A. Banez, Ph.D. Cleveland Clinic Children's Hospital for Rehabilitation, 2801 MLK Jr. Drive/CR11 Cleveland, Ohio 44104. T: 216-448-6253; F: 216-448-6207 http://my.clevelandclinic.org/childrens-hospital	110	8-21	+	+	+	+	+	0	+	0	+	+	0	interdiscip. inpatient/ day rehab CRPS, headache, fibromyalg. Abd. pain.

Pain Center Locator For the latest updated list of Centers go to http://americanpainsociety.org/uploads/get-involved/PediatricPainClinicList_Update_2.10.15.pdf

+ =AVAILABLE EXPERTISE 0 =Not available

		#/yr.	Age Elig.	Multidisci.	BioPsySoc.	PT	Psy	Comp. Rx	NPsy	Exprt	Interv. Proc.	Rehab-in	Rehab-out	Trials	Comments
OH	Dr. Ibrahim Farid Dr. Bradley Riemenschneider, Akron Children's Hospital Medical Center. Akron, Ohio 44308 T: 330-543-8503 *ifarid@chmca.org; briemenschneider@chmca.org*	120	0-21	+	+	+	+	+	0	+	+	+	+	0	
OH	Dir.: Ken Goldschneider MD, Pediatric Pain Management Center, Cincinnati Children's Hospital Medical Center, 3333 Burnet Avenue, ML #2001 Cincinnati, OH 45229 T: 513.636.7768: F:513.636.292 *kenneth. goldschneider@cchmc.org www.cincinnatichildrens.org/service/p/pain/ default*	270	0-21	+	+	+		0	0	+	+	+	0	0	Ehlers-Danlos Epidermo-lysis Bullosa, Inpatient pain Rehab
OK	Klanci McCabe PhD Pediat Pain Mgmt, Children's Hospital at OU Medical Center 825 NE 10th St., 2nd Floor, Suite 2300,Oklahoma City, OK 73104 *www.oumedicine.com/childrens* T: 405-271-7255 F: 1,405 271-4015														
OR	Jeffrey Koh MD,Dir., Anna Wilson PhD, Pain Psychology Services; Ped Pain Mngmt Center OHSU Doernbecher Childr.Hospital, 3181SW Sam Jackson Park Rd., Portland, OR 97239 T: 503.418.5188 *LONGANN@OHSU.EDU www.ohsu.edu/xd/health/services/clinics/ PainManagementCenterPediatrics.cfm*	150	0-17	+	+	+	+	+	0	0	0	0	0	+	

PAIN CENTER LOCATOR

Pain Center Locator For the latest updated list of Centers go to *http://americanpainsociety.org/uploads/get-involved/PediatricPainClinicList_Update_2.10.15.pdf*

+ = AVAILABLE EXPERTISE 0 = Not available

		#/yr.	Age Elig.	Multidisci.	BioPsySoc.	PT	Psy	Comp. Rx	NPsy	Exprt	Interv. Proc.	Rehab-in	Rehab-out	Trials	Comments
PA	James Mooney MD Virginia Thompson Peds Chronic Pain Clinic Penn State Milton Hershey Children's Hospital 500 University Dr. UPCII, Suite 1100 Hershey, PA 17033 T: 717-531-6834 F: 717-531-4143; *www.pennstatehershey.org/web/anesthesia/patientcare/services/pediatric-chronicpain*	100	0-18	+	+	+	+	0	0	0	+	0	0	+	
PA	Prog. Dir.: David D. Sherry MD Children's Hospital Philadelphia, 34th & Civic Center Blvd. Philadelphia, PA 19104 *www.StopChildhoodPain.org* ampsprogram@email.chop.edu T: 215-590-7234 F: 251-590-4750	250	4-17	+	+	+	+	0	+	+	+	+	+	+	Amplified pain: CRPS, fibromyalgia, abdomin. & head pain.
PA	Prog. Dir.: F. Wickham Kraemer MD Children's Hospital of Philadelphia, 3401 Civic Center Blvd. Philadelphia, PA 19104. T: 215-590-1409 *www.chop.edu/centers-programs/pain-management-program*	NR	0-18	+	+	+	+	+	+	+	0	+	0	0	All chronic pain
TX	Dir.: Artee Gandhi MD, Medical Pain Mngmnt Cook Children's Hospital Dodson Specialty Clinics, Department Neurosciences, 1500 Cooper St., Fort Worth,TX 76104, Appts: T: 682-885-7246, Nurse Coord: T: 682-885-4549 *www.cookchildrens.org www.cookchildrens. org/SpecialtyServices/Pain%20Management/ Contact%20Us/Pages/default.aspx*	200	0-21	+	+	+	+	+	+	+	+	+	0	0	CRPS, Fxnal pain palliative care, In-patient rehab program

Pain Center Locator For the latest updated list of Centers go to *http://americanpainsociety.org/uploads/get-involved/PediatricPainClinicList_Update_2.10.15.pdf*

+ =AVAILABLE EXPERTISE 0 =Not available

	Center	#/yr.	Age Elig.	Multidisci.	BioPsySoc.	PT	Psy	Comp. Rx	NPsy	Exprt	Interv. Proc.	Rehab-in	Rehab-out	Trials	Comments
TX	Dir.: Alan C. Farrow-Gillespie MD, Lynn Clark, CPNP, Pediatric Pain Management Center at Children's Health System of Texas, 1935 Medical District Drive, Dallas, Texas 75235. T: 214-456-8131 *www.childrens.com/specialties-services/specialty-centers-and-programs/pain-management*	200	0-17	+	+	+	+	+	0	+	+	0	+	+	Headache, Abdominal Pain
WA	Prog. Dir.: Gary A. Walco, PhD, ABPP Seattle Children's Hospital, 4800 Sand Point Way NE; P.O. Box 5371, M/S MB.11.500.3 Seattle, WA 98145-5005	398	3-18	+	+	+	+	+	+	+	+	+	+	+	Intensive rehab program.
DC-Wash	Julia Finkel MD; DC Washington Complex Pain Management Center (outpatient program) Children's National Medical Center/111 Michigan Ave., NW Wash, DC 20010 T: 202 476- 3273 *www.childrensnational.org*	-	-		+	+	+	+	+	+	+	+	0	0	
WI	Steven J. Weisman MD Dir. Jane B. Pettit Pain & Headache Center, Children's Hospital Wisconsin, 9000 W Wisconsin Ave MS 792. Milwaukee, WI 53226 Contact: T: 414-266-2775 F: 414-266-1761 *webmaster@chw.orgwww.chw.org/medical-care/pain-management-program* ;	1100	0-18	+	+	+	+	+	+	+	+	0	0	+	-CRPS -Headache -Functional pain disorders -Analgesics

PAIN CENTER LOCATOR

Pain Center Locator   For the latest updated list of Centers go to *http://americanpainsociety.org/uploads/get-involved/PediatricPainClinicList_Update_2.10.15.pdf*
+ =AVAILABLE EXPERTISE 0 =Not available

		#/yr	Age Elig.	Multidisci.	BioPsySoc.	PT	Psy	Comp. Rx	NPsy	Exprt	Interv. Proc.	Rehab-in	Rehab-out	Trials	Comments
CANADA	Dir.: Stephen Brown MD Pain Prog Dept. Anesthesia/Pain Mgmt. Hospital for Sick Children, 525 University Ave.# 925; Toronto, ON,M5G 1X8. T:416-813-6975 F: 416-813-7646 *http://www.sickkids.ca/chronicpainclinic*	150	2-18	+	+	+	+	0	0	0	+	0	0	+	
CANADA	Dir.: Pablo M. Ingelmo MD, Chronic Pain Service. Montreal Children's Hospital.1001 Decaire Blvd. B04 2427, Montreal (QC) H4A3J1 Canada T: +514 412-4400 Ext 24886 *mchchronicpainclinic@muhc.mcgill.ca* *www.thechildren.com*	100	0-18	+	+	+	+	+	+	0	+	0	0	+	Tertiary care program
CANADA	IWK Health Centre – Pediatric Complex Pain Clinic, 5850 University Ave., Halifax, NS B3K 6R8, Canada, T: 902-470-8769 *allen.finley@iwk.nshealth.ca*	60	0-17	+	+	+	+	0	0	+	+	0	0	0	
CANADA	Dir: Dr. Christine Lamontagne Med Children's Hospital, Eastern Ontario Chronic Pain Clinic. 401 Smyth road, Ottawa, ON K1H 8L1; T:613-737-7600 x3792 *clamontagne@cheo.on.ca*	96	0-17	+	+	+	+	0	0	0	+	0	0	0	

Pain Center Locator For the latest updated list of Centers go to http://americanpainsociety.org/uploads/get-involved/PediatricPainClinicList_Update_2.10.15.pdf

+ = AVAILABLE EXPERTISE 0 = Not available

	#/yr.	Age Elig.	Multidisci.	BioPsySoc.	PT	Psy	Comp. Rx	NPsy	Exprt	Interv. Proc.	Rehab-in	Rehab-out	Trials	Comments
CANADA Dir.: Mark Simmonds MB, Stollery Children's Hospital Pediatric Chronic Pain Prog. 8440–112 St Edmonton AB T6T1C5. Contact: Kathy Reid, NP. Kathy.reid@albertahealthservices.ca T: 780-407-1363 F: 780-407-8529 http://www.albertahealthservices.ca/services.asp?pid=service&rid=1019352	60	0-18	+	+	+	+	0	+	0	0	0	0	0	
CANADA Tim Oberlander MD, BC Children's Hospital, Complex Pain Program, 4480 Oak Street, Vancouver BC, Canada, V6H 3V4 T: 604-875-5108; F: 604-875-2767 Contact: srandhawa3@cw.bc.ca www.bcchildrens.ca/services/painservice	93	0-18	+	+	+	+	0	+	+	+	+	+	0	Headache, abdominal, CRPS, pain developmental disabilities
CANADA The Vi Riddell Children's Pain and Rehabilitation Centre, Alberta Children's Hospital. 2888 Shaganappi Trail NW Calgary, Alberta, Canada,T3B-6A8.T: 403-955-7430	117	0-18	+	+	+	+	+	+	+	+	0	+	0	
UK Dr Hannah Connell, Clinical Lead. Bath Centre for Pain Children's Services ; Royal United Hospitals Bath, Royal National Hospital for Rheumatic Diseases, Upper Borough Walls, Bath BA1 1RL, UK. www.bathcentreforpainservices.nhs.uk T: +44 1225 473 427	100	0-29	+	+	+	+	0	0	+	0	+	+	0	3 wk. residence program & child/ adolescent specialist services.

Pain Center Locator For the latest updated list of Centers go to *http://americanpainsociety.org/uploads/get-involved/PediatricPainClinicList_Update_2.10.15.pdf*

+ =AVAILABLE EXPERTISE 0 =Not available

		#/yr.	Age Elig.	Multidisci.	BioPsySoc.	PT	Psy	Comp. Rx	NPsy	Exprt	Interv. Proc.	Rehab-in	Rehab-out	Trials	Comments
UK	Dr Ewan Wallace MBChB FRCA, Paediatric Chronic Pain services, Royal Hospital for Children, 1345 Govan road, Glasgow G51 4TF ewan.wallace@ggc.scot.nhs.uk T: +441414524316	100	0-20	+	+	+	+	+	0	0	+	+	0	0	chronic fatigue syn inpatient/ no formal pain mmmt program
UK	Dr P M Rolfe MA MB. Outpatient Pain Service Box 215 Addenbrooke' Hospital Cambridge University Hospitals.NHS Foundation Trust Hills Road Cambridge CB2 0QQ UK T: +44 1223 217796	75-100	0-18	+	+	+	+	0	+	+	+	0	0	0	Complex pain of any type
UK	Lead: Dr Thanthullu Vasu MBBS MD; Pain Mgmt Multidiscip.Paediatric Chronic Pain Service, Univ.Hospitals of Leicester NHS Trust, Leicester General Hospital, Gwendolen Road, Leicester LE5 4PW. UK T: +44 116 258 4720/ 258 8253 email: thanthullu.vasu@uhl-tr.nhs.uk	75	0-18	+	+	+	+	+	+	+	+	0	0	+	Pain mngmt Program (4 weeks after school)
UK	Dir.: Elaine Wilson-Smith FRCA Pain Mngmt Service, Sheffield Children's Hospital, Western Bank, Sheffield S10 2TH; T: 44 1142660843 http://www.sheffieldchildrens.nhs.uk/our-services/pain-management/chronic-pain.htm Elaine.Wilson-Smith@sch.nhs.uk	200	0-18	+	+	+	+	+	+	+	+	+	0	+	Occupational Therapy

Pain Center Locator For the latest updated list of Centers go to *http://americanpainsociety.org/uploads/get-involved/PediatricPainClinicList_Update_2.10.15.pdf*

+ =AVAILABLE EXPERTISE 0 =Not available

		#/yr.	Age Elig.	Multidisci.	BioPsySoc.	PT	Psy	Comp. Rx	NPsy	Exprt	Interv. Proc.	Rehab-in	Rehab-out	Trials	Comments
UK	Dr Sachin Rastogi FRCA Pediatric Pain Clinic. Great North Children's Hospital,Newcastle upon Tyne ,NHS Foundation Trust, Queen Victoria Road, Newcastle upon Tyne NE1 4LP T: +44 191 2821596	50	0-18	+	+	+	+	+	+	+	+	+	0		
UK	Dr Alison Bliss MB ChB MSc Clinical lead: Children's Pain Service, Leeds Children's Hospital, Leeds General Hospital, Great George Street, Leeds, LS1 3EX T: 0113 3925466	84	0-18	+	+	+	+	+	0	+	+	+	+	0	Pain mnmgmt programme teenagers, younger child/parent
AU-NSW	Prog. Dir.: John Collins PhD MD. Children's Hospital at Westmead, Hainsworth Street, Westmead NSW 2145 AUSTRALIA. Contact: *natasha.haynes@health.nsw.gov.au* T: +612 9845 2573 *http://www.schn.health.nsw.gov.au/ parents-and-carers/our-services/pain-medicine/chw*	200	0-18	+	+	+	+	0	0	0	+	+	+	0	Telehealth available. TAME Your Pain Day Program. CRPS/head-ache hyper mobility/Complex Pain
AU-NSW	Prog. Dir.: Dr.Matthew Crawford, Sydney Children's Hospital, High Street, Randwick, NSW 2032 AUSTRALIA. Contact: *david.anderson@health.nsw.gov.au* T: +612 9382 1817	45	3-18	+	+	+	+	0	0	0	0	0	0	0	
AU-WA	Anna Hilyard	Program Coord Complex Pain, Princesss Margaret Hospital, 431 Godfrey House, PMH, Subiaco WA 6008, PERTH. T: +618 9340 7391; *anna.hilyard@health.wa.gov.au*	120	0-15	+	+	+	+	+	0	+	+	0	+	+	cognitive behavioural framework. Six wk CBT Emphasis on self-mangmt

APPENDIX B
GLOSSARY-USEFUL PAIN TERMINOLOGY[84]

Arthralgia. Arthritis-like pain that occurs in joints but without any noticeable inflammation. For example, arthralgias occur during flu, even though there is no actual inflammation of the joints.

Arthritis. An inflammatory condition of the joints associated with joint pain, such as juvenile rheumatoid arthritis (JRA).

Asperger's Syndrome (AS). A developmental condition characterized by social interaction problems, difficulty reading nonverbal cues, difficulties with transitions or changes, preference for routine and rituals, clumsiness, unusual preoccupations, and normal language development. (see also Autism Spectrum Disorder)

Autism spectrum disorder (ASD). A developmental condition characterized by a delay in the acquisition of language, repetitive mannerisms and interests, a strong preference for routines and rituals, lack of imaginative play, severe social difficulties, poor eye contact, and a lack of interest in others.

Autonomic nervous system (ANS). The portion of the nervous system that regulates involuntary body functions, including those of the heart and intestine. Controls blood flow, digestion and temperature regulation.

Clinical Trials. Carefully planned and monitored experiments to test a new drug or treatment. Many clinical trials involve children. Some of the pediatric pain programs in the appendix can be contacted to see if they have clinical pain trials for children

Cognitive Behavioral Therapy (CBT). A treatment strategy used to teach a child how to identify things and situations that stress him, and how to control anxiety associated with those stressors. It strives to replace anxiety producing thoughts and behaviors with new ones until the stressors no longer make the child anxious.

Central Nervous System (CNS). The brain, spinal cord, and spinal nerves. It serves as the main "processing center" for the whole nervous system, and thus controls all the workings of the body.

---

84 Adapted from "Conquering your Childs Pain". Lonnie Zeltzer MD. Harper Collins. New York. 2005.

PAIN IN CHILDREN AND YOUNG ADULTS

Complementary and Alternative Medicine (CAM). Approaches to medical treatment outside of mainstream medical training. (acupuncture, meditation, aroma therapy, Chinese medicine, dance therapy, music therapy, massage, herbal medicine, therapeutic touch, yoga, osteopathy, chiropractic treatments, naturopathy, homeopathy).

Complex regional pain syndrome (CRPS) A neuropathic pain condition (also called reflex sympathetic dystrophy or RSD) in which sensory nerves to a certain, regional, part of the body get "turned on" and that area becomes super sensitive, so that even light touch can be painful.

Computerized tomography (CT scan). An X-ray technique that uses a computer to construct cross-sectional images of the body.

Electrical stimulation. Application of currents to induce pain relief, such as transcutaneous electrical nerve stimulation (TENS).

Endorphins. Naturally occurring molecules made up of amino acids. Endorphins attach to special receptors in the brain and spinal cord to stop pain messages. These are the same receptors that respond to morphine.

Enkephalins (en-KEF-uh-lins). Naturally occurring molecules in the brain. Enkephalins attach to special receptors in your brain and spinal cord to stop pain messages. They also affect other functions within the brain and nervous system.

Fibromyalgia. A disorder characterized by fatigue, stiffness, joint tenderness, and widespread muscle pain. Juvenile fibromyalgia is different than adult onset fibromyalgia, in that children with juvenile fibromyalgia can outgrow this condition.

Functional abdominal pain (FAP). A functional gastrointestinal (GI) condition with belly pain (no other GI symptoms) caused by disordered brain-gut nerve signaling.

Functional dyspepsia. A painful functional GI condition in the mid-upper abdomen (ulcer location but no ulcer) caused by disordered brain-gut nerve signaling.

Functional pain. Pain that is not derived from infection, inflammation, injury, or structural damage. It is related to the abnormal and disordered function of nerve signals that send increased pain messages to the brain.

Gastroenterology. The branch of medicine dealing with the study of disorders affecting the stomach, intestines, and associated organs.

General anesthesia. A state of unconsciousness induced by a medication that eliminates pain perception.

Headaches. Pain in the head. Tension (muscular) headaches can feel like pressure or throbbing; Migraines are often throbbing and can be associated with nausea and visual disturbances.

346

GLOSSARY

Individualized Educational Plan (IEP). Parents of a student with physical, emotional, or learning disabilities can submit a "Request for Special Education Assessment." An evaluation is then made to see whether the student qualifies for special accommodations and modifications under an Individualized Educational Plan (IEP). IEP students usually have serious academic or learning problems that prevent them from meeting the standards of the class.

Inflammatory bowel disease (IBD). Intestinal disease related to inflammation and associated with diarrhea, bleeding, cramping, obstruction (a blockage of the intestine), malabsorption (failure of the intestines to absorb minerals and nutrients), and weight loss or poor weight gain (e.g. ulcerative colitis and Crohn's disease).

Irritable bowel syndrome (IBS). A functional GI condition with belly pain, and nausea, vomiting, bloating, diarrhea, or constipation, and caused by disordered brain-gut nerve signaling.

Juvenile rheumatoid arthritis (JRA). An autoimmune condition in children that involves primarily pain and inflammation in the joints. There are a number of differences between juvenile rheumatoid arthritis and adult rheumatoid arthritis.

Limbic center. The portion of the brain that produces emotions. This is the core of the "emotional brain."

Magnetic resonance imaging (MRI). A technique used in a medical setting to produce high quality images of the inside of the body.

Musculoskeletal. Relating to or involving the muscles and the skeleton.

Myofascial pain. Pain and tenderness in the muscles & adjacent fibrous tissues (fascia) with sensitive areas known as trigger/ tender points, located in the muscles.

Nervous System. Generally refers to three body systems: 1) the central nervous system, which is the brain and spinal cord; 2) the peripheral nervous system, which is the cervical, thoracic, lumbar, and sacral nerve trunks leading away from the spine to the limbs, and 3) the autonomic nervous system (ANS), which has cell bodies alongside the spinal cord with nerves that travel back and forth to internal organs, the body's periphery, and to a central area in the brain stem.

Neuromodule. Pain circuits within the cortical (conscious) areas of the brain.

Neurotransmitters. The naturally occurring chemicals in human beings and animals that relay electrical messages between the nerve cells. Three neurotransmitters we are most familiar with are serotonin, norepinephrine, and dopamine.

Nociceptors (no-sih-SEP-turs). Special small nerve fibers that carry pain or negative sensory messages.

347

PAIN IN CHILDREN AND YOUNG ADULTS

Neuropsychology. The study of brain behavior relationships. Neuropsychologists have extensive training in the anatomy, physiology, and pathology of the nervous system and in how these systems affect thinking and emotions. Clinical child neuropsychologists evaluate cognitive (thinking and performing) function in children and make recommendations for treatment to improve function based on the testing results and their observations of the child. Cognitive testing can be helpful for children with suspected learning disabilities or uneven IQ.

Opioids. Prescription medications that relieve pain by binding to specialized receptors in the brain and spinal cord. Some are derived from opium, others are synthetic (same as **Narcotics).** (For natural opioids, see **enkephalins.**)

Pain. An unpleasant sensory and emotional experience associated with actual or potential tissue damage or described in terms of such damage (International Association for the Study of Pain).

Pain associated disability syndrome (PADS). A condition in which a child with chronic pain functions less and less well over time (e.g. not attending school, sleeping poorly, not playing with friends, not physically active).

Parasympathetic nervous system (PNS). The part of the autonomic nervous system responsible for restorative functions like digestion.

Patient controlled analgesia (PCA). A computerized system allowing a patient to control the amount of pain medicine he receives. The patient pushes a button and a machine delivers a pre-set dose of pain medicine into the blood stream through a vein.

Peripheral nerves. Nerves that run from your spinal cord to all other parts of your body. They transmit messages from the spinal cord and the brain to and from other parts of your body, and send sensory signals back to the spinal cord and brain.

Perseverative. Tending to stay with one thing and not let go. It is often used to describe children with pervasive developmental disorders (PDD) such as Autism.

Pervasive developmental disorder (PDD). A neurological condition associated with a broad range of cognitive and behavioral abnormalities, but always including a deficit in social perception and interaction (problems with emotional intelligence).

Phantom pain. Pain or discomfort following amputation that feels as if it comes from the missing limb or organ.

Physical therapy. A treatment in which muscles and ligaments are stretched, balanced, and strengthened.

348

GLOSSARY

Placebo. A supposedly inert/inactive substance (e.g. sugar pill, saline injection), psychological, or behavioral treatment that is used in clinical studies as control factors to help determine the efficacy of active treatments. However, more recent research has shown that "placebos" can also have active effects.

Recurrent pain. Pain that occurs or appears again or repeatedly.

Rehabilitation. A treatment aimed at restoring function.

Relaxation. A condition in which muscles are loose, stress hormones are low, heart rate, breathing rate, and blood pressure are normal or low, and the body feels warm and comfortable. Relaxation techniques are strategies to attain relaxation.

Selective serotonin reuptake inhibitors (SSRIs). Medications used to relieve depression and anxiety. May work by increasing the availability of a brain chemical that helps to regulate mood (serotonin).

Side effects. Unwanted changes produced by medication or other treatment, ranging from minor and temporary, such as dry mouth, to more serious, such as gastrointestinal bleeding.

Spinal cord. A cordlike bundle of nerves that extends from the base of the brain to the small of the back. The dorsal part (outer part towards the back) of the spinal cord carries the nerve fibers that relay pain messages to the brain.

Sympathetic nervous system (SNS). Part of the autonomic nervous system responsible for fight or flight reactions (speeds up heart, breathing, sweating, etc.).

Symptom. What your child tells you he is feeling such as reported feelings of pain, nausea, or vomiting. (This is as opposed to a **sign** of pain which is what a doctor notices in a patient, such as a heart murmur, an enlarged liver, or a rash.)

Tricyclic antidepressants. A group of drugs used to relieve symptoms of depression in high doses and can help to relieve certain types of pain in low doses (e.g. IBS, neuropathic pain).

Trigger point. A hypersensitive area or site in muscle or connective tissue at which touch or pressure will elicit pain. Also called "tender point."

349

APPENDIX C
SAMPLE LETTERS & TRACKING FORMS

- Sample Letters to School (3)
- Medication tracking form,
- Medical bill tracking form
- Insurance Records

SAMPLE LETTERS (3) FROM THE PROFESSIONAL TO THE SCHOOL (ABOUT CRPS)

To whom it may concern:

I am a clinical psychologist, physician, nurse who is working with patient _____ through UCLA's pediatric pain program. _____ has a joint/nerve disorder in her knee called complex regional syndrome, which causes extreme pain. The condition also causes discomfort when the area is touched by others. Therefore, most people with CRPS are very cautious around others and try to protect the area from being bumped. _____ has been working hard in physical therapy to recover from this condition. She has made a great deal of progress in her ability to walk, but she is still very slow, and she continues to be cautious about others touching her knee. We are confident that she will continue to gradually improve throughout the year.

_____'s treatment, in addition to the physical therapy, includes distraction from the pain. One of the best ways to distract her and help her become normal again is to treat her normally. This is best achieved by teachers, staff and students refraining from asking _____ questions about her knee and commenting on how she seems to be doing. Of course it is acceptable and nice for people to greet _____ when she returns to school and tell her that it is nice to have her back, but the fewer questions and comments that can be directed towards her about her knee, the faster she will recover. We are trying to help her return to seeing herself as a normal child. Thanks so much for your help with this transition back to school. Please do not hesitate to contact me if you have any questions.

Sincerely, your name, title

SAMPLE LETTERS & TRACKING FORMS

A SAMPLE LETTER EXPLAINING CHRONIC PAIN TO PEERS

Dear Teachers,

My name is _____ and I am a student in one of your classes. I have been diagnosed with _____. I have been and will remain in ongoing treatment for my _____ through the Pediatric Pain Program at UCLA. My chronic pain is a constant presence, and though I can participate just as well as any other student in your classroom, there may be times when my pain will cause some complications. The pain switches off and on constantly, and I know that causes people confusion—it's confusing to me, as well! Some days, I might seem completely normal and pain free, whereas other days I might be in excruciating pain.

I am a very conscientious, dedicated student and am frustrated by the impact that my pain has on my daily life. There are some accommodations that would help me focus better on my academics in order for the pain to interfere as little as possible. Although it is nice for people to ask about my pain, this brings unwanted attention to the pain and can even cause the pain to increase. Therefore, it is helpful for people to refrain from talking to me about my pain. Sometimes my pain causes me to walk slowly. Please know that if I am late for class, this is the reason. Carrying heavy books also increases my pain. Thus, it would be extremely helpful if I could store an extra set of books for your class at your desk.

Throughout the school year, I will be working hard to cope and break free from my chronic pain, and I am grateful in advance to all of you for understanding and helping me work towards my goal of being pain free.

Thanks, and I look forward to the year.

PAIN IN CHILDREN AND YOUNG ADULTS

A SAMPLE LETTER TO STUDENTS THAT A 3RD GRADER PLUS MIGHT READ TO THE CLASS AFTER BEING ABSENT FOR A WHILE

This 3rd grade student chose to read a speech to her class during the first week of the new school year:

My name is _____. Most of you know that I broke my right foot in second grade. I had to use a wheel chair and crutches sometimes. I am much better now. I have something called Complex Regional Pain Syndrome. You cannot catch this from me! The doctors don't know why I got this, but I am much better now. I am allowed to run, play and do everything that you can do. But please be a little careful with my foot, and don't kick it or anything.

Sometimes my foot might cause me to be in pain because the pain can come and go. This is part of my syndrome. I might feel fine one day and be in pain the next, or I might be fine in the morning and start feeling pain an hour later. And then, it can go away again. This is part of the illness, too. It doesn't always make sense. It's kinda like when you have a tummy ache one day, and you don't know why. And then the next day, your tummy feels fine.

I really appreciate it when you ask me about my pain and how I'm doing, but the questions make me think about the pain. It's kinda like this: When you ask me about my pain, my brain tells me to open up my pain drawer and to feel pain. I try to keep my "brain pain drawer" shut. It would help me if you don't ask me about my pain or my foot. When I am distracted from the pain, I can do everything that you can do.

Thank you for listening to me, and if you have any questions right now, I am happy to answer them. Please remember though, that after this, I wanna keep my "pain drawer" shut, so let's not talk about it. Thank you!

352

SAMPLE LETTERS & TRACKING FORMS

FORMS TO KEEP YOU ORGANIZED

Table C.1 Medications Tracking Form					
My child's Allergies: 1. 2.			3. 4.		
Pharmacy 1 :			Phone number _____ _____		
Pharmacy 2 :			Phone number _____ _____		
Date Started	Date stopped	Medication Name	Dose	Times given	Rx by Dr._____

Date	Provider	Service-Hospital dates	Charges	Insurance payment	We owe	Date paid

SAMPLE LETTERS & TRACKING FORMS

Table C.3   Insurance Coverage and Funding Sources:
Insurance Company
Policy Number
Contact Person
Address
Phone
Insurance Company
Policy Number
Contact Person
Address
Phone
SSI Supplemental Security Income Contact Person Address Phone

APPENDIX D
SELECTED READING

1   Pain in America. IOM Report 2011. *www.iom.edu/Reports/2011/*
    Relieving-Pain-in-America-A-Blueprint-for-Transforming-Prevention-Care-
    Education-Research.aspx

2   Yunus MB, Masi AT. Juvenile primary fibromyalgia syndrome. A clinical
    study of thirty-three patients and matched normal controls. Arthritis &
    Rheumatism 1985;28:138-45.
    Kashikar-Zuck S, Ting TV. Juvenile fibromyalgia: Current status of research
    and future developments. Nature Reviews Rheumatology 2013; 10:89-96
    Kashikar-Zuck S, Ting TV, Arnold LM, et al. Cognitive behavioral therapy
    for the treatment of juvenile fibromyalgia: A multisite, single-blind,
    randomized, controlled clinical trial. Arthritis Rheum 2012;64:297-305.
    Stephens S, Feldman BM, Bradley N, et al. Feasibility and effectiveness
    of an aerobic exercise program in children with fibromyalgia: results of a
    randomized controlled pilot trial. Arthritis Rheum 2008;59:1399-406.
    Kashikar-Zuck S, Cunningham N, Sil S, et al. Long-term outcomes of
    adolescents with juvenile-onset fibromyalgia in early adulthood. Pediatrics
    2014;133 (3):e592-e600.

3   Per Kjaer, PT, MSc, PhD, Charlotte Leboeuf-Yde, DC, MPH, PhD, Joan
    Solgaard Sorensen MD, Tom Bendix, MD, PhD. Spine. 2005; 30(7):798-
    806An Epidemiologic Study of MRI and Low Back Pain in 13-Year-Old
    Children.

4   *www.gastrojournal.org/article/S0016-5085%2814%2900279-0/abstract*

5   Kappelman MD, Moore KR, Allen JK, Cook SF. Recent trends in the
    prevalence of Crohn's disease and ulcerative colitis in a commercially
    insured U.S. population. Dig Dis Sci. 2013;58:519–525.

6   Pain Management". Nalamliang, MF,. Lotstein,DS, Zeltzer PM, *A Parent's
    Guide to Enhancing Quality of Life in Children with Cancer* by Ruth I.
    Hoffman, MPH & Sandra E. Smith, 2014.
    Edited by Ruth I. Hoffman, MPH & Sandra E. Smith

SELECTED READING

7   Stuber Ml, Kazak AE, et al. "Predictors of Posttraumatic Stress Symptoms in Childhood Cancer Survivors. Pediatrics 1997;100;958-964.

8   Paul Zeltzer, Brain Tumors – Finding the Ark – Meeting the Challenges of Treatment Choices, Side Effects, Healthcare Costs and Long Term Survival (Encino, CA: Shilysca Press, 2004). Refer to Chapter 24: Managing Costs, Benefits and Healthcare with Insurance, HMOS and More

9   Adapted from J.S. Schneider, PhD: *www.tbts.org/virtual_html/Internetsearch.htm*

10 Taddio Al, Katz J. The effects of early pain experience in neonates on pain responses in infancy and childhood. Paediatr Drugs. 2005;7(4):245-57.

11 Hathway GJ1, Koch S, Low L, Fitzgerald M. The changing balance of brainstem-spinal cord modulation of pain processing over the first weeks of rat postnatal life. J Physiol. 2009 Jun 15;587(Pt 12):2927-35. doi: 10.1113/jphysiol.2008.168013. Epub 2009 Apr 29.

12 LaPrairie JL1, Murphy AZ. Long-term impact of neonatal injury in male and female rats: Sex differences, mechanisms and clinical implications. Front Neuroendocrinol. 2010 Apr;31(2):193-202. doi: 10.1016/j.yfrne.2010.02.001. Epub 2010 Feb 6.

13 *http://www.susankaisergreenland.com/*

14 Explain Pain. David Butler (Author), G. Lorimer Moseley *http://www.amazon. com/Explain-Pain-David-Butler-ebook/dp/B00IP7AXR0*
    Ezendam, D., et al, Systematic review of the effectiveness of mirror therapy of the upper extremity, Disability and Rehabilitation, 2009;
    Moseley, G.L., Graded motor imagery is effective for long-standing complex regional pain syndrome: a randomized controlled trial, Pain, 2004; 108: 192-198

15 Erpelding, N., et al.. (2014). Rapid treatment-induced brain changes in pediatric CRPS. Brain Structure and Function, 1-17.
    Gaughan, V., Logan, D., Sethna, N., & Mott, S. (2014). Parents' Perspective of Their Journey Caring for a Child with Chronic Neuropathic Pain. Pain Management Nursing, 15(1), 246-257.
    Logan, D. E., et al. (2012). A day-hospital approach to treatment of pediatric complex regional pain syndrome: initial functional outcomes. The Clinical journal of pain, 28(9).

PAIN IN CHILDREN AND YOUNG ADULTS

Logan, D. E., et al.. (2012). Changes in willingness to self-manage pain among children and adolescents and their parents enrolled in an intensive interdisciplinary pediatric pain treatment program. PAIN®, 153(9), 1863-1870.

Logan, D. E., et al.. (2015). Changes in sleep habits in adolescents during intensive interdisciplinary pediatric PR Journal of youth and adolescence, 44(2), 543-555.

Simons, L. E., et al (2012). What does it take? Comparing intensive rehabilitation to outpatient treatment for children with significant pain-related disability. Journal of pediatric psychology, jss109.

Simons, L. E., et al. (2012). Fear of pain in the context of intensive PR among children and adolescents with neuropathic pain: associations with treatment response. The Journal of Pain, 13(12), 1151-1161.

Simons, L. E., et al. (2014). The responsive amygdala: Treatment-induced alterations in functional connectivity in pediatric complex regional pain syndrome. PAIN®, 155(9), 1727-1742.

16 Girsberger, W., Bänziger, U., Lingg, G.,et. Al. Heart rate variability and the influence of craniosacral therapy on autonomous nervous system regulation in persons with subjective discomforts: a pilot study. *Journal of Integrative Medicine* 2014; 12(3):156–161.

17 Mataran-Penarrocha, G.A., Castro-Sanchez, A.M., Carballo Garcia, G., et.al. Influence of craniosacral therapy on anxiety, depression, and quality of life in patients with fibromyalgia. *Evidence-Based Complementary and Alternative Medicine* 2011; article ID 178769.

18 Haller, H., Lauche, R., Cramer, H., et.al.. Craniosacral therapy for the treatment of chronic neck pain: a follow-up study. *Journal of Alternative & Complementary Medicine* 2014; 20(5).

19 Townsend, C.S., Bonham, E., Chase, L. et.al. Comparison of still point induction to massage therapy in reducing pain and increasing comfort in chronic pain. *Holistic Nursing Practice* 2014; March/April.

20 Jäkel, A., & von Hauenschild, P. A systematic review to evaluate the clinical benefits of craniosacral therapy. *Complementary Therapies in Medicine* 2012; 20:456—465.

21 Kendall P.C. et al. Considering CBT with Anxious Youth? Think Exposures in *Cognitive and Behavioral Practice* 12, 136-150, 2005

SELECTED READING

22 Francisco J. Ruiz . Acceptance and Commitment Therapy versus Traditional Cognitive Behavioral Therapy: A Systematic Review and Meta-analysis of Current Empirical Evidence. International Journal of Psychology & Psychological Therapy, 12, 2, 333-357, 2012

23 Lance M. McCracken, Chris Eccleston. Coping or acceptance: what to do about chronic pain? Pain 105 (2003) 197–204

24 Adams D, Dagenais S, Clifford T, et.al. Complementary and alternative medicine use by pediatric specialty outpatients. Pediatrics, 2013; 131(2): 225-32 Birdee GS, Phillips RS, Davis RB, et.al. Factors associated with pediatric use of complementary and alternative medicine. Pediatrics, 2010; 125(2): 249-56 Young L and Kemper KJ. Integrative care for pediatric patients with pain. J Altern Complement Med, 2013; 19(7): 627-32

25 Eisenberg DM, et al. Trends in alternative medicine use in the United States, 1990-1997: results of a follow-up national survey., JAMA. 1998 Nov 11;280(18):1569-75.

26 Evans, S., Sternlieb, B., Zeltzer, L., et.al. (2013). Iyengar yoga and the use of props for pediatric chronic pain: A case study. Alternative Therapies in Health and Medicine 19(5), 66-70.

27 Coda: Psychoanalysis and Music in the Psyche and Society. J. J. Nagel, Samuel Bradshaw. *http://onlinelibrary.wiley.com/doi/10.1002/aps.1357/abstract*

28 Scientific research points to significant activation of the 'emotion' centers of the brain while listening to and engaging in music, including decreased anxiety and stress (Labrague & McEnroe-Petitte, 2014; Longhi & Pickett, 2008; Rasco, 1992; Wang et al., 2014), decreased measured heart rate and blood pressure (Tse, Chan, & Benzie, 2005), increased oxygen saturation, reduced pain perception and dependence on pain medication (Cochrane Review, 2006; Hatem, et al., 2006; Siegel, 1983; Tse, Chan, & Benzie, 2005) improved mood (Burrai, Micheluzzi, Bugani, 2014; Radstaak, Geurts, Brosschot, & Kompier, 2014) and increased immunity (i.e. decreased cortisol levels) (Field et al., 1998).

29 Melchart D, et al. Results of five randomized studies on the immunomodulatory activity of preparations of echinacea. Journal of Alternative and Complementary Medicine. 1995;1(2):145-159. 9

30 Grimm, W. A randomized controlled trial of the effect of fluid extract of echinacea purpura on the incidence of severity of colds and respiratory infections. The American Journal of Medicine. 1999;106(2):138-143.

31 Hoheisel, O. Echinagard. Treatment shortens the course of the common cold: a double-blind, placebo-controlled clinical trial. European Journal of Clinical Research. 1997;9:261-268.

32 P.L. 94-142 and Section 504 of the Rehabilitation Act and the more recent passage of P.L. 99-457 and P.L. 101-476 *https://en.wikipedia.org/wiki/ Education_for_All_Handicapped_Children_Act*

33 (adapted in part from Sarah McDougal Indiana University, December 11, 1997.) Accessed February 1, 2016: *www.acor.org/ped-onc/cfissues/backtoschool/cwc.html*

34 Katz, E.R. (1980). Illness impact and social reintegration. In J. Kellerman (Ed.), Psychological aspects of childhood Chronic pain. Springfield, IL: Charles C. Thomas.

35 Katz, E.R., et al.. (1988). School and social reintegration of children with Chronic pain. Journal of Psychosocial Oncology, 6, 123-140.

36 Chekryn, J., Deegan, M., & Reid, J. (1987). Impact on teachers when a child with Chronic pain returns to school. Children's Health Care, 15, 161-165.

37 Zebrack B. Reflections of a Chronic pain survivor/research scientist. Cancer.2003 Jun 1;97(11):2707-9.

38 Eimear Kinsella, Paul Zeltzer, et al.. Safety of summer camp for children with chronic and/or life threatening illness. European Journal of Oncology Nursing 2006 Ms. No. YEJON-D-05-00040R1

39 Zeltzer LK, et al. Psychosocial outcomes and health-related quality of life in adult childhood cancer survivors: a report from the Childhood Cancer Survivor Study. Cancer Epidemiology, Biomarkers and Prevention, 2008 Feb;17(2):435-46 Zeltzer LK, et al. Psychological status in childhood cancer survivors: a report from the Childhood Cancer Survivor Study. J Clin Oncol. 2009 May 10;27(14):2396-404.

40 I am indebted to Ted Schreck Chief Exec. Officer, University of Southern California University Hospital for this advice.

Acknowledgments

There are many people we would like to acknowledge for their contributions. First and foremost, we would like to thank our many patients and their parents who contributed content, reviewed, and critiqued the book to strengthen and make it more helpful. We also thank our patients and their families who, over the years, have contributed by sharing their stories and their lives with us. Their willingness to share such intimate details has made us become better physicians.

We thank members of our Whole Child LA and UCLA Pediatric Pain Program team for their important clinical contributions to our programs. Because of the sharing by these excellent clinicians, our pain program is greater than the sum of its parts. They have all contributed to the book directly through their writing, reviewing, providing case histories, or guiding the book in other ways. These individuals include psychologists Samantha Levy, PhD, Shelley Segal, PsyD, Diana Taylor, PhD, and Bruce Levine, PhD, who also is one of our biofeedback experts, as well as psychotherapist and art therapist Azita Sachmachian, MFT, and Esther Dreifuss-Kattan, PhD, psycho-oncologist, psychoanalyst and art therapist. We thank child psychiatrist Ryan Davis, MD, and psychopharmacology guidance from UCLA child psychiatrist Mark DeAntonio, MD. We appreciate the many years of ongoing support and collaboration from acupuncturist Michael Waterhouse, MA, OMD, LAc, hypnotherapist Kathryn dePlanque, PhD, and Iyengar yoga and Vipassana meditation instructor Beth Sternlieb, MA. We are indebted to our outstanding physical therapists Sean Hampton, MPT, Celia Demayo, PT, MA, OCS, and Diane Poladian, DPT, OCS, who also is a biofeedback clinician. We thank our program music therapist Vanya Green, MA, our craniosacral therapists Karen Axelrod, MA, CST-D, and Hillary Bedell, who is also an energy therapist, and our massage therapists Cara Amenta and Erin Wilson.

We so appreciate the UCLA Pediatric Pain and Palliative Care Program psychologists Elana Evan, PhD, Jennie Tsao, PhD, Subhadra Evans, PhD, and Laura Payne, PhD, and our nurse practitioner M. Michaela Nalamliang, RN, MA, CPNP.

We are indebted to author Georgia Huston and Professor Amy Kenny, PhD for their reviewing, critiquing, and contributing in countless other ways. We also wish to thank the following clinical and scientific experts whose written contributions to this book have helped to make it the "state of the science" in pediatric chronic pain. While we include their details in contributed sections, we acknowledge them here with gratitude: Paul Abend, Joan R Asarnow, Margaret Baumann, Richard G Boles, Tim Buie, Jacqueline Casillas, Thomas D Coates, Christopher

Eccleston, Leah Ellenberg, G Allen Finley, Joe Garcia, Stacey Garcia, Christopher C. Giza, Kenneth R Goldschneider, Susan Kaiser Greenland, Harvey Karp, Susmita Kashikar-Zuck, Kathi Kemper, Elliot Krane, Jason Lerner, Deirdre Logan, William L Oppenheim, Tanya Palermo, Shervin Rabizadeh, Andrea Rapkin, Ricki Robinson, Laura E Schanberg, Neil Schechter, Robert Shulman, Kathleen Sluka, Lorraine Stern, Jorge Vargas, Carl vonBaeyer, Gary Walco, Steven Weisman, Shahram Yazdani, Tracy Zaslow, and David Ziring.

INDEX

READERS NOTE

Page numbers followed by f indicate a figure. Page numbers followed by t indicate a table.

A

abdominal pain
  autistic spectrum disorder and, 121–126
  gender and prevalence of, 171
  pathophysiology and management, 66–74
Abend, Paul (D.O.), 118–121
abortive medications, headache management, 62–64
acceptance and commitment therapy (ACT), 234–235
acetaminophen, 298–299
  headache management, 63–64
ACT. *See* acceptance and commitment therapy
acupuncture, 23, 256–259
  menstrual pain management, 77–79
  sickle cell disease and, 100–101
acute pain, chronic pain *vs.,* 16–18
adalimumab /Humira™, 90
addiction
  opioid use and, 287–290
  stereotypes of sickle-cell disease patients at risk for, 99–106
adolescents
  back pain in, 57–58
  cancer pain and bone marrow transplantation in, 107–111
  chronic fatigue syndrome in, 79
  cognitive-behavioral therapy for, 231–233
  dialectical behavioral therapy for, 233–234
  irritable bowel syndrome in, 68–74
  juvenile fibromyalgia and, 55–56
  pain medication in, 284–285
  personal trainers for, 223–226
  school re-integration for, 304–311
  sickle cell disease in, 99–100
  sports injuries in, 45–46
  yoga therapy for, 262–264

adrenalin, pain control and, 22
Adriamycin, mucositis from, 108
Advil™, 23
African-Americans, sickle cell disease (SCD) in, 98–106
age, chronic pain management and role of, 183
alexithymia, 170, 177–178
alleviation of pain, tips for, 37t
allodynia, 47, 49–50
alpha-galactosidase A deficiency, 130–131
Alpha lipoic acid, mitochondrial dysfunction and, 83
Amenta, Cara, 218–220
American College of Sports Medicine, 209
Amitriptyline (Elavil™), 62, 85, 130, 291–293
amygdala
  autism and, 115f
  pain control mechanisms in, 22
analgesics, 23
  non-prescription/over-the-counter analgesics, 298–299
  patient-controlled analgesics (PCAs), 288–289
Ankenmann, Ralph, 119
anterior cingulate cortex, pain activation in, 23
anti-anxiety medications, 175, 293–294
antibiotics, pseudotumor cerebri from, 61
anticonvulsants, 294
  juvenile fibromyalgia, 55–56
anti-depressants. *See also* specific medications
  anxiety treatments and, 175
  guidelines for using, 290–293
  irritable bowel syndrome and, 73
  juvenile fibromyalgia, 55–56

363

menstrual pain management, 79
mitochondrial disorders and, 84–85
systemic lupus emphysematous and, 286
anti-emetics, 62
anti-inflammatory drugs, inflammatory bowel
disease, 94–95
anti-oxidant supplements
botanicals, 276–278
mitochondrial dysfunction and, 80–85
anxiety
in autism, 116
chronic pain and, 171–173
classification of, 173–175
medications for, 175, 293–294
POTS and, 286
aquatic (water) therapy, 214–216
Arena Fitness Training Center, 223–226
arthritis
other conditions with, 90
pathophysiology and management, 88–92
types of pain with, 24
art therapy, 272–273
Asarnow, Joan (Dr.), 234
ASD. *See* autism spectrum disorder
assessment
of care team guidelines for, 140–142,
141t
learning disabilities in bright children,
186
questions to consider, 34t
"auras," in migraine headaches, 62
autism spectrum disorder (ASD)
biology of, 123–126
common physical illnesses and, 124–126
gastrointestinal symptoms and abdominal
pain with, 121–126
pain and, 114–126
social skills deficits and, 177–178
Autism Think Tank of New Jersey,
118–121
autonomic (unconscious) nervous system,
19–21
anxiety and, 171–173
sickle cell disease and, 101
Axelrod, Karen, 220–223
Ayurvedic medicine, 276–277

B
Babikian, Talin, 119
backpacks, back pain linked to, 57–58
back pain
massage therapy for, 220
pathophysiology and treatment, 57–58
in sickle cell disease, 99–100
Banez, Gerard A. (PhD), 337
basal ganglia, autism and, 115f
Bauman, Margaret (Dr.), 119, 123–126
Beck, Jennifer J., 126–128
Becker, David K. (Dr.), 331
Bedell, Hillary, 124–126
behavioral cues
children's chronic pain and, 33–34
family-based psychotherapy and, 237–238
illness and behavioral interactions,
123–126
pain in autistic patients and, 121–126
behavioral plans, family therapy and,
239–240
beliefs and thoughts, impact on pain, 21
Bentley, Katherine (Dr.), 334, 337
benzodiazepines, limitations and side-effects
of, 293–294
Berde, Charles (Dr.), 335
beta-blockers, for POTS, 285–286
biofeedback, chronic pain management with,
264–267
biological pain process, 12–15
memory and, 21, 180–181
biologics, arthritis therapy, 90
bio-psycho-social treatment model, 5, 226
integrative approach based on, 227–229
Birmingham, Patrick K. (Dr.), 333
Bliss, Alison (Dr.), 344
blood tests, record of, 157–159
body reactions
in autistic spectrum disorder, 116–117
to exercise, 209–210
pain in autistic patients and, 122–126
symptoms and signs of pain and, 37–38
therapeutic yoga and, 260–264
body-up approach, juvenile fibromyalgia
therapy, 54–56
Boles, Richard (Dr.), 81–85

INDEX

bone marrow transplantation
  pain management in, 107–111
  sickle cell disease and, 101
bone pain, 109
Boston Children's Hospital, pediatric pain
  rehabilitation program, 216–218
botanicals, complementary therapy with,
  276–279
brain
  acupuncture and opioid production by, 257
  autism and structures of, 115–118, 115f
  biofeedback and responses of, 266–267
  complex regional pain syndrome and role
    of, 46–53
  Geo-location system, 18f
  impact of chronic pain on, 208–210
  music therapy and, 274–275
  pain control mechanisms in, 21–23
  pain perception in, 13–15, 14f, 23
  pain signals pathway to, 13f
  sensory and motor areas of, 18–21
  signaling pathways to, 15–16
  sports injuries and, 208
  turn off, top-down system in, 16f
brain-down treatment, juvenile fibromyalgia,
  54–56
brain-gut axis, irritable bowel syndrome and,
  68–74, 69f
brain stem, autism and, 115f
brain tumors, headaches and, 60
breathing exercises
  cognitive-behavioral therapy and, 231
  practice tips for, 193–196
Brown, Stephen (Dr.), 341
Budapest Criteria, complex regional pain
  syndrome, 50–51
Buie, Tim (Dr.), 119, 121
B vitamins, mitochondrial dysfunction and,
  84

C

calendar, guidelines for maintenance of, 160
cancer pain
  pathophysiology and management of,
    107–111

strategies for reducing, 107t
carnitine deficiency, mitochondrial
  dysfunction and, 83–84
"carpentry" approach to pain management,
  44, 46–47
Carter, Bryan (PhD), 334
case managers for insurance benefits,
  guidelines for dealing with, 326–328
Casillas, Jacqueline (Dr.), 109–111
catastrophizing of pain, 21–23
  cognitive-behavioral therapy and, 231–233
CBT. *See* cognitive-behavioral therapy
central nerve blocks, complex regional pain
  syndrome, 52
central nervous system, 19f
  anatomy, 19
  anxiety and, 172–173
  juvenile fibromyalgia, 54–56
cerebellum, autism and, 115
cerebral cortex, autism and, 115f
cerebral palsy (CP), pain in, 126–128
cerebrospinal fluid (CSF)
  back pain and, 58
  headaches and, 61–66
chat rooms, guidelines for using, 149–150
chemotherapy, mucositis with, 107–108
chest pain, 74–75
Chiari malformation, 58, 133–134
Child Life Services, 110–111
children's descriptions of chronic pain, 31–33
  behavioral cues, 33–34
chiropractic care, 223
chronic fatigue syndrome, 79
  complementary therapies for, 278
chronic pain
  ABC's care for, 329–330
  acute pain *vs.,* 16–18
  in cerebral palsy, 127–128
  children's descriptions of, 31–33
  chronology of child's journey through,
    157–161
  conditions related to, 42–44
  difficulty of diagnosis, 4–5
  emotions and memory and, 18–21
  as family pain, 241–244
  incidence and prevalence, 4–5, 10

365

ineffective medications or procedures for, 27

measurement of, tools for, 39–40

mitochondrial dysfunction in, 80–85

non-medical management of, 21–23

Pain Center Locator, 331–344

physical *vs.* psychological pain, 12–15

physicians' dilemma in assessment of, 139–140

real *vs.* imaginary pain, 10–11

under-treatment of, 25–27

unpredictability of, 5–7

Chronic Widespread Pain (CWP). *See* juvenile fibromyalgia

CIH. *See* complementary and integrative health

Clark, Lynn (CPNP), 340

classroom preparation, school re-integration and importance of, 310

clinical trials

denial of coverage in, 325–326

information sources about, 162–163

Coates, Tom (Dr.), 98–106

Coenzyme Q10 therapy

complementary medicine and, 278

mitochondrial dysfunction, 83–85

cognitive-behavioral therapy (CBT)

for anxiety, 175

case studies involving, 230–233

irritable bowel syndrome and, 73

juvenile fibromyalgia, 55–56

juvenile idiopathic arthritis, 88

cognitive disabilities

children's descriptions of pain and, 32–33

depression and, 179

Collins, John (PhD), 344

common physical illnesses, autism spectrum disorder and, 124–126

communication disorders, pain in, 126–128

communication with children

listening and observation, 35–37

pain in autistic patients and, 121–126

parental expectations and, 38–39

problems and dysfunction in, 170, 177–178

compensating behavior, hidden learning disabilities and, 183–185

complementary and integrative health (CIH), 251–254

complementary therapies (CT). *See also* specific therapies

acupuncture, 256–259

basic principles, 251

biofeedback, 264–267

botanicals and natural products, 276–279

diseases and conditions treated with, 254f

evaluation of, 270–275

hypnotherapy, 267–270

internet resources for, 280–281, 280t

major areas of, 250–251, 250t

mind-based techniques, 270–275

practitioner selection and assessment, 275, 281t

practitioners in WCLA and UCLA pain programs, 255–256

risk and limitations of, 255

yoga, 260–264

complex regional pain syndrome (CRPS)

children's descriptions of, 31–33

diagnosis and treatment approaches to, 48–53

gender and prevalence of, 171

neuropathic pain with, 24

physical therapy for, 211–212

sample letters and tracking forms concerning, 350–355

symptoms and mechanisms, 46–53

transcutaneous electrical nerve stimulation for, 212–213

concussion, diagnosis and management, 64–66

Connell, Hannah (Dr.), 342

Conroy, Caitlin (Psy.D), 216–218

constipation

in autistic patients, pain from, 122–126

irritable bowel syndrome and, 68–74

consultation reports, record of, 159

coping mechanisms for chronic pain, age, developmental level and skill in, 183

core strength, back pain and, 57–58

corpus callosum, autism and, 115f

cost issues

INDEX

hidden costs of second opinion, 143–145,
  327–328
insurance coverage and funding sources
  tracking, 161, 355t
medical bill records, 161, 354t
tax deductions for medical expenses, 328
couples' therapy, 245–247
craniosacral therapy (CST)
  autism spectrum disorder and, 124–126
  definition and basic principles, 220–223
  practitioner selection guidelines, 222–223
Crawford, Matthew (Dr.), 344
Crohn's disease, 25, 93–96
CRPS. See complex regional pain syndrome
CST. See craniosacral therapy
CT. See complementary therapies (CT)
cues to pain
  in autistic spectrum disorder, 116–117
  behavioral cues, 33–34
  children's descriptions of pain and, 31–33
  communication with children and, 35–37
  in migraine headaches, 62
  parents' awareness of, 30–31
  questions to consider, 34
curcumin. See turmeric

D

DBT. See dialectical behavioral therapy
DeMayo, Celia Sabin, 214–216
denial of insurance coverage, guidelines for
  challenging, 144t, 145t, 322–326, 326t
dependence on drugs, opioids and risk of,
  287–290
De Planque, J. Kathryn (Ph.D), 268–270
depression
  pain and brain chemistry in, 179
  St. John's wort for, 277–278
  suicide and, 235–236
Descartes, René, 13–14
desensitization, cognitive-behavioral therapy
  and, 230–231
developmental levels
  autistic spectrum disorder and, 114–118
  coping mechanisms for pain and, 183
  pain in disorders of, 126–128

diagnosis, chronic pain and difficulty with,
  4–5, 139–140
dialectical behavioral therapy (DBT),
  233–234
diarrhea, irritable bowel syndrome and,
  68–74
diet. See also nutrient therapies
  eosinophilic esophagitis and modifications
    to, 98
  headache management and, 63
  mitochondrial dysfunction and, 80, 84–85
  pain in autistic patients and, 122–126
  parent/child conflicts over food and,
    241–244
dietary supplements, 252–254. See also
  botanicals
disability law, legal rights of children with
  chronic pain and, 304–306
disease, back pain linked to, 57–58
distraction, pain management and, 35–36,
  180
  ideas for, 35t
divorced parents, issues for, 246–247
Dreifuss-Kattan, Esther (PhD), 273–274
drug-seeking behavior, sickle cell disease
  patients accused of, 99–106
dysmenorrhea. See menstrual pains
  (dysmenorrhea)
dyspepsia, 71, 277
dysphagia, eosinophilic esophagitis and,
  96–97

E

Ear Pull technique, 125–126
"eat to treat" technique, pain in autistic
  patients and, 122–126
Eccleston, Christopher (Dr.), 30–31
ECG. See electrocardiogram
Echinacea, 278–279
economic burden of chronic pain in children,
  320–321
EDS. See Ehlers-Danlos syndrome
Ehlers-Danlos syndrome (EDS), 129–130
electrical signaling mechanisms
  complex regional pain syndrome, 46–47

367

juvenile fibromyalgia, 54–56
electrical stimulation techniques
  complex regional pain syndrome, 52
  menstrual pain management, 77–79
"electrician" approach to pain management,
  44, 46–47
  functional abdominal pain, 68–74
electrocardiogram (ECG), 291
Ellenberg, Leah (Dr.), 186
emergency care, record of, 159
emotions
  chronic pain and, 18–21
  memory and, 180–181
  psychological therapy and, 230–231
  yoga and, 262–264
empirical treatment, pain in autistic patients
  and, 122–126
endogenous pain relief system, 209
endometriosis, 76–79
endorphins
  acupuncture and release of, 257
  pain management and, 23
endoscopy, eosinophilic esophagitis
  diagnosis, 96–97
energy (Qi), acupuncture and, 256–259
energy therapy
  assessment of, 274
  autism spectrum disorder and, 124–126
enkephalins, acupuncture and release of, 257
environmental stimuli
  autistic spectrum disorder and, 116–117
  pain management and, 168–169
enzyme replacement therapy (ERT), 131–132
eosinophilic esophagitis, 93–94, 96–98
ERT. See enzyme replacement therapy (ERT)
esophageal sensitivity and spasm, chest pain
  and, 74–75
etanercept/ Enbrel™, 90
Evans, Subhadra (PhD), 262–264
exercise. See also physical therapy; yoga
  arthritis and, 90
  chronic pain management and, 208–212
  juvenile fibromyalgia, 55–56
  menstrual pain management, 77–79
  mitochondrial dysfunction and, 84–85
  physical body changes from, 209–210

in Traditional Chinese Medicine, 258–259
extremities
  complex regional pain syndrome and
    swelling of, 50
  myofascial pain, 53

F

Fabry disease, pathophysiology and
  treatment, 130–133
Family and Medical Leave Act (FMLA),
  314–316, 314t
family-based psychotherapy, 236–244
family issues
  children's chronic pain as family pain,
    241–244
  fathers' participation and, 247
  marital (couples) issues and, 245–247
  pain management and, 168–169
  parent/child conflicts over food and,
    241–244
  re-integration of chronic pain patient and,
    311–312
  school re-integration and, 308–311
  siblings of chronic pain patients, 312
  in sports injuries, 46
FAP. See functional abdominal pain
Farid, Ibrahim (Dr.), 338
Farrow-Gillespie, Alan C. (Dr.), 340
fathers, inclusion in management of chronic
  pain plan, 247
fatigue, diagnosis and management of, 79
favorite place relaxation technique, 200,
  269–270
Federal Law P.L. 94-142 (1975), 304–306
fibromyalgia, 278
  juvenile fibromyalgia distinguished from,
    54–56
"fight or flight" warning and protection
  system, 19–21
  autism and, 117
  biofeedback and, 265–267
  in sickle cell disease patients, 101
Finkel, Julia (Dr.), 340
Finley, G. Allen (Dr.), 15
fitness screening and assessments, 224

INDEX

FIT Teens (Fibromyalgia Integrative Training for Teens) program, 56
Fitzgerald, Maria, 180
504 Plans, 306
FMLA. *See* Family and Medical Leave Act
focus of attention, pain and interruption of, 179–180
follow-up notes to care, record of, 159
Food and Drug Administration (FDA), medication approval by, 289–290
Friebert, Sarah (Dr.), 337
Friedrichsdorf, Stefan (Dr.), 336
functional abdominal pain (FAP), 68–74
    medication for, 284–285, 290–293
functional/autonomic-related (FAR) disorders, 82–85
functional pain, 12
    mitochondrial disorders and, 81–85

G

GAD. *See* generalized anxiety disorder
Gandhi, Artee (Dr.), 339
Garcia, Joe, 223–226
Garcia, Stacey, 225–226
gastroenteritis, irritable bowel syndrome and, 24
gastroesophageal reflux
    autism spectrum disorder and, 114, 120–126
    chest pain and, 75
    eosinophilic esophagitis and, 96–98
    yoga therapy for, 263–264
gender
    chronic pain and, 75–76
    perception of pain and differences in, 170–171
generalized anxiety disorder (GAD), 173
generally recognized as safe (GRAS) criteria, 276–279
gene therapy, sickle cell disease, 102, 106
Giardia, 93
Giza, Chris (Dr.), 64–66
Gold, Jeffrey I (PhD), 332
Goldschneider, Kenneth R. (Dr.), 290, 338
GRAS. *See* generally recognized as safe
Green, Vanya, 274–276

grief, management of, 175–176
group sites on internet, guidelines for using, 149–150
Gulur, Padma (Dr.), 332

H

Haiken, Sheri, 119
headaches
    gender and prevalence of, 171
    massage therapy for, 218–219
    migraine, 61–64
    pathophysiology and treatment, 60–66
    prevention, 64
    in sickle cell disease, 99–100
head banging, pain in autistic patients and, 122–126
head trauma, diagnosis and management, 64–66
healthcare providers, contact information for, 157
health fraud, internet and, 152–153
Health Insurance Portability and Accountability Act (HIPAA), 316–317
health maintenance organizations (HMO)
    guidelines for navigating, 322–323
    strategies for expert care from, 143–145
health-medical teamwork, 224–225
Health Questionnaire, 224
heating pads, menstrual pain management, 77–79
Helicobacter *Pylori* infection, 93
Henry, Charles, 119
herbal medicine, 258–259
Hilyard, Anna, 344
HIPAA. *See* Health Insurance Portability and Accountability Act
hip pain, in sickle cell disease patients, 100
hippocampus, autism and, 115f
Hispanic Americans, sickle cell disease (SCD) in, 98–106
home exercise programs, 45, 212
    denial of coverage for, 327
hormonal contraceptives, menstrual pain management, 77–79
hormone levels, menstrual pain and, 75–79

369

hospital discharge summaries, record of, 159

hospital resources, cancer pain management, 109–111

hydrocephalus, diagnosis and treatment, 61

hydroxyurea, sickle cell disease and, 101

hypnotherapy, 267–268

hypo-verbal communication, pain in autistic patients and, 123–126

I

IBD. *See* inflammatory bowel disease

IBS. *See* irritable bowel syndrome

IEPs. *See* individual education plans

imagery therapy, 269–270
  neuropathic pain, 100–101

imaging studies of brain
  acupuncture points and, 257
  headaches and, 61–66
  pain activity and, 23
  record of, 158

indigestion, turmeric for, 277

individual education plans (IEPs), 305–307

Individuals with Disabilities Education Act (IDEA), 304–306

inflammation, pain and, 25

inflammatory bowel disease (IBD), 25
  arthritis and, 90
  experts' discussion of, 94–98
  pathophysiology and treatment, 92–94
  regional enteritis, ulcerative colitis & eosinophilic esophagitis, 93–94

information resources
  guidelines for managing volume of, 148
  medical dictionary and other books, 161
  record of, 160

Ingelmo, Pablo M. (Dr.), 341

Institute of Medicine (IOM), bio-psycho-social model of chronic pain and, 5

insurance benefits
  coverage and funding sources tracking, 355t
  denials of coverage, guidelines for appealing, 322–326
  frequently asked questions about, 326–328
  negotiation tips for, 322–323

rules for obtaining, 318–323, 318t
  tracking form for, 355
  web resources for, 328t

integrative medicine
  bio-psycho-social model of chronic pain and, 227–229
  complementary and integrative health (CIH), 251–254

International Association for the Study of Pain (IASP), 49–50

Internet resources. *See also* websites
  chat rooms and groups, 149–150
  chronic pain websites, 6
  on complementary medicine practitioners, 281t
  for complementary therapies, 280t
  consulting with physicians about, 154
  health fraud on, 152–153
  for insurance benefits and health care, 328
  risk and limitations of, 255
  truthfulness of, 150–151
  volume of information on, 148

intracranial pressure (ICP), 60–61

IQ tests, 186

irritable bowel syndrome (IBS), 12
  inflammatory bowel disease *vs.*, 93
  massage therapy for, 219–220
  neural pathways in, 69f
  pathophysiology and management, 66–74
  peppermint for symptomatic relief, 276
  reconditioning in adolescents with, 225–226
  types of pain with, 24
  yoga therapy for, 263–264

IWK Health Center-Pediatric Complex Pain Clinic, 341

Iyengar yoga, chronic pain therapy using, 260–264

J

Jerman, Jonathan (Dr.), 331

JFM. *See* juvenile fibromyalgia

JIA. *See* juvenile idiopathic arthritis

Joint Legal Custody, parental rights and responsibilities and, 247

INDEX

Joseph, Michael (Dr.), 337

journaling, self-care for parents of children with cancer and, 110–111

Journal of Pediatrics, 179

juvenile fibromyalgia (JFM)
complementary therapies for, 278
gender and prevalence of, 171
pathophysiology and treatment, 54–56

juvenile idiopathic arthritis (JIA), 88–92
other diseases with, 90–92

K

Kaiser-Greenland, Susan, 202, 271–272

Karp, Harvey (Dr.), 190–192

Kashikar-Zuck, Susmita (Dr.), 54–56, 192–193

Kemper, Kathi J. (Dr.), 218–219, 252–254

Kent, Sheryl (PhD), 333

Koh, Jeffrey (Dr.), 338

Kohn, Donald (Dr.), 106

Kost-Byerly, Sabine (Dr.), 335

Kraemer, F. Wickham (Dr.), 339

Krane, Elliot (Dr.), 48, 288–289, 332

L

Lactaid™, 93

lactose intolerance, 93

Lamontagne, Christine (Dr.), 341

laughter, distraction from pain and, 35–36

learning disabilities
autistic spectrum disorder and, 117
children's descriptions of pain and, 32–33
compensation for, 183–185
recognition in bright children, 185–186
subtle learning disorders, 306–308

legal rights of children with chronic pain, 304–306
Family & Medical Leave Act and, 314–316
insurance benefits, rules for obtaining, 318–323
privacy rights, 316–317

Lerner, Jason (Dr.), 62–66

Levine, Bruce (PhD), 264–267

Levy, Samantha (Dr.), 228–229, 246–247

L-Glutamine, sickle cell disease and, 101

licensing, of acupuncture practitioners, 258–259

Lidoderm™ patches, 297

Life Force in energy therapy, 274

lifestyle changes
headache management and, 63
menstrual pain and, 78–79
sleep problems and, 191–192

lifetime coverage limits in insurance, chronic illness patients risk of exceeding, 322

light, sleep problems and, 191

listening, pain assessment and, 35–37

LISTSERVs, guidelines for using, 149–150

Logan, Deidre (Dr.), 216–218

lysosomal storage diseases, 130–131

M

managed care plans, guidelines for navigating, 322–323

Managing Your Child's Chronic Pain (Palermo), 233

marital (couples) issues, 245–247

massage therapy
application of, 23
autism spectrum disorder and use of, 124–126
definition and basic principles, 218–220
neuropathic pain and, 100–101
practitioner selection guidelines, 219–220
in Traditional Chinese Medicine, 258–259

mastoid process compression, 126

Mayo Clinic Pediatric Pain Rehab Center, 336

Mayo Family Pediatric Pain Rehabilitation Center (PPRC), 217–218

McCabe, Klanci (Ph.D), 338

measurement of pain, tools for, 39–40

mechanisms of pain, targeted treatment and, 24–25

medical dictionaries, 161

medical/insurance bills and correspondence, records of, 161

medical notebook
guidelines for creating, 156–163

371

insurance information and, 323
medication records in, 290
medical resource notebook, creation and
content recommendations for, 156–161
medications. *See also* specific medications,
e.g., anti-depressants
anticonvulsants, 55–56, 294
for anxiety, 175, 293–294
arthritis, 90–92
for chronic pain management, overview of,
284–285
complex regional pain syndrome and,
51–52
for Ehlers-Danlos syndrome, 129–130
FDA approval, 289–290
headache management, 63–64
ineffective choices of, 27
inflammatory bowel disease, 94–96
insurance coverage for, 319–320,
324–326
juvenile fibromyalgia, 54–56
limitations and side effects of, 23
migraine headaches, 62
muscle relaxants, 294–295
nausea and vomiting, 297
neuroleptics, 295–297
non-prescription/over-the-counter
analgesics, 298–299
off-label drugs, 289–290
opioids, 23, 27, 286–290
pseudotumor cerebri from, 61
record of past and present meds and doses,
159–160
for syringomyelia, 133–134
topical agents, 297
tracking form for, 353t
meditation. *See also* yoga
neuropathic pain and, 100–101
melatonin therapy, 278
memory, chronic pain and, 21, 180–181
menstrual pains (dysmenorrhea), 75–79
Mental Health Parity Law, 319–320
methotrexate
arthritis therapy, 90–92
mucositis from, 108
Miele, Laure (RN), 333

migraine headaches, 61–64
Millspaugh, Dan (Dr.), 336
mind-based techniques
assessment of, 270–275
chest pain management, 74–75
complex regional pain syndrome, 48
irritable bowel syndrome, 70–74
juvenile fibromyalgia, 54–56
mindfulness meditation, 200–202, 270–272
The Mindful Child (Kaiser-Greenland), 202,
271–272
mirror therapy, 211
Mirtazapine (Remeron™), 291
mislabeling, dietary supplements, 252–254
mitochondria, structure of, 80f
mitochondrial disorders, 81–85
mitochondrial dysfunction, chronic pain and,
80–85
monoamine oxidase, 277–278
Mooney, James (Dr.), 339
motor nervous system, 19
movement-based training systems, 224
mucositis, 107–108
Murray, Katherine, 121–126
muscle relaxant medications, 294–295
muscle relaxation techniques, 196–199
muscle tension, headaches and, 61
music therapy, 274–275
myofascial pain
exercise therapy for, 209–210
pathophysiology and treatment, 53

N
Nalamliang, Michaela, 109
National Center for Complementary and
Alternative Medicine (NCCAM), 251
National Center for Complementary and
Integrative Health (NCCIH), 251
natural products, in complementary therapy,
276–279
nausea and vomiting
headaches and, 60
medications for, 297
migraine headaches, 62
signs and symptoms of pain and, 37–38

372

INDEX

nerve blocks, complex regional pain
  syndrome, 52
nervous system
  electrical connectivity in, 17–18, 22, 116
  pain control mechanisms in, 21–23
  subdivisions of, 18–21
neural signaling mechanisms
  complex regional pain syndrome and role
    of, 48–53
  irritable bowel syndrome and, 68–74
  pain and depression, 179
neuroanatomy of pain, 18–21
neurobiology, 228
neurochemical pain processes, 12–15
  depression and, 179
  stress and, 21
neuroleptic medications, 295–297
neuromuscular training
  juvenile fibromyalgia and, 56
  massage therapy and, 220
neuropathic pain, 46
  Coenzyme Q10 for, 278
  in complex regional pain syndrome, 48–53
  Fabry disease, 131–132
  inflammatory bowel disease and, 94
  in sickle cell disease, 100
  targeted treatment of, 24–25
neuropsychological testing
  learning disabilities recognition in bright
    children, 185–186
  school re-integration for chronic pain
    patients and, 307
neurotransmitters
  medications targeted to, 23
  pain control mechanisms, 21–23
  pain perception and, 13–15
nociceptive pain, 24–25, 46
non-medical pain management, 21–23. *See
  also* mind-based techniques
  complementary therapies (CT), 250–251
  hospital resources for cancer pain, 109–111
  juvenile fibromyalgia, 55–56
  sickle cell disease, 100–101
non-prescription analgesics, 298–299
nonsteroidal anti-inflammatory drugs
  abdominal pain and intake of, 93

arthritis, 90–92
  headache management, 63–64
  menstrual pain management, 76–79
  non-prescription/over-the-counter
    analgesics, 298–299
non-verbal communication, pain in autistic
  patients and, 123–126
nutritional therapies, 253–254, 253t. *See also*
  botanicals
  in Traditional Chinese Medicine, 258–259

O

Oberlander, Tim (Dr.), 342
observation, pain assessment and, 35–37
obsessive-compulsive disorder (OCD),
  173–174
occupational therapy, complex regional pain
  syndrome, 51
OCD. *See* obsessive-compulsive disorder
off-label drugs, 289–290
opioids
  acupuncture and release of natural opioids,
    257
  limitations and side effects in children with
    use of, 23, 27, 286–290
  as mucositis therapy, 108
  neuropathic pain and, 100–101
  post-operative pain management, 108
Oppenheim, William L. (Dr.), 126–128
organ structure, chronic pain and, 17–18
osteoarthritis
  pathophysiology and management, 88–92
  turmeric for, 277
over-the-counter analgesics, 298–299
oxidative stress, mitochondrial dysfunction
  and, 80–85
OxyContin™, 23

P

Pain Center Locator, 331–344
pain suffering, brain area related to, 23
Palermo, Tanya (PhD), 231–233
pancreatitis, medications for, 288–289
panic disorder, 173

373

breathing exercises, 193–196

parasympathetic nervous system (PNS), 19–21, 20f

anxiety and, 172–173

Parent-Pain Burnout Syndrome (P-PBS), 10–11

parents

of arthritis patients, 91–92

assessment of care team, guidelines for, 140–142, 141t

of autistic children, 114–121

awareness of children's cues about pain by, 30–31

of cerebral palsy patients, 125–128

as children's' models, 181

expectations of, with chronic pain patients, 38–39

of Fabry disease patients, 132–133

family-based psychotherapy for, 236–244

individual issues for, 245

of irritable bowel syndrome patients, 70–74

leadership role in diagnosis and recovery, importance of, 27–28

marital (couples) issues for, 245–247

mindfulness meditation for, 200–202, 270–272

parent/child conflicts over food and, 241–244

principles for helping children with chronic pain, 182

questions concerning pain assessment for, 34t

relaxation breathing exercise for, 193–196

school re-integration for chronic pain patients and, 304–311, 307t

self-behavior checklist for, 238t

self-care for parents of cancer patients, 110–111

siblings of chronic pain patients and, 312

of sickle cell disease patients, 102–106

sleep problems and role of, 188–192

sources of help for, 138

support for, 161–163

yoga therapy for, 262–264

paroxysmal orthostatic tachycardia (POTS), 73

patient-controlled analgesics (PCAs), 288–289

patient stories about chronic pain, 42–44

PCAs. *See* patient-controlled analgesics

pediatric pain expert/treatment center, strategies for finding, 142

pediatric pain rehabilitation (PPR), 216–218

peer support for chronic pain patients, school re-integration and, 309–311

peppermint, in complementary therapy, 276

perception of pain

in autistic spectrum disorder, 116

brain function and, 13–15, 14f

chronic pain's impact on, 18

gender differences in, 170–171

perfectionism, hidden learning disabilities and, 183–185

performance-based training systems, 224

peripheral verve blocks, complex regional pain syndrome, 52

personal trainers, 223–226

phantom pain, 16, 180–181

phobias, chronic pain and, 174–175

phono-phobia, 61–62

photo-phobia, 61–62

physical pain, 12–15

physical therapy

aquatic (water) therapy, 214–216

chest pain, 74–75

complex regional pain syndrome, 51

definition and basic principles, 208

juvenile fibromyalgia, 55–56

pain sensitivity and, 44

resources for locating therapists, 213–214, 226, 226t

sports injuries, 45

for syringomyelia, 133–134

traditional PT, 208–212

transcutaneous electrical nerve stimulation (TENS) units, 77–79, 212–213

physicians

consulting about internet research with, 154

contact information for, 157

374

INDEX

dilemma concerning children's chronic pain, 139–140

parents' communication with, 32–33

second opinion discouraged by, 143

point-of-service (POS) plans, 322–323

post-operative pain management, 108

post-traumatic stress disorder (PTSD), 174

unresolved grief or trauma and, 175–176

postural orthostatic tachycardia (POTS), 73, 82, 129, 285–286

posture, back pain and, 57–58

POTS. *See* postural orthostatic tachycardia

prefrontal cortex

juvenile fibromyalgia, 54–56

pain control mechanisms in, 22–23

premenstrual dysphoric disorder (PMDD), 77–78

premenstrual syndrome (PMS), 77–78

prepaid health plans, strategies for using, 143–145

prevention of pain

in cerebral palsy patients, 127–128

stresses and warning signs, 202–203

privacy rights of chronic pain patients, 316–317

progressive muscle relaxation technique, 196–197

prostaglandin production, menstrual pain and, 77–79

proton pump inhibitors, gastroesophageal reflux and, 114, 120–121

pseudo-addiction

opioids and, 287–290

sickle-cell disease and misdiagnosis of, 99–106

pseudotumor cerebri, 60–61

psoriasis, arthritis and, 90

psychological issues

aquatic (water) therapy and, 214–216

depression and suicide, 235–236

insurance coverage for treatment of mental conditions, 319–320

pain management and, 168–169

in sickle cell disease patients, 99–106

in sports injuries, 46

psychological pain, 12–15

psychological therapy. *See also* specific techniques, e.g. cognitive behavioral therapy

categories of, 230–235

couples' therapy, 245–247

definition and basic principles, 229–235

family therapy, 236–244

therapist selection guidelines, 247

psychosomatic pain, 12

psychotropic drugs, mitochondrial disorders and, 85

pulse assessment, signs and symptoms of pain and, 37–38

Q

questions and answers, record of, 160

R

Rabizadeh, Shervin (Dr.), 94–95

radiation

mucositis with, 107–108

XRT for bone marrow transplantation, 108

Rapkin, Andrea (Dr.), 76

Rastogi, Sachin (Dr.), 344

reactive oxygen species (ROS), mitochondrial dysfunction and, 83–85

reflex neurovascular dystrophy (RND), 49

reflex sympathetic dystrophy (RSD), 49

regional enteritis, 93–94

rehabilitation programs, 216–218

relative rest, 45

relaxation/muscle contraction, 197–198

relaxation techniques, 192–202

breathing exercises, 193–196

favorite place technique, 200

mindfulness meditation, 200–202

muscle relaxation techniques, 196–199

rest, ice, compression and elevation (RICE) regimen, 45

Revivo, Gadi (DO), 334

Riemenschneider, Bradley (Dr.), 338

Risperidone, 295–297

Robinson, Riki (Dr.), 114–118

375

role-playing, cognitive-behavioral therapy
and, 231
Rolfe, P. M. (Dr.), 343

S
Sachmachian, Azita (MFT), 230–231, 236–237, 245
Sadun, Rebecca (Dr.), 89–92
St. John's wort, 277–278
Salamon, Katherin S. (PhD), 333
sample letters and tracking forms, 350–355
SCD. *See* sickle cell disease
Scemama, Pascal (Dr.), 335
Schanberg, Laura E. (Dr.), 89–92
Schechter, Neil (Dr.), 243–244, 335
Schmitz, Michael (Dr.), 331
school re-integration for chronic pain patients
504 Plans and, 306
individual education plans and, 305–307
legal rights of children with chronic pain
and, 304–306
managing transition back to school, 304
parental tips for, 307t
resources for, 310–311
roadmap for, 304t
sample letters and tracking forms for,
350–355
subtle learning disorders, 306–308
Schrock, Charles (Dr.), 336
Scott, Eric (PhD), 334
second opinion
denial of coverage for, 145, 145t, 323–326
guidelines for seeking, 142
health plan coverage of, 144–145
hidden costs of, 143–145, 327–328
preparations for seeking, 143
selective norepinephrine reuptake inhibitors
(SNRIs)
chronic pain management and, 84–85
juvenile fibromyalgia, 55–56
selective serotonin reuptake inhibitors
(SSRIs)
anxiety treatments and, 175
chronic pain management and, 84–85,
291–293

irritable bowel syndrome and, 73
juvenile fibromyalgia, 55–56
menstrual pain management, 79
mitochondrial disorders and, 84–85
self-behavior checklist for parents, 238t
self-care for caregivers, 110–111
self-help tools
biofeedback, 264–267
bio-psycho-social treatment model and,
228
self-injury, pain in autistic patients and,
122–126
sensory nervous system, 19
autism and, 116–117
Sethna, Navil, 335
Sherry, David D. (Dr.), 339
shingles, neuropathic pain with, 24
Shulman, Robert (Dr.), 71–74
sickle cell disease (SCD), 98–106
autonomic (unconscious) nervous system
and, 101
crises in, 101–102
hypnotherapy for, 267–268
patients' experiences with, 102–106
signs of pain, 37–38
in sports injuries, 45–46
Simmonds, Mark (MB), 342
single event multilevel (SEML) surgery, 128
skills development
dialectical behavioral therapy and, 234
pain coping mechanisms, 183
sleep hygiene, steps for improvement of,
191–192
sleep problems
causes of, 85, 189, 189t
chronic fatigue syndrome and, 79
depression and, 179
parental assessment of, 188–192, 188t
in syringomyelia, 133–134
Slover, Robin (Dr.), 333
Sluka, Kathleen (PT, PhD), 208–210
small-fiber polyneuropathy, juvenile
fibromyalgia, 56
Smith, Timothy P. (Dr.), 337
social phobia (social anxiety disorder), 174
social skills deficits, 177–178

INDEX

school re-integration and, 307–308

Sole Legal Custody, parental rights and responsibilities and, 247

somatic pain, 24

spasticity, in cerebral palsy patients, 127–128

specialists, guidelines for selecting, 142, 144, 144t

"Special Place" imagery, 269–270

sports injuries
in children, 44–46
headaches and, 61
pain with, 13
psychological/family issues with, 46
surgery for, 45

SS-type sickle cell disease, 101, 105–106

stem cell transplantation, pain management in, 107–111

Stern, Lorraine (Dr.), 139–140

Sterni, Lynne (Dr.), 336

Sternlieb, Beth, 260–264

steroids
arthritis therapy, 90–92
back pain linked to, 57–58
for POTS, 286

stool tests, record of, 157–158

stress. *See also* anxiety
biofeedback and, 265–267
hidden learning disabilities and, 183–185
pain and, 21
sickle cell disease and management of, 101
signs and symptoms of, 37–38
warning signs and pain prevention, 202–203

suicide, depression and, 235–236

support groups, for parents and children, 162–163

surgery
in cerebral palsy patients, 127–128
complex regional pain syndrome, 52
memory of pain during, 180–181
record of, 159
for sports injuries, 45

sweating, signs and symptoms of pain and, 37–38

sympathetic nervous system (SNS), 19–21, 20f

anxiety and, 172–173

biofeedback and, 265–267

complex regional pain syndrome and, 52

pain control mechanisms in, 22

POTS and, 286

symptoms of pain, 37–38
complex regional pain syndrome, 46–53
in sports injuries, 45–46

syringomyelia, 58
pathophysiology and treatment of, 133–134

systemic lupus erythematosus (SLE), 286

T

Tachdjian, Raffi, 119

Taddio, Anna, 180

Tarique, Sarah (Dr.), 331

tax deductions for medical expenses, 328

teachers, school re-integration for chronic pain patients and, 310–311

teenagers. *See* adolescents

temporal lobe compression, autism spectrum disorder, 125–126

tender point examination, juvenile fibromyalgia, 54–55

tension headaches, POTS and, 286

tertiary medical experts, autism spectrum disorder and, 120–121

testing procedures, record of, 157–161

tetracycline, pseudotumor cerebri from, 61

Thomas, Suresh (Dr.), 335

thought-stopping technique, 231

tolerance of medications, opioids and, 287–290

topical agents, 297

toxicity, dietary supplements, 252–254

Traditional Chinese Medicine (TCM), 258–259

transcutaneous electrical nerve stimulation (TENS), 209–210, 212–213
menstrual pain management, 77–79

transition roadmap for chronic pain students returning to school, 304t

Transverse Facial Membrane Release, 125–126

trauma, management of, 175–176

377

traumatic brain injury (TBI), 64–66
tricyclic anti-depressants (TCAs), 84–85,
  290–293
  abdominal pain and irritable bowel
    syndrome, 66–67
  complex regional pain syndrome, 50, 52
trigger point injections. *See also* acupuncture
  myofascial pain, 53
triptans, headache management, 62–64
Tumor Necrosis Factor (TNF) inhibitor,
  arthritis therapy, 90–92
TUMS™, 74
turmeric, as complementary therapy, 276–277
Tylenol™, 23

U
ulcerative colitis, 25, 93–96
  turmeric for, 277
ulcer-type pain, 93
under-treatment of pain, 25–27
unhelpful behaviors checklist, 239–240, 239t
unpredictability of chronic pain, 5–7
Upledger, John (Dr.), 125–126
urine tests, record of, 157–158
USCF Benioff Children's Hospital Integrated
  Pediatric Pain/Palliative Care Clinic, 331
uveitis, 277

V
"values-based living," acceptance anc
  commitment therapy and, 234–235
Vargas, Jorge (Dr.), 96–98
vaso-occlusive pain crisis, 101–102
Vasu, Thanthullu (Dr.), 343
Venable, Claudia (Dr.), 333
ventriculo-peritoneal (VP) shunt, 61
Vicodin™, 23
viral infection, irritable bowel syndrome and,
  24
Vi Riddel Children's Pain and Rehabilitation
  Centre, 342
visceral pain, 24
vital signs, pain assessment and, 38
Vitamin C, mitochondrial dysfunction and, 83

vitamin D, chronic pain and, 253–254
Vitamin E, mitochondrial dysfunction and, 83
vomiting. *See* nausea and vomiting
Von Baeyer, Carl (Dr.), 35, 182

W
Walco, Gary A. (PhD), 340
Wallace, Ewan (Dr.), 343
warning signs of pain, stresses and, 202–203
Waterhouse, Michael, 256–259
websites
  for complementary therapies, 280t
  evaluation of sources on, 151–152
  for insurance benefits and health care, 328t
  list of helpful pain websites, 153t
  truthfulness of content on, 150–151
Wechsler Intelligence Scale for Children,
  Fifth Edition, 186
Weisman, Steven (Dr.), 200–202, 340
Weiss, Karen E. (PhD), 336
"whole child" paradigm, chronic pain
  management and, 170
Wilson, Anna (PhD), 338
Wilson-Smith, Elaine (FRCA), 343

X
XRT treatments, for bone marrow
  transplantation, 108

Y
Yadzani, Shahram (Dr.), 128–134
Yin/Yang, acupuncture and, 257–259
yoga. *See also* exercise; meditation
  as chronic pain therapy, 260–264

Z
Zaslow, Tracy (Dr.), 44–46
Zeltzer, Lonnie (Dr.), 119, 332
Zeltzer, Paul (Dr.), 332
Zempsky, William T. (Dr.), 333
Ziring, David (Dr.), 95–96

THE AUTHORS

Lonnie Zeltzer, M.D. is Distinguished Professor of Pediatrics, Anesthesiology, Psychiatry and Biobehavioral Sciences at David Geffen School of Medicine at UCLA and Director of UCLA's Pediatric Pain and Palliative Care Program. She co-authored the Institute of Medicine report on *Transforming Pain in America* and is a member of the national steering committee providing directions for pain research at NIH. She has received, among other awards, the Mayday Pain and Policy Fellowship and 2005 Jeffrey Lawson Award for Advocacy in Children's Pain Relief from the American Pain Society (APS). Her UCLA integrative pediatric pain program received the 2009 Clinical Centers of Excellence in Pain Management Award from APS and a 2012 award from the Southern California Cancer Pain Initiative. She is also a member of the national Autism Think Tank. Her research includes yoga, mindfulness, hypnotherapy, and other self-help interventions, including mobile technologies, to help children and adolescents who have chronic pain, as well as understanding pain mechanisms in irritable bowel syndrome, cancer, sickle cell disease, headaches and dysmenorrhea. She has over 350 research publications on childhood pain and complementary therapies, has written more than 80 book chapters. Her book "*Conquering Your Child's Pain*, for parents on chronic pain in childhood (HarperCollins, 2005) had been the most popular in its niche.

Dr. Zeltzer. M.D. is a neuro-oncologist, educator, brain cancer researcher, author and entrepreneur whose medical career spans 35 years with expertise in the areas of Neuro-Oncology, immunotherapy. Dr. Zeltzer previously directed two National Cancer Institute-sponsored clinical trials for leukemia and brain tumors, was the funded Principal Investigator for seven years at University of Texas Health Science Center at San Antonio, PI at University of California at Irvine. He edited two major text books in Oncology and Neuro-Oncology and authored over 130 publications on the molecular biology, treatment results, and long-term outcomes of cancer. His expertise in the field of immunotherapy includes early investigations using antigen-presenting cells (at UCI) and dendritic cell-based immune-therapy while at Cedars-Sinai Hospital and UCLA Department of Neurosurgery in Los Angeles. He is a Consultant to the Medical Board of California. Dr. Paul Zeltzer was the recipient of the 2012 Southern California Pain Initiative Award for 2012. Dr. Zeltzer founded two web/ mobile-based ventures: GoMed Solutions Inc, a mobile interface that connects medical applications and all mobile wireless devices (two US patents), & *www.NavigatingCancer.com* a comprehensive website and novel search engine that links patients having specific types/ stages of cancer with the medical experts in that area. He served as Medical Director, Northwest Biotherapeutics Inc, focused on developing personalized vaccines to harness the body's natural defenses to create cancer therapies for brain cancer. He completed two books for the lay public: *"Brain Tumors: Leaving the Garden of Eden."* (2006) & *"Brain Tumors: Finding the Ark"*. He is an inventor and has approved US patents: *System and Method for Storing Information on a Wireless Device. The GoMed Application* (US patent 6,970,827B2 11-10-2005). He has given medical advice to several Television series including: "The Bold Ones" (1969-70) and "SCRUBS" (2002-2009). He acts with Ving Rhames in "Caged Animal" on DVD (2010).

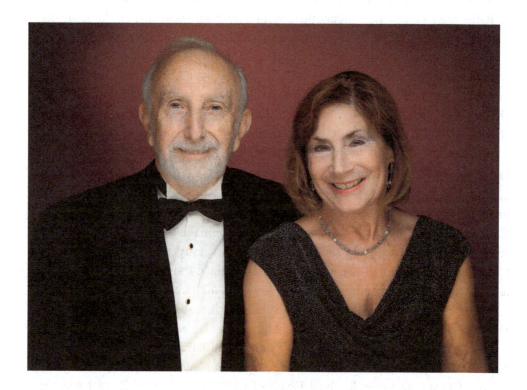